Home Cage Monitoring in Rodents: A Global Effort

Stefano Gaburro • Silvia Mandillo
Editors

Home Cage Monitoring in Rodents: A Global Effort

Springer

Editors
Stefano Gaburro
Tecniplast Spa
Buguggiate, Italy

Silvia Mandillo
Institute of Biochemistry and Cell Biology
National Research Council
Monterotondo, Roma, Italy

Editorial contact: Annette Klaus-Brusola

ISBN 978-3-032-19780-1 ISBN 978-3-032-19781-8 (eBook)
https://doi.org/10.1007/978-3-032-19781-8

This Springer imprint is published by the registered company Springer Nature Switzerland AG
The registered company address is: Gewerbestrasse 11, 6330 Cham, Switzerland

Foreword

Automated home-cage monitoring has become one of the most significant technological and methodological advancements in laboratory animal science over the last decade. By enabling continuous, automated, and minimally invasive observation of rodents in their familiar environments, it provides unprecedented opportunities to improve both the quality of research and animal welfare, thus directly addressing the principles of 3Rs. These technologies allow for capturing richer behavioural and physiological data, enhance reproducibility, and reduce the confounding effects caused by handling of the animals and observing them for too short time under possibly stressful conditions.

The COST Action TEATIME (2021–2025) has united an international network of researchers in behavioural neuroscience and laboratory animal science, veterinarians, technology developers, and data scientists, to exchange expertise, promote harmonisation, and establish best practices for automated monitoring in biomedical research with rodents.

This book, *Home Cage Monitoring in Rodents: A Global Effort*, will cover the scientific, operational, and ethical dimensions of home-cage monitoring. The chapters explore experimental design, data handling, and statistical approaches alongside practical considerations such as training, communication, and the development of "do-it-yourself" systems. Together, these contributions demonstrate how the integration of technology, welfare, and good experimental design can refine research practices and enhance translational relevance.

This book stands as both a summary of current achievements and a guide for future progress. It exemplifies what can be accomplished through international collaboration and interdisciplinary engagement—hallmarks of the TEATIME initiative. These insights will serve as a valuable reference for researchers seeking to advance robust, ethical, and innovative animal-based science.

Vootele Voikar

Chair of the COST Action CA20135—Improving biomedical research by automated behaviour monitoring in the animal home-cage (TEATIME)

This book is based upon work from COST Action CA20135 TEATIME, supported by COST (European Cooperation in Science and Technology). COST (European Cooperation in Science and Technology) is a funding agency for research and innovation networks. Our Actions help connect research initiatives across Europe and enable scientists to grow their ideas by sharing them with their peers. This boosts their research, career, and innovation.

EUROPEAN COOPERATION IN SCIENCE & TECHNOLOGY

Funded by the European Union

Preface For Stefano Gaburro

In October 2024, Springer invited me to author a book on the digitalisation of preclinical research. As an active member of COST Action TEATIME, I discussed the idea with the chair, Vootele Voikar, and, from the very beginning, worked closely with Silvia to shape the concept and structure of the volume. Together with the other lead authors, we decided to create a comprehensive and practical reference on home cage monitoring, bringing together global experts from science, veterinary medicine, technology, and data analysis. The result is a collaborative book that not only describes HCM technologies but also supports real-world decisions on systems, study design, data handling, welfare, and translation.

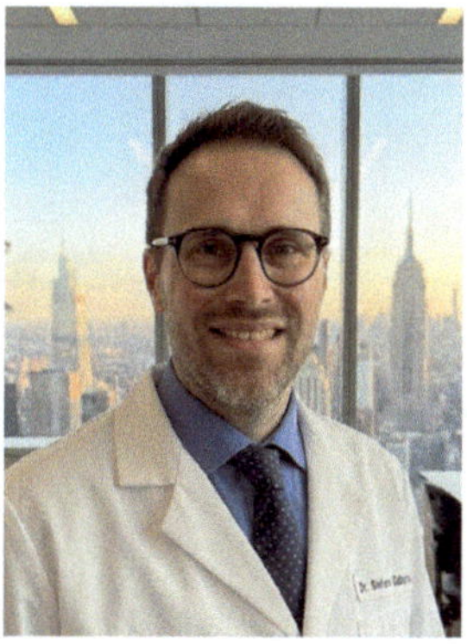

I am deeply grateful to Silvia, to Vootele and to all contributors, as well as to the wider TEATIME community and the Springer team for their support. I also warmly thank Tecniplast S.p.A., and in particular its owner, who shared this passion and consistently supported my activities leading to this book. My deepest thanks and love go to my wife Katharina and to my family, whose patience and encouragement allowed me to push my boundaries. This book reflects a conviction that the digitalisation of preclinical research, together with advanced analytics and synthetic data, will reshape how we generate and interpret evidence. In that vision, home cage monitoring becomes a conduit between the everyday lives of laboratory animals and the broader digital ecosystem of research, helping us align better data, better welfare, and better translation.

Buguggiate, Italy　　　　　　　　　　　　　　　　Stefano Gaburro

Preface For Silvia Mandillo

Since 2021, I have had the privilege of helping shape the COST Action TEATIME "Improving biomedical research by automated behaviour monitoring in the animal home-cage", as a proposer, co-chair, and faculty member. Towards the last year of the Action, Stefano Gaburro and Vootele Voikar invited me to contribute as a co-author to some chapters of this book and, eventually, to join the editorial team. I gladly accepted and embarked on this journey of writing, supporting, advising, and finally reviewing the chapters that now form this well-deserved compendium on the development of automated home-cage monitoring in rodents.

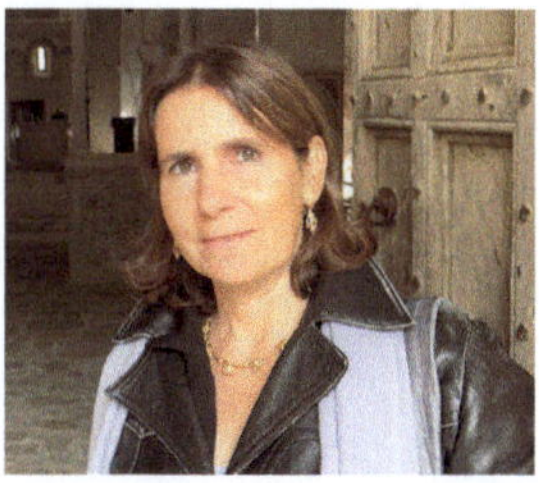

This volume stands as a testimony to the remarkable work accomplished over the 4 years of TEATIME. It brings together the collective expertise, creativity, and dedication of an extraordinary network of colleagues, who have become not only collaborators but also friends. We hope the book will serve as a guide and inspiration for future generations who are as committed and enthusiastic about home-cage monitoring as we, the editors and authors, have been.

I want to emphasise the wealth of knowledge we have been able to gather in this emerging field, made possible only through the passionate contributions of this international community. It is my sincere hope that these collaborations will continue to flourish, advancing this rapidly growing area of research and helping us meet future scientific challenges for the benefit of the research community, animal welfare, and the health of our world.

Monterotondo, Rome, Italy — Silvia Mandillo

Contents

Home Cage Monitoring: Where We Are and What We Need?

Anna Kiryk, Aleksandra Bartelik, Sara Wells, and Hilary Gates

Abstract

This book presents the first comprehensive overview of Home Cage Monitoring (HCM) in rodents, examining how these technologies may contribute to addressing some of the key challenges in animal research. HCM systems provide a method for continuous, automated observation of laboratory animals within their home environment, allowing for reduced handling and environmental disruption. This approach supports efforts to improve data quality and reproducibility in behavioural and physiological research and aligns with the principles of Replacement, Reduction, and Refinement (3Rs). To facilitate knowledge exchange and methodological alignment among researchers using HCM systems, the COST TEATIME Action (CA20135) was established.

This chapter presents the collective work of TEATIME Working Groups and includes:

- A definition of HCM, developed through a structured conceptual framework.
- A literature review covering publications from 1974 to 2024.
- A catalogue of available HCM systems, both commercial and self-made.

A. Kiryk (✉)
Nencki Institute of Experimental Biology, Polish Academy of Sciences, Warsaw, Poland
e-mail: a.kiryk@nencki.edu.pl

A. Bartelik
Institute of Microbiology of the Czech Academy of Sciences, Prague, Czech Republic
e-mail: aleksandra.bartelik@biomed.cas.cz

S. Wells · H. Gates
Mary Lyon Centre at MRC Harwell, Oxford, UK
e-mail: s.wells@har.mrc.ac.uk; h.gates@har.mrc.ac.uk

S. Gaburro, S. Mandillo (eds.), *Home Cage Monitoring in Rodents: A Global Effort*,
https://doi.org/10.1007/978-3-032-19781-8_1

- An international survey of 279 professionals across research, facility management, animal care, and technology development.

  Survey and literature findings indicate growing interest in HCM, but also highlight common limitations, including high setup costs, challenges with group housing, and data management workload. Despite this, continued development and standardisation efforts are likely to drive wider adoption and application of HCM technologies in basic and preclinical research.

Keywords

HCM · Animal research · Welfare · Reproducibility · Survey

1 Introduction: Can HCM Systems Improve the Reproducibility of Animal Research?

Since the seminal work *The Principles of Humane Experimental Technique* by W.M.S. Russell and R.L. Burch in 1959, the 3Rs principles (Replacement, Reduction, and Refinement) have become a foundational ethical and methodological framework in animal-based scientific research. These principles guide researchers not only in minimising animal suffering but also in enhancing the quality, reliability, and applicability of scientific outcomes (Tannenbaum and Bennett 2015).

Yet, as we entered the twenty-first century, a major challenge to the credibility of biomedical research began to surface: concerns about reproducibility and replicability. Alarmingly, studies have demonstrated that between 75% and 90% of basic and preclinical experiments fail to be successfully replicated across laboratories. Although this issue is often highlighted in the context of translational research, it originates much earlier in the research pipeline. Basic research forms the intellectual and experimental foundation upon which further translational and preclinical studies are built. Without robust and reproducible early-stage findings, the entire process of biomedical innovation is at risk (Begley and Ioannidis 2015).

Several interrelated factors contribute to this reproducibility crisis. These include insufficient experimental transparency, poor study design, suboptimal data quality, and inadequate reporting of methods and results. Each of these elements can severely hinder the ability of other scientists to reproduce the findings (Cobey et al. 2024).

In animal research, the issue is compounded by a frequent lack of understanding of species-specific behaviour. Misinterpreting natural behavioural patterns can lead to flawed models of disease or treatment effects. Moreover, even in well-designed studies, behavioural variation between litters of mice can significantly influence outcomes, sometimes overshadowing the effects of experimental interventions themselves (Begley and Ioannidis 2015).

Moreover, even in well-designed studies, biological variability, such as litter effects in young rodents or strain, sex, and environmental factors in adults, can significantly influence outcomes, sometimes overshadowing the effects of the interventions themselves (Begley and Ioannidis 2015).

This book presents the first comprehensive overview of Home Cage Monitoring (HCM) in rodents, examining how these technologies may contribute to addressing some of the key challenges in animal research. By enabling continuous, automated observation of animals in their home environment, HCM reduces stress linked to environmental disruption and human handling (Voikar and Gaburro 2020). These systems support long-term behavioural monitoring, generating rich datasets that can increase both the sensitivity and reproducibility of behavioural measurements in laboratory rodents (Kahnau et al. 2023; Bains et al. 2023; Kohler et al. 2022; Singh et al. 2019).

However, the benefits of HCM, not only in the context of the reproducibility crisis, depend strongly on appropriate implementation. The use of poorly chosen behavioural tests or analysis strategies can lead to the collection of large, but ultimately uninformative datasets, and may inadvertently increase the number of animals required. To address this, comprehensive training in experimental design, methodology, and data interpretation is essential, and should also include knowledge of the physiology and natural behaviours of the species studied, while keeping in mind individual variability.

Recognising these challenges, the COST Action "CA20135—Improving biomedical research by automated behaviour monitoring in the animal home cage (TEATIME)" created a collaborative European network for researchers in this field (2021–2025). Its primary aim was to foster knowledge exchange and skill development among scientists working with HCM systems, particularly in the context of rodent behaviour. The initiative played a central role in building a network of behavioural scientists, promoting collaboration and the exchange of expertise across the field. It actively organised workshops and training sessions, both in-person and online, including webinars that were made available through platforms such as the "*COST TEATIME YouTube channel*," to ensure broad accessibility for participants worldwide (see Chap. 11 for more details). Alongside these activities, comprehensive guidelines for HCM system users were developed, encompassing complementary protocols and standardised formats for data analysis and presentation of results (see Chap. 8 for more details). The initiative also assessed current needs for the development of new bioinformatics tools and identified key stakeholders, establishing effective communication channels. Platforms like "The Behaviour Forum" were leveraged as additional spaces for discussion of experimental methods in animal behaviour, facilitating continuous knowledge exchange (see also Chaps. 9 and 12). Through these combined efforts, the initiative significantly enhanced the transfer of knowledge and experience, empowering users to implement best practices more effectively and with greater confidence (Fig. 1).

2 HCM Definition

An essential step in fostering productive collaboration within the international network was to establish a shared language and an objective, common understanding of what constitutes HCM. Although the term is widely used, its interpretation varies depending on the research context, system type, and institutional practices. To address this ambiguity, the

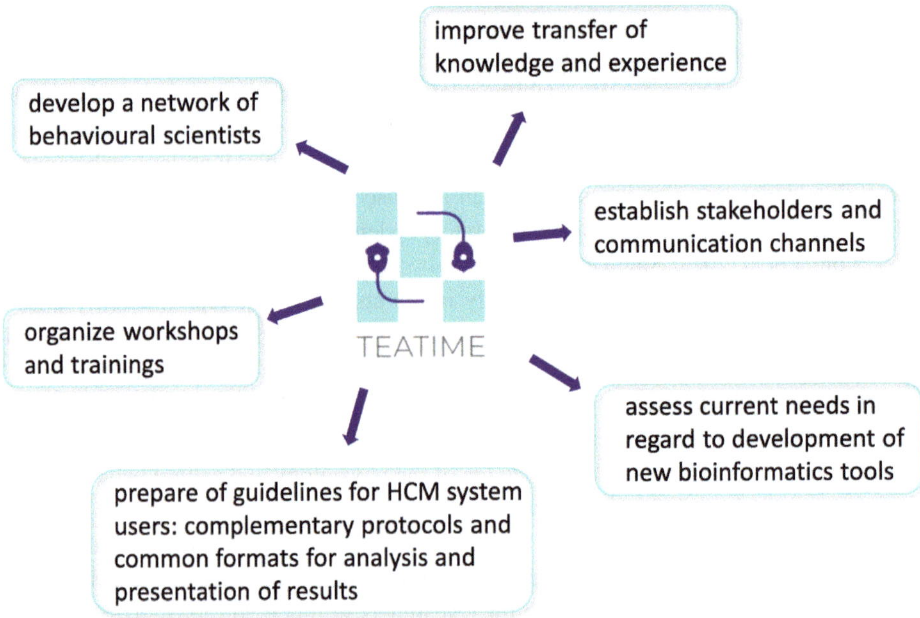

Fig. 1 Aims of the COST TEATIME Action 2021–2025

TEATIME network proposed a conceptual clarification of the term, aiming to build a foundation for consistent communication and methodological alignment across disciplines and scientists.

A useful tool for this purpose, which allows for collaborative editing, adding references, and refining explanations, is the theoretical category-based knowledge representation model, Olog, described by Spivak and Kent (2012). Using this model, we constructed a conceptual framework for the definition of HCM, which can be summarised as:

> A system that collects information on an animal which lives inside an enclosure that provides food, water, social contacts, safety from threat, and environmental enrichment.

The detailed nuances and clarifications that provide a more complete picture of HCM are shown in the graphical representation (Fig. 2).

Fig. 2 (continued) communicates with software to capture or elicit the behaviour, or physiology of an animal inside the enclosure. Hardware contains a sensor and an actor. These two elements may not necessarily be present at the same time; "Behaviour and Physiology": Behaviour is defined as a collection of visible movements, while physiology may be any collection of biological processes (e.g. heart rate, respiration); "Interval of time": Animals must be housed in the HCM for at least 24 h in order for the system to be able to capture a circadian rhythm; "Limited Human Interaction": A key property of all HCM systems is the limited human-animal interaction they provide. The animal is left undisturbed for protracted stretches of time, in order to allow the system to capture natural behaviour

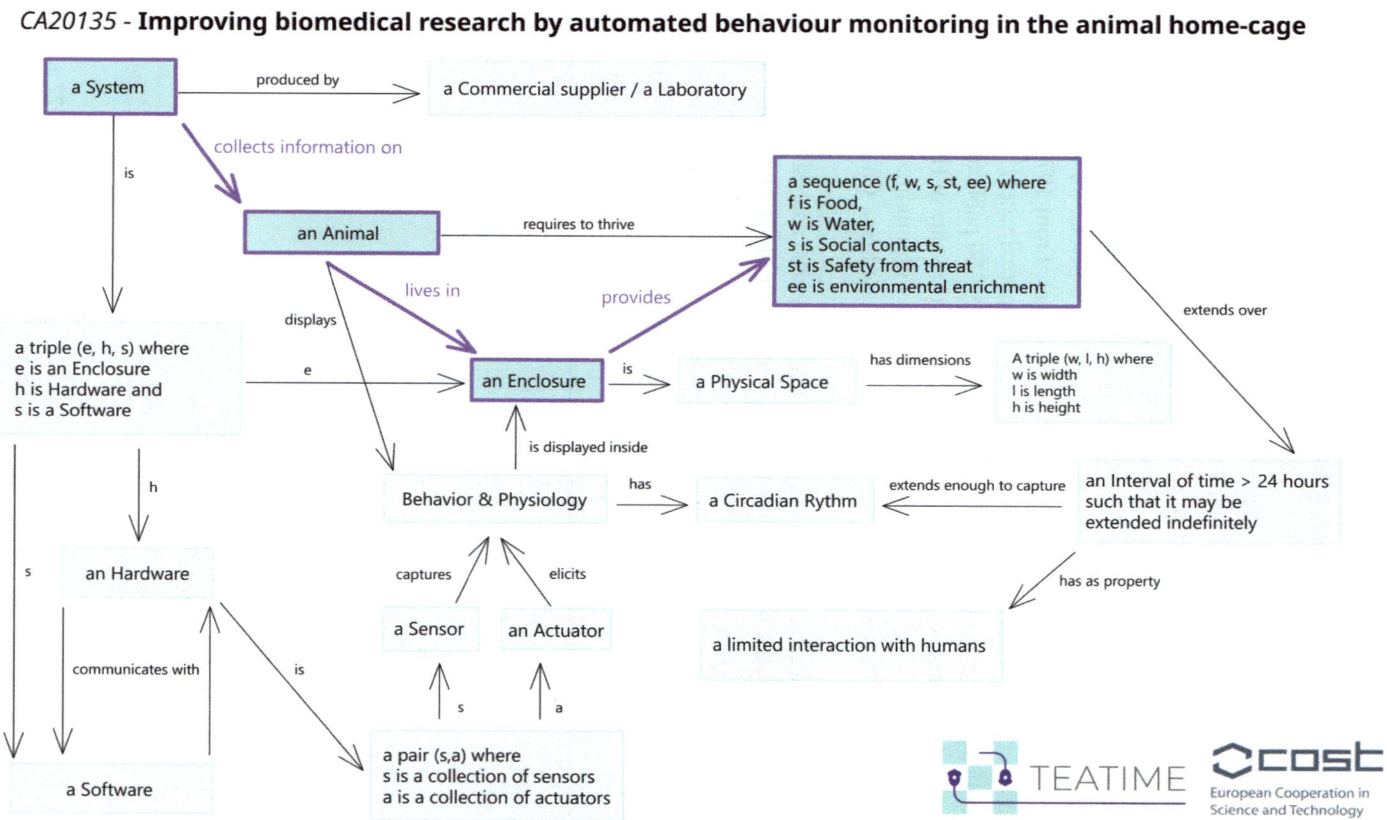

Fig. 2 Definition of HCM created using the Olog model, developed under the lead of Dr. Leonardo Restivo (TEATIME member). Additional detailed information: "An Animal": Any animal that can be observed either in a laboratory setting or in a farm setting; "An Enclosure": Enclosure is a physical place delimited by walls, floor, and optionally ceiling. It has physical dimensions that must be reported in papers; "Food, Water, Social contracts, Safety from threats, Environmental enrichment": All these elements are necessary for an animal to thrive when living inside an enclosure; "Enclosure, Hardware and Software": This is the definition of an analytical system used to capture behaviour and physiology. It consists of an enclosure, hardware, and software; "Hardware": Any piece of equipment that

3 Knowledge to Date About HCM

3.1 Evolution of HCM Technologies and Their Scientific Applications

The interest in HCM systems for the continuous and automated assessment of animal behaviour has grown markedly over time. Early studies, particularly before the 2000s, relied heavily on manual testing procedures, involving the physical transfer of animals to a novel test arena and labour-intensive scoring of behaviour. Monitoring was typically short, often less than 12 h, which limited the ability to capture circadian patterns or subtle, long-term changes in activity. However, the 2000s brought a pivotal shift toward 24-h monitoring and increasing adoption of automated technologies. From 1974 to 2024, the absolute number of HCM-related publications increased approximately 26-fold, from about 1–2 publications per year in the mid-1970s to around 50–60 publications annually by 2024 (Fig. 3). As awareness of animal welfare has grown, the value of HCM in capturing complex, spontaneous behaviour over extended periods with minimal disruption to animal life ("refinement" 3R rule) has become widely increased (see Chap. 3 for more details).

Moreover, in the last decade, advances in sensor technology, data analysis, and artificial intelligence have accelerated the development and application of HCM. Modern HCM systems integrate a variety of sensors, including passive infrared (PIR) detectors, depth cameras, radar-based motion sensors, and even microwave-based detectors, enabling the capture of a wide range of behavioural and physiological parameters without disturbing

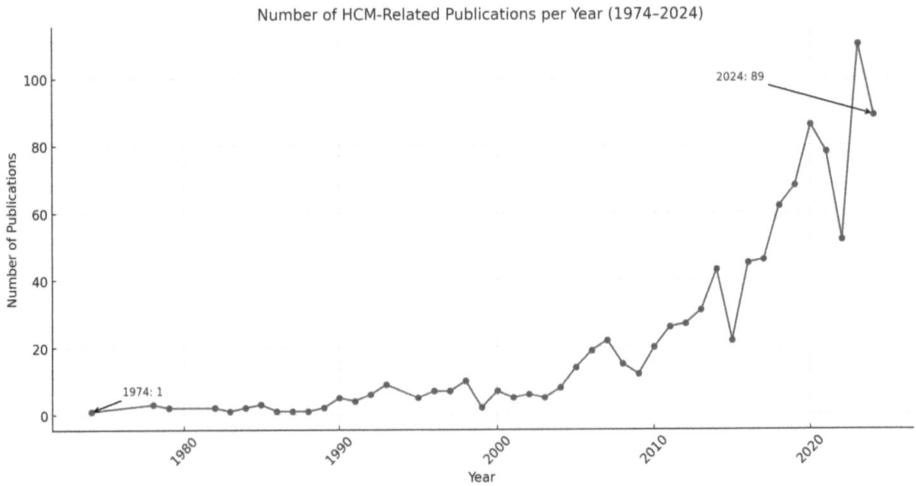

Fig. 3 Trends in the use of HCM in rodent research. The decline in publications in 2022 and the rebound-peak in 2024 may reflect delayed research and publication timelines caused by the COVID-19 pandemic. PubMed search with keywords "home cage monitoring" AND "mice" OR 'rats' (record date 06 June 2025)

Table 1 HCM application areas

Application Domain	Examples and Authors
Disease modelling	Colitis (Zentrich et al. 2021) Epilepsy (Jankovic et al. 2019) Fragile X (Bonasera et al. 2017) Huntington's and Alzheimer's (Bains et al. 2023; Ho et al. 2023) LPS-induced sickness (Hasriadi et al. 2021) Narcolepsy (Piilgaard et al. 2023)
Drug testing	Paroxetine effects and discontinuation (Collins et al. 2023)
Ageing and frailty	Age-related decline and frailty index (Ruby et al. 2023)
Neurobehavioural phenotyping	Circadian patterns, sleep behaviour, cognitive function, and locomotor activity in transgenic and wild-type mice (Steel et al. 2022; Voikar and Gaburro 2020; Murphy et al. 2020)
Welfare assessment	Quantifying stress responses to husbandry procedures such as timed mating and cage changes (Fuochi et al. 2023; Moore and Brook 2022)

the animals. For instance, video-based platforms like MouseVUER (Salem et al. 2024) and AI-powered systems such as RodentWatch (Hsieh et al. 2024) demonstrate how real-time tracking of position, posture, and body temperature can be achieved using a single camera paired with edge computing and deep learning algorithms. These systems not only automatically recognise behaviours, such as drinking, resting, or climbing, but also provide high-throughput data collection, significantly enhancing scalability and minimising the need for human intervention. Since 2020, more than 70 articles on HCM have been published annually, reflecting continued rapid growth and establishing HCM as a key tool for behavioural phenotyping and animal welfare assessment in rodent research.

Between 1974 and 2024, HCM systems have been applied across diverse research domains. Table 1 provides a representative selection of these application areas and the studies within them.

Unlike traditional behavioural tests that remove animals from their familiar environment and can introduce stress or bias, HCM allows for:

- Uninterrupted, long-term monitoring (Ho et al. 2023; Bonasera et al. 2017).
- Reduction of handling stress (Moore and Brook 2022; Zentrich et al. 2021).
- Naturalistic behaviour tracking (Bains et al. 2023; Balzani et al. 2018).
- High-throughput and scalable phenotyping (Murphy et al. 2020; Singh et al. 2019).

The range of behavioural and physiological parameters that can be assessed using HCM is summarised in Fig. 4.

3.2 Current Limitations of HCM Systems

Despite its many advantages, HCM faces several limitations that can impact its broader adoption and effectiveness, based on a review of 521 publications identified in the literature search to date (Kahnau et al. 2023). One key limitation is the variability introduced by

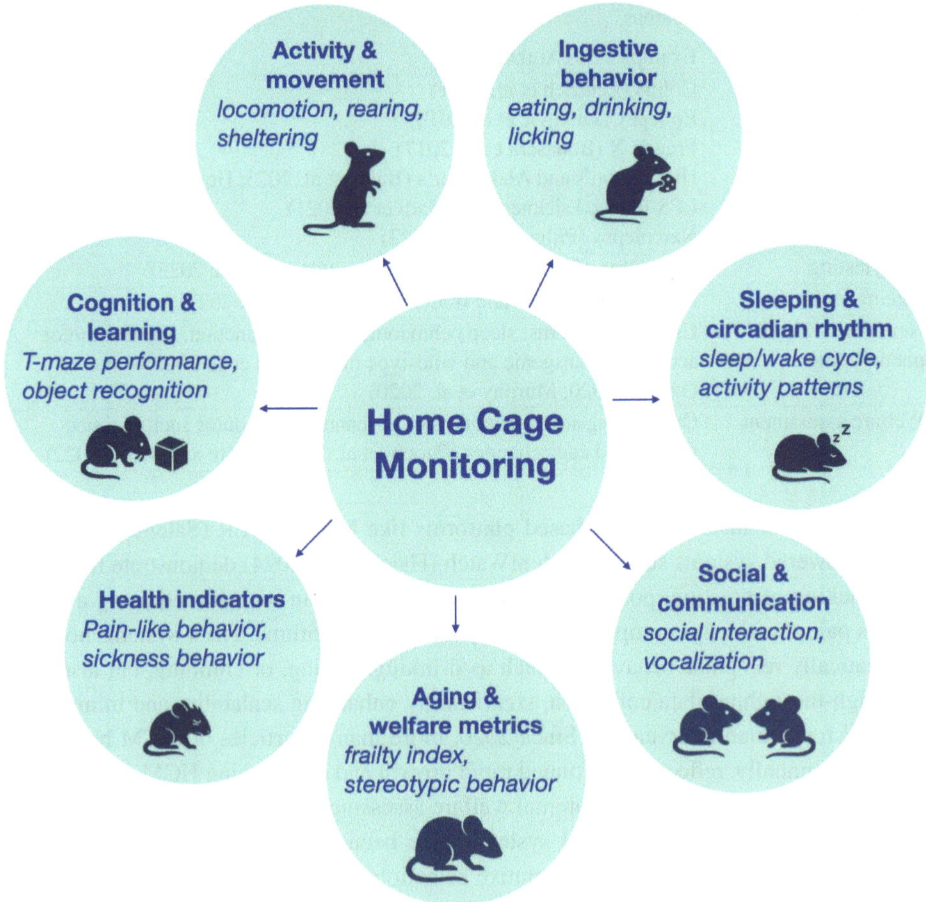

Fig. 4 Key behavioural and physiological parameters measured by HCM

environmental factors such as cage position and lighting conditions, which can influence activity patterns and circadian rhythms in rodents (Steel et al. 2022).

HCM studies have traditionally favoured male rodents, largely due to concerns that the female estrous cycle may introduce unwanted variability (Kahnau et al. 2023). However, this exclusion limits the scope and relevance of research, as many physiological and behavioural traits differ between sexes. Recent efforts increasingly include female animals to improve the translational value and completeness of behavioural phenotyping.

Individual housing has been commonly used in HCM to simplify tracking and data analysis, but it neglects the social nature of many rodent species and can introduce stress-related artefacts (Kahnau et al. 2023). Group housing better reflects natural living conditions and improves welfare, yet presents technical challenges, such as distinguishing individuals during continuous monitoring. New technologies like radio-frequency identification (RFID) and AI-based tracking are beginning to overcome these limitations, enabling more accurate group-housed data collection.

Additionally, while automated data collection reduces experimenter bias and stress on animals, it also limits the detection of subtle behaviours, especially those related to external appearance or infrequent events, which often still require manual observation. Furthermore, high setup costs and the need for specialised hardware or proprietary systems can be barriers for smaller laboratories, although open-source solutions are beginning to address this gap (Singh et al. 2019).

Lastly, while artificial intelligence and machine learning have enhanced data analysis, these approaches require technical expertise and robust validation to ensure accuracy and reproducibility across different research settings.

4 Guide to HCM Systems: A Catalogue of Commercial and Self-Made Solutions

Given the large number of HCM systems currently available for behavioural research, and each utilising different data acquisition technologies and offering varying capacities to capture behaviour, members of Working Group 2 of the TEATIME COST Action undertook the task of compiling a structured catalogue of currently existing systems. The aim was to create a resource that enables easy identification and comparison of equipment based on key features such as:

- The underlying technology (e.g. RFID, video tracking, photosensors, DeepLabCut-based pose estimation),
- The categories of behaviour they monitor (e.g. activity, memory, learning, feeding, social behaviour, temperature, heart rate, and more),
- The system implementation (hardware, software, or both),
- The animal species for which the system is optimised,
- The type of cage the system supports (standard or modified).

The catalogue includes both commercially available systems and custom-built setups developed by researchers for their specific experimental needs. It functions as an interactive database with a filter system and includes links to additional resources. Contact details for expert users, who have agreed to share their knowledge and expertise, are also included. The complete, interactive version of the catalogue is available at (thebehaviourdatabase.org). For a more detailed description of available HCM technologies, see Chap. 7.

As this compilation clearly shows, no single system currently captures the full range of behavioural and physiological parameters in a comprehensive way. Therefore, it is essential that researchers selecting a system do so based on the type of data needed to answer their specific scientific questions (and this is where the catalogue is an essential resource). Moreover, as mentioned earlier, automated recording enables long-term experiments that generate enormous amounts of data. This presents a further challenge for behavioural scientists: how to manage, analyse, and interpret such complex datasets. The following chapters of this book aim to support that process by offering perspectives and reflections on methodology to aid in a deeper understanding of the topic (Chaps. 7, 8, 9, and 10).

To further support the scientific community, researchers involved in the TEATIME consortium have also created an open-access platform TheBehaviourForum.org, where users can share their knowledge and experience, ask questions, and seek guidance related to behavioural monitoring systems and experimental design.

5 Exploring HCM: Results from an International Survey

Members of Working Group 1 of the COST Action TEATIME conducted an international survey to examine the current use, perceived benefits, limitations, and future potential of HCM technologies. The survey was disseminated through networks linked to the TEATIME in 2022, receiving 279 responses from 37 countries (31 European, 3 Asian, 2 North American, and 1 South American). Questions were tailored to professional groups: researchers, facility managers, animal caretakers and welfare specialists, and equipment/technology developers. These groups correspond to the role categories provided in the survey, from which each respondent was asked to select the one that best reflected their professional identity or responsibilities. The complete list of questions is attached as Appendix 1.

Survey Results

Out of 279 survey respondents, the majority (72%) identified as researchers. Animal caretakers and welfare specialists constituted 14%, facility managers 11%, and equipment/technology developers 3%. This indicates a predominance of input from the research community.

Nearly all respondents (99%) worked with rodents. Among these, 51% used only mice, 8% used only rats, and 40% used both species. This suggests that rodents and particularly mice were mainly used in laboratory research involving HCM systems.

5.1 Perceived Demand for 24/7 HCM

A majority of all respondents (77%) reported seeing a demand for 24/7 HCM (Fig. 5). However, only 42% used HCM systems in 2022 (Fig. 6).

Among the 58% who did not use HCM, 73% anticipate a future need to adopt the technology. Among HCM users, nearly all (98%) foresaw continued use, and 90% anticipated expanding their use. These findings suggest a strong and growing interest in HCM technologies despite current limitations in adoption (see Table 2).

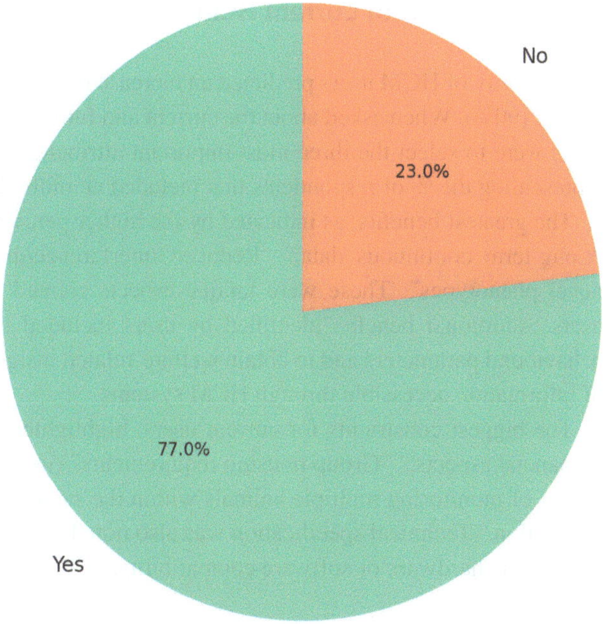

Fig. 5 Perceived demand for 24/7 HCM (279 respondents)

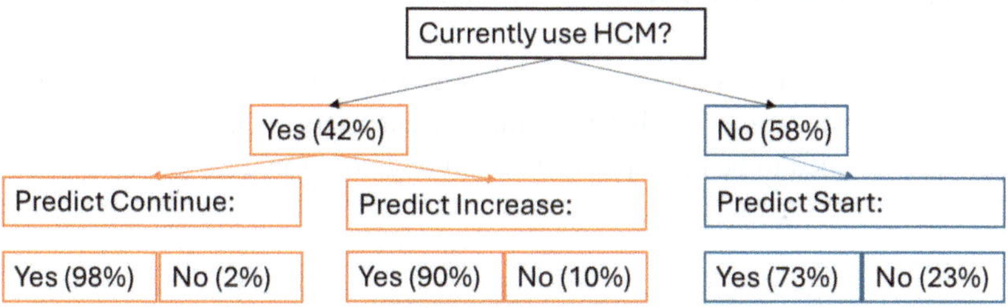

Fig. 6 Current use and anticipated demand for HCM systems

Table 2 The limitations of HCM ranked as % of responses from non-users ($n = 161$)

Limitations of HCM systems (non-users)	% of respondents
Cost of ownership	67%
Technical and IT support/data management support	47%
Acceptance of new testing methods	35%
Facility space	32%
IT infrastructure limitations	30%
Awareness of capabilities	20%

5.2 Opinions of Current HCM Users

The majority of HCM users predicted an increase in demand in coming years for this technology (90%). When asked about the current and future benefits of HCM systems, respondents were to select the three most important attributes of HCM. The data are displayed representing the % of respondents that included an individual answer in their selections.

The greatest benefits, as indicated by the higher percentage in green (Fig. 7), included "Long-term continuous data," "Reduced interference/disturbance," and "Discovery of novel phenotypes". These were unique aspects created by HCM according to current users. Additional benefits identified by users included the capacity to record multiple behavioural parameters and to obtain welfare-related insights, thereby extending the scope of information accessible through HCM systems.

The biggest constraints for current users, highlighted in red (Fig. 7), were primarily "Financial aspects," "Group housing requirements" (i.e. the technical and logistical challenges of monitoring multiple animals within the same cage), "Data analysis" and "Data integration." Technical specification was also noted as a limitation, for example, the need for specific hardware or software compatibility.

5.3 Opinions of Non-Users of HCM Systems

For non-users, the main concern was "Cost of ownership," marked by 67% of respondents (Table 2). There was some overlap with the current users' concerns about "Financial aspects," but it seemed to be more pronounced among non-users.

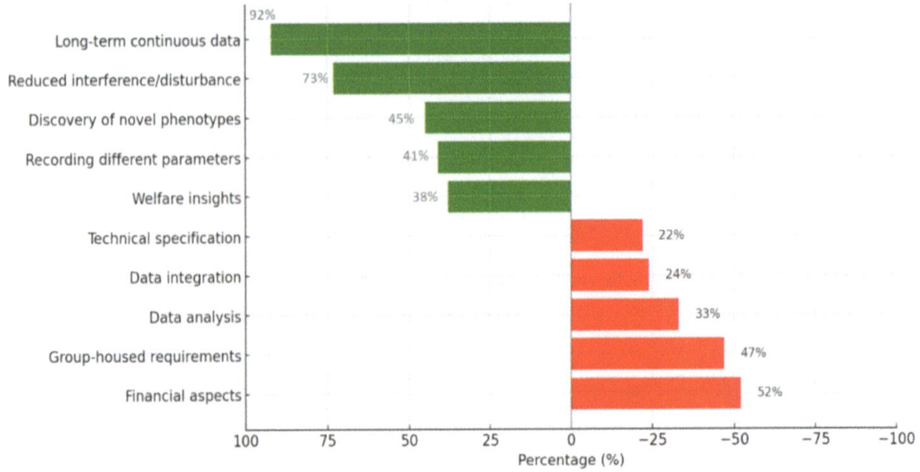

Fig. 7 Current and future benefits (green) and limitations (red) of using HCM as % of responses from current users

"Technical and IT support/data management support" was the second most significant constraint for non-users, mentioned by 47%, which may correlate with the "Data analytics" (33%) and "Data integration" (24%) issues identified by current users, albeit at a lower percentage level.

"Acceptance of new testing methods" at 35% and "Facility space" at 32% were further unique concerns among non-users, suggesting hesitancy in adopting new technologies and practical limitations of space.

"IT infrastructure limitations" and "Awareness of capabilities" (understanding what HCM systems can actually do and their potential benefits) at 30% and 20% respectively, were less important to non-users compared to other factors.

In summary, both users and non-users recognised the challenges associated with financial, analytical, and technical support. Additionally, non-users emphasised acceptance of the new method and the practical limitations of the facility, pointing out the obstacles associated with implementing new research methods. Despite these concerns, 62% of non-users predicted that they would start to use HCM systems.

It should be noted that these projections may be influenced by the fact that the survey was conducted among a community potentially already familiar with HCM concepts, and therefore may not fully reflect the broader behavioural research community.

5.4 Assessment of the Suitability of Existing Out-of-Cage Systems

Respondents were asked to assess how the existing "out-of-cage" tools (conventional behavioural testing methods conducted outside the animals' home environment, such as open field tests or maze-based arenas) satisfy their current needs in different types of research (including toxicology, multi-morbidities, long-term studies, disease progression, and translational data). A significant proportion of both HCM users and non-users reported that the out-of-cage methods suited their studies "well" or "very well" (41% and 47% for users and non-users, respectively).

However, it appears that there is significant room for improvement (Fig. 8). 22% of HCM non-users and 27% of users indicated poor performance and around 30% of both users and non-users indicated only a moderate suitability.

5.5 Research Needs Identified for HCM Systems

When asked what additional research data respondents would like to collect, there was again no significant difference between current users and non-users of HCM systems. These can be grouped into three main categories:

A. *Social and behavioural monitoring*:
  - Social interactions (61%)
  - Data of individual mouse in social context (60%)

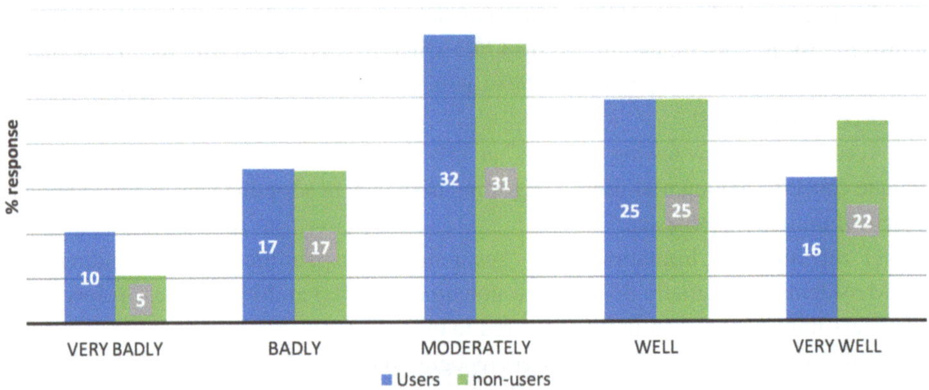

Fig. 8 How did the existing out-of-cage tools satisfy research needs? This figure shows the reported performance of out-of-cage tools as % of all responses ($n = 279$)

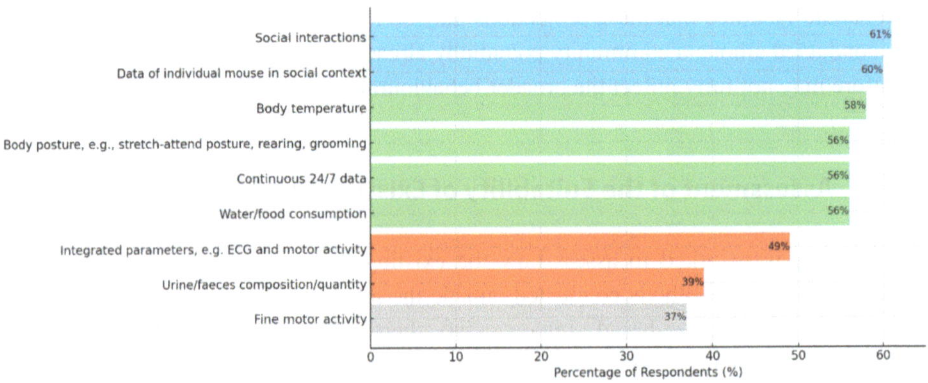

Fig. 9 Additional parameters wish list as % of respondents ($n = 279$). Bar colours indicate how often each parameter was selected: blue = most frequent, green = frequent, orange = moderate, grey = least frequent

- Body posture (e.g. stretch-attend posture, rearing, grooming) (56%)
- Fine motor activity (37%)

B. *Physiological and health indicators*
- Body temperature (58%)
- Water/food consumption (56%)
- Urine/faeces composition and quantity (39%)
- Integrated physiological parameters (e.g., ECG and motor activity) (49%)

C. *Monitoring continuity*
- Continuous 24/7 data collection (56%)

The highest priorities were related to understanding social dynamics and individual behaviour in group settings (Fig. 9).

6 Discussion

The survey results highlight strong interest in expanding the use of HCM, but limited by concerns about financial and infrastructure barriers. Despite current limitations, most respondents, including those who do not use these technologies, anticipate wider adoption of HCM technologies. The data suggest a need for validation of HCM systems, meaning formal studies that demonstrate their reliability, accuracy, and relevance for specific scientific or welfare-related applications. Additionally, efforts should focus on cost-reduction strategies, and increased awareness of the benefits of HCM systems (see Table 3).

Mice are the predominant species in HCM use

The majority of survey respondents identified as researchers working with rodents, with most current users of HCM systems employing them in mouse-based studies rather than in rat models. This pattern appears to reflect the trajectory of HCM technologies, which have been primarily tailored for mouse studies. In contrast, the development of HCM methods for other species remains limited (see Chap. 13 for more details). These findings suggest an opportunity to broaden the application of HCM technologies beyond their current scope, particularly in areas such as animal welfare assessment, husbandry practices, agricultural research, and studies involving alternative species, including rats, fish, chickens, and larger laboratory animals. Expansion into these areas may be supported by continued technological advancements and targeted dissemination efforts (see Chap. 12 for more details).

Out-of-cage methods are considered adequate by less than half of the respondents

The survey results highlighted dissatisfaction with the adequacy of existing non-HCM tools to meet current research needs. More than 20% of participants rated such tools poorly, and less than half considered them well-suited to their work. Both HCM users and non-users expressed a desire for systems capable of capturing a wider range of behavioural and physiological data, including social interactions, body attitudes, and welfare-related indicators such as body temperature and food and water intake. These needs indicate a demand for high-resolution, continuous monitoring of individual animals in a social context—an application that remains technically challenging in standard cage configurations.

However, the ability of HCM systems to meet these needs may support the partial replacement of certain out-of-cage tests, particularly those associated with poor reproducibility, limited interpretability, and elevated stress responses. For example,

Table 3 Examples of current and potential efforts to overcome barriers to HCM adoption

Barrier	Example of Ongoing or Potential Efforts
High initial costs	Modular, lower-cost systems; open-source hardware/software
Institutional barriers	Cross-institutional training, outreach, and shared HCM platforms
Reluctance to adopt new methods	Case studies demonstrating scientific benefits; user networks for knowledge exchange

standard open field tests often produce variable results due to their sensitivity to environmental conditions and handling-related stress. While such methods are not necessarily obsolete, their utility may be enhanced by integrating them into a home-based behavioural framework. In this context, HCM technologies may offer a complementary or, in some cases, preferable alternative, depending on the research question and experimental design.

Cost is the primary barrier to HCM wider adoption

Financial constraints emerged as the most frequently cited barrier to adoption of HCM systems, reported by both current users and non-users. Respondents noted that the initial investment required for HCM, especially for high-end systems, can exceed the cost of conventional cages or phenotyping equipment, placing a significant cost burden on institutions. Despite this, comparisons between HCM and out-of-cage methods can overlook the additional scientific value offered by continuous cage monitoring. In addition to financial concerns, HCM non-users highlighted a broader reluctance to adopt new testing methods, suggesting cultural or institutional resistance to change. In particular, current users emphasised the advantages of HCM in enabling 24-h, minimally disruptive monitoring and detection of subtle or previously unobservable phenotypes. These perspectives suggest that HCM systems may offer significant scientific advantages that are not fully accounted for in cost-based comparisons with out-of-cages methods. Approaches to overcoming challenges related to the implementation and management of HCM are explored in the context of animal facilities (Chap. 2), scientific research (Chap. 4), and the pharmaceutical sector (Chap. 5).

Data management and technical demands limit HCM adoption

Data management emerged as the second most frequently reported challenge to the effective use of HCM systems. Respondents noted that the large volume and complexity of data generated, including behavioural, physiological, and environmental parameters, can be difficult to store, process, and analyse. These logistical burdens can be a barrier to wider adoption, especially for institutions without dedicated infrastructure or expertise. This technical challenge may also contribute to a general reluctance to adopt new testing methods, as the high-throughput data obtained with HCM often requires scientists to adapt their analytical and statistical processes. Such changes go beyond routine adjustments and may be a difficult learning curve for some laboratories. Expanding collaboration among institutions and user communities can facilitate collaborative learning and validation, and support scalable integration of HCM across diverse research settings.

7 Conclusions

The survey conducted by COST TEATIME Action among diverse professional groups has shed light on the usage and perceived usage (for non-users) of HCM systems and their anticipated future trends:

- 42% of respondents were users of HCM (mainly Researchers using mice).

- 58% of respondents did not use HCM (mainly Animal Care and Welfare Specialists, Facility Managers, respondents using rats only).
- Benefits of HCM systems focus on improving research quality and ethical standards by comprehensive rodents' longitudinal data collection, minimising interference, discovering new behavioural features, recording various experimental parameters, and gaining insights into animal well-being.
- Less favourable aspects were mainly financial and technical support, housing requirements, data analysis, and integration issues. Non-users emphasised their concerns about adopting new methods and the practical limitations of the facility's space, pointing out the obstacles associated with implementing new research methods.
- Despite these concerns, 62% of non-users predict that they would start to use HCM systems and 90% of current users foresaw an increased demand for HCM systems in the forthcoming years.
- The existing out-of-cage tools only moderately meet the current needs of respondents, indicating significant room for improvement.
- Potential future needs include the ability to study social behaviour and physiological parameters using HCM systems.

Currently, HCM systems are recognised as significantly improving scientific rigour and animal welfare in rodent research, which has led to growing popularity. To fully realise their potential, future solutions must overcome existing barriers related to cost and technical support. HCM systems must also expand capabilities to meet new needs for monitoring physiological and social behaviours.

Appendices

Appendix 1: TEATIME-Home-Cage-Monitoring-Survey-Report-12-June-2024

A1.1 Exploring the Present and Future of Home Cage Monitoring: A Comprehensive Survey

A1.1.1 Introduction

This survey was designed to explore the interest in Home Cage Monitoring (HCM) technologies for animal monitoring in their natural environment, aiming to identify the potential benefits and challenges for the biomedical community. The survey was sent to members of the EU COST Action (TEATIME: https:/www.cost-teatime.org/) and further shared through their networks, including various animal associations, scientific societies, and mailing groups. It gained additional exposure at conferences like FELASA 2022, where presentations and fliers helped spread the word. The survey ran for several months, attracting 279 responses from 37 countries, with a diverse representation from Europe, Asia, North America, and South America.

A1.1.1.1 Survey Methodology

Work Group 1 of COST Action (20,135 TEATIME) created the survey to identify the prevalence and use of HCM systems in science, application of the 3Rs and well-being principles, views on current and future use, barriers to adoption, and the need to improve HCM for scientific and welfare aims. The questions were developed by 11 WG1 members during a face-to-face meeting in May 2022, and 20 WG1 members attending online.

Five to six questions were developed for four target groups:

1. Researchers
2. Facility managers
3. Animal care and welfare specialist
4. Equipment/technology developer

The complete list of questions is attached at Appendix 2. The survey was open for about 5 months, from 10 June 2022 (launched at the FELASA conference) to 31 October 2022.

Invitations for the survey were sent to TEATIME Action participants and their wider network, promoted via social media (Twitter and LinkedIn), and further distributed through emails from Action members to various institutions, researchers, and relevant stakeholders. Additionally, it was featured in newsletters from LASA forum, EARA, and The North American 3Rs Collaborative.

The survey (available at Google platform) received 279 responses, which were analysed in Excel. For multiple entries from the same person, only the latest response was included in the analysis.

A1.1.2 Surveyed Community

A1.1.2.1 Survey Respondent Distribution by Target Groups

The data collection from this survey was extensive, yet not all answers delivered clear indications about the trends or opinions of the whole community. We have used further categorisation in the analyses of some of the data to ensure that the responses from as many people as possible were included in this report. This includes the roles of the participants (Fig. 10). Unless stated specifically, the numbers reported within the results below do not differ according to roles or laboratory animal species.

These categories indicate a diverse range of professional backgrounds among survey respondents. The distribution of survey respondents is shown in Fig. 10. The majority of respondents categorised as researchers (72%), with animal care and welfare specialists and facility managers forming 14% and 11% and a small number of equipment and technology developers (3%).

A1.1.2.2 Use of Laboratory Animals Species

Species used by the population surveyed: 99% used rodents of these 51% used mice only, 8% rats only and 40% used both mice and rats (Fig. 11).

The results of the survey indicate that HCM is mainly used in rodent (predominantly mouse) research, as evidenced by the distribution of roles and species.

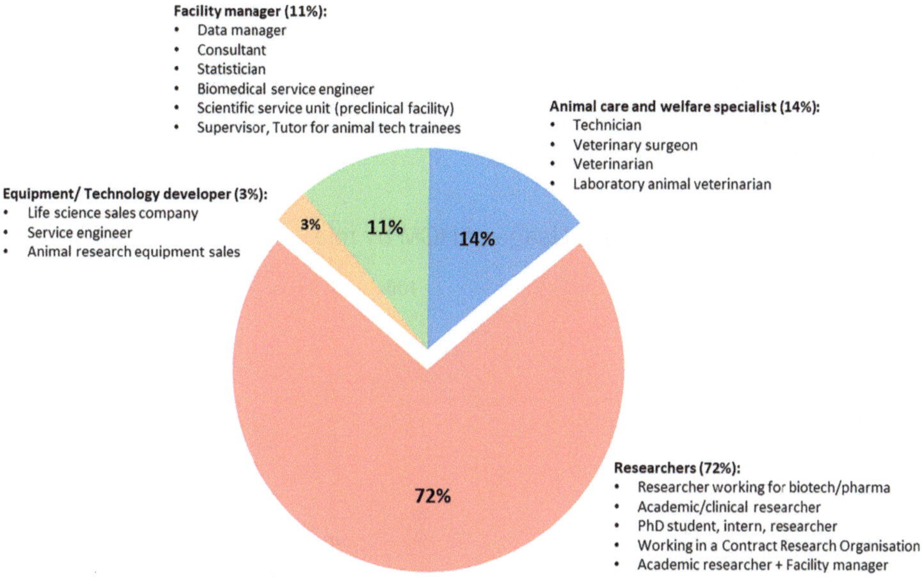

Fig. 10 Survey respondents by professional groups

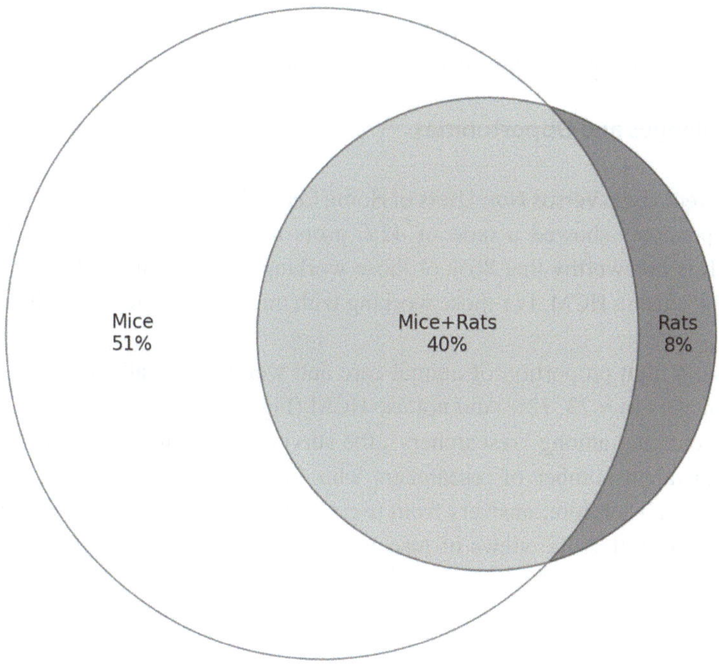

Fig. 11 Rodent species used by survey respondents (researchers)

Table 4 Users versus non-users of HCM systems

Home Cage Monitoring systems	Users (%)	Non-Users (%)
Overall respondents	42%, 118 individuals	58%, 161 individuals
Working with mice only	53%	47%
Working with rats only	14%	86%

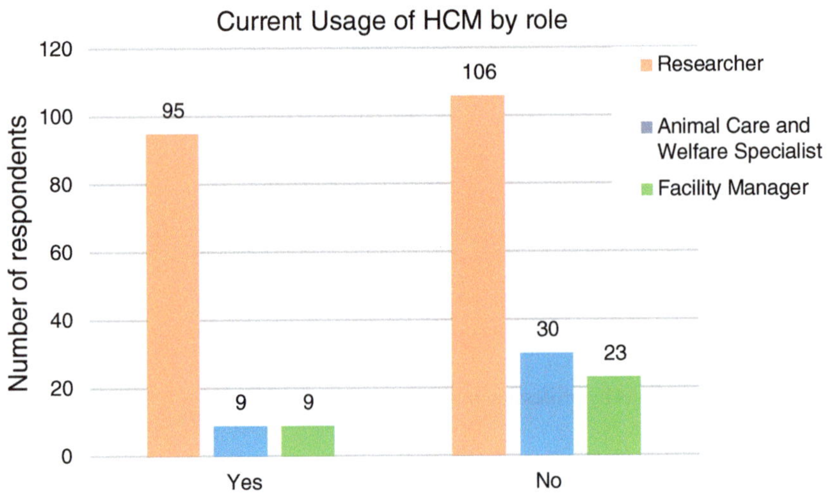

Fig. 12 Number of users/non-users of HCM systems by professional group (numbers on the top of each bar represent total number of individuals of each role)

A1.1.3 Challenges and Opportunities

A1.1.3.1 Current Users Versus Non-Users of Home Cage Monitoring Systems

Survey respondents showed a ratio of 42% users to 58% non-users of HCM systems (Table 4). It is noteworthy that 86% of those working with rats alone did not use HCM, with only 14% using HCM. For those working with mice, 53% were using HCM and 47% were not.

Likewise, a high proportion of animal care and welfare specialist ($n = 30$, 77%) and facility managers ($n = 23$, 72%) did not use HCM (Fig. 12).

It is of note, that among "researchers", the survey successfully collected information from an equivalent number of researchers who "use" ($n = 95$, 47%), or "do not use" ($n = 106$, 53%). Therefore, answers from users of HCM systems in this report are more likely to closely reflect the views of researchers who make up 81% of the current user respondents.

A1.1.3.2 Opinions of Current HCM Users

The results in this section are mainly based on the responses of researchers, who accounted for 81% of HCM users. Therefore, answers from users are more likely to closely reflect the views of researchers.

Current users selected three most important advantages/limitations of HCM systems from a pre-defined list. The data shows the percentage of respondents who selected each attribute (Fig. 13).

The greatest benefits, as indicated by the higher percentage in green, include "Long-term continuous data", "Reduced interference/disturbance", and "Discovery of novel phenotypes". These are unique aspects created by HCM according to current users.

The biggest constraints for current users, highlighted in red, are primarily "Financial aspects", "Group housing requirements", "Data analysis" and "Data integration".

Despite these limitations, the majority of current HCM predicted an increase in demand in coming years for HCM technology (90%).

A1.1.3.3 Opinions of Non-Users of HCM Systems

For non-users, the main concern is "Cost of ownership", marked by 67% of respondents (Table 5). There is some overlap with the current users' concerns about "Financial aspects", but it seems to be more pronounced among non-users.

"Technical and IT support/data management support" is the second most significant constraint for non-users, mentioned by 47%, which may correlate with the "Data Analytics" (33%) and "Data Integration" (24%) issues identified by current users, albeit at a lower percentage level.

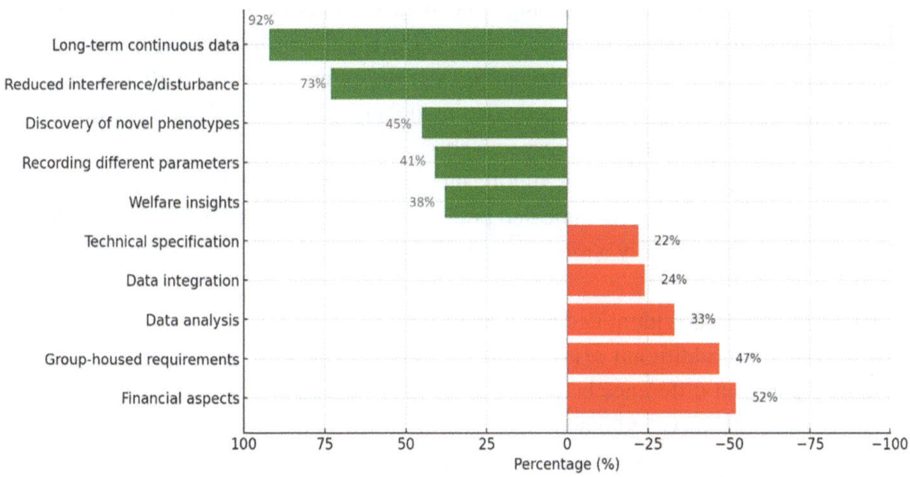

Fig. 13 Current and future benefits (green) and limitations (red) of using HCM as % of responses from current users

Table 5 The limitations of HCM ranked as % of responses from non-users ($n = 161$)

Limitations of HCM systems (non-users)	% of respondents
Cost of ownership	67%
Technical and IT support/data management support	47%
Acceptance of new testing methods	35%
Facility space	32%
IT infrastructure limitations	30%
Awareness of capabilities	20%

"Acceptance of new testing methods" at 35% and "Facility space" at 32% are further concerns among non-users, suggesting hesitancy in adopting new technologies and practical limitations of space.

"IT infrastructure limitations" and "Awareness of capabilities", at 30% and 20%, respectively, are less important to non-users compared to other factors. They may imply difficulties in understanding the technical aspects and potential of the systems.

In summary, both users and non-users recognise the challenges associated with financial and technical support. Additionally, non-users emphasise acceptance of the new method and the practical limitations of the facility, pointing out the obstacles associated with implementing new research methods. Despite these concerns, 62% of non-users predicted that they would start to use HCM systems.

A1.1.4 Requirements, Needs, and Opportunities

A1.1.4.1 Suitability of Existing Out-of-Cage Systems

When asked to assess how the existing "out of cage" tools satisfy their current needs in different types of research (including toxicology, multi-morbidities, long-term studies, disease progression, and translational data), a significant proportion of both users and non-users thought that the out-of-cage methods suited their studies "well" or "very well" (41% and 47% for users and non-users, respectively).

However, it appears that there is significant room for improvement (Fig. 14). With 22% of non-users and 27% of users indicated poor performance and around 30% of both users and non-users indicated only a moderate suitability.

A1.1.4.2 Research Needs Identified for HCM Systems

When asked what additional research data respondents would like to collect, there was again no significant difference between current users and non-users of HCM systems.

The community surveyed noted many parameters which they would like to include in their studies, including behavioural parameters such as social interactions with individual animals in a social context and physiological indicators such as body temperature and food/water consumption, as selected from a pre-defined list (results in Fig. 15).

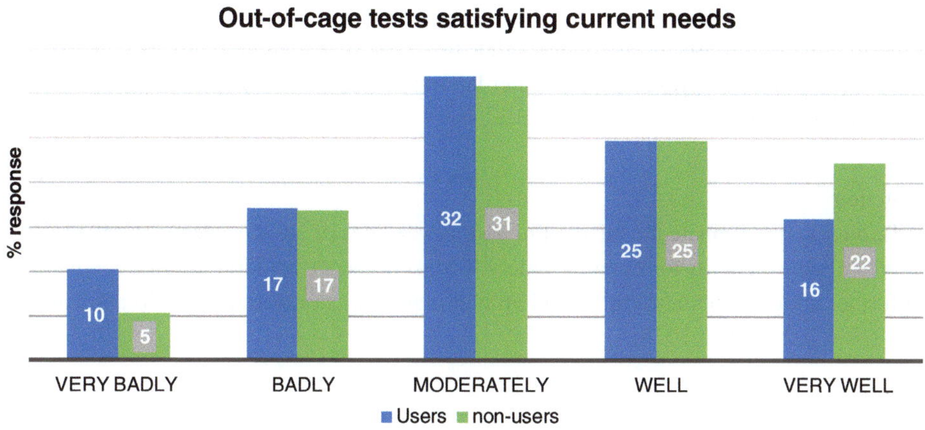

Fig. 14 How does the existing out-of-cage tools satisfy current needs? This figure shows performance of out of cage tools as % of all responses ($n = 279$)

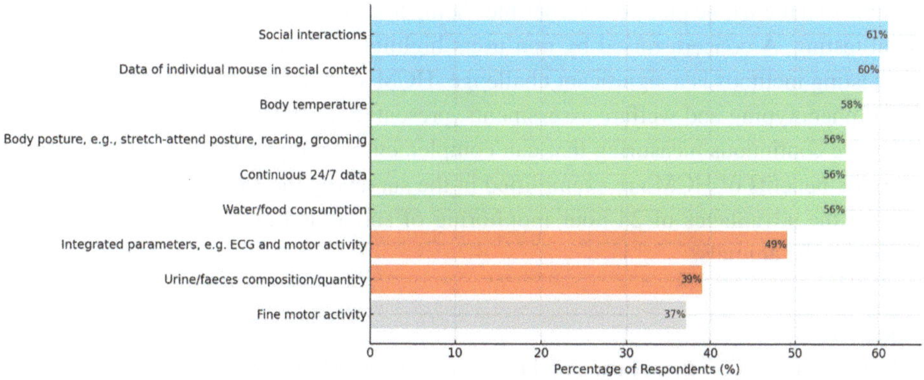

Fig. 15 Additional parameters wish list as % of respondents ($n = 279$)

A1.1.5 Discussions and Further Opportunities

Action

Continue to proactively target other communities including welfare sector and those working with species other than mice for interaction with the TEATIME network over Years 3 and 4 of the ACTION (Nov 2023 to Oct 2025).

The majority of the respondents to this survey worked as researchers using rodents, with the majority of those already using HCM working with mice, not rats. This reflects the current state of HCM systems which have focussed their development for mouse research purposes, while other fields are not necessarily seeing the same level of growth in uptake.

There is a clear opportunity, especially with some of the developing technologies, to continue to expand the use of HCM into other fields such as welfare analysis (see below), husbandry, agricultural research, and other laboratory models including rats, fish, chicken, and larger species.

Action

Explicitly disseminate the huge number of advantages of HCM systems, with examples of their benefits to research widely to stakeholders (including funding bodies), further targeting both scientific and animal management meetings over Years 3 and 4 (Nov 2023 to Oct 2025).

The number one and most significant challenge from current users and non-users of HCM systems is the financial challenge of setting up a new system. Indeed, some sophisticated systems are priced higher than existing caging/phenotyping equipment and represent a significant strategic outlay for institutes, universities, and companies. However, it is possible that the whole picture is sometimes being lost in a comparison with more conventional testing. A concern raised by non-users highlighted that the lack of acceptance of new testing methods is a significant challenge. HCM systems are additive to other methods of phenotyping and welfare assessments, presenting a whole new range of long-term and more continuous measuring that can complement phenotyping efforts. The potential scientific benefits of HCM are exemplified in the survey by the HCM current users highlighting the advantages of 24-hour monitoring of subtle and novel phenotypes without disturbing the animals.

Action

Expansion of WG3 to include a collaborative framework specifically to link up users of similar systems or those analysing similar datasets to promote validation of HCM systems in order to associate HCM indices with hard-core biological relevant data.

The second most significant challenge identified by this survey is that of data management. The vast array of different parameters which can be measured by the HCM systems is daunting, as well as logistically difficult, with some systems including high volumes of data collection and processing prior to any biological analysis. TEATIME Working Group 3 has been focussing on some of the issues relating to current and further development of HCM, in terms of data handling and analyses. Expanding the network to other potential users and offering the opportunity of collaborative working with laboratories already embracing these systems should be a future goal.

This survey indicates many opportunities that development and further adoption of HCM systems could fulfil in the future. A significant proportion of responses indicated a great dissatisfaction in the suitability of existing non-HCM systems (over 20%) with less than 50% indicating that their current tests worked well in meeting the current needs of their studies.

Respondents, both current "users" and "non-users" of HCM systems, indicated a wish to collect a range of behavioural indices and physiological parameters. The leading needs related to collecting 24/7 data from individual mice in social context, including social behaviours, body postures, but also welfare indicators, like body temperature and water/food consumption.

This is clearly the most demanding technical challenge to overcome within the settings of standard home cage rearing. Nevertheless, this may allow reduction of the use of some of the currently used "out of the cage" tests that appear to be not suitable tools for phenotyping because of low replicability, high interpretational ambiguity, and/or high sensitivity to unspecific stressors. However, this does not apply to all "out of the cage" tests, although novelty-induced exploration can also be assessed when starting out from a home base to better assess the organisation/progression of behavioural exploration (commonly as more deterministic than stochastic) as reported for open field exploration.

A1.1.6 Concluding Remarks

The survey conducted by COST TEATIME Action among diverse professional groups has shed light on the current usage of HCM systems and their anticipated future trends:

- 42% of respondents are current users of HCM (mainly Researchers using mice).
- 58% of respondents do not use HCM (mainly Animal Care and Welfare Specialists, Facility Managers, respondent using rats only).
- Current and future benefits of HCM systems focus on improving research quality and ethical standards by comprehensive rodents' longitudinal data collection, minimising interference, discovering new behavioural features, recording various experimental parameters, and gaining insights into animal well-being.
- Less favourable aspects are mainly financial and technical support, housing requirements, data analysis, and integration issues. Non-users emphasise their concerns about adopting new methods and the practical limitations of the facility's space, pointing out the obstacles associated with implementing new research methods.
- Despite these concerns, 62% of non-users predict that they would start to use HCM systems and 90% of current users foresee an increased demand for HCM systems in the forthcoming years.
- The existing out-of-cage tools only moderately meet the current needs of respondents, indicating significant room for improvement.
- Potential future needs include the ability to study social behaviour and physiological parameters using HCM systems.

Further Information

- Behavioural forum—https://www.cost-teatime.org/about/thebehaviourforum/
- HCM catalogue—https://www.cost-teatime.org/about/technologies/
- YouTube channel—https://www.youtube.com/@cost_teatime

Acknowledgement
This article is based upon a survey and work from COST Action TEATIME "Improving biomedical research by automated behaviour monitoring in the animal home-cage", CA20135, (www.cost-teatime.org) supported by COST (European Cooperation in Science and Technology).

Appendix 2: TEATIME Home Cage Monitoring Survey Questions

1

Which of the following best describes your role?

- ○ Academic/clinical researcher
- ○ Researcher working for biotech/pharma
- ○ Equipment/technology developer
- ○ Animal care and welfare specialist
- ○ Facility manager
- ○ Data manager
- ○ Working in a Contract Research Organisation
- ○ Other:

Asked to all

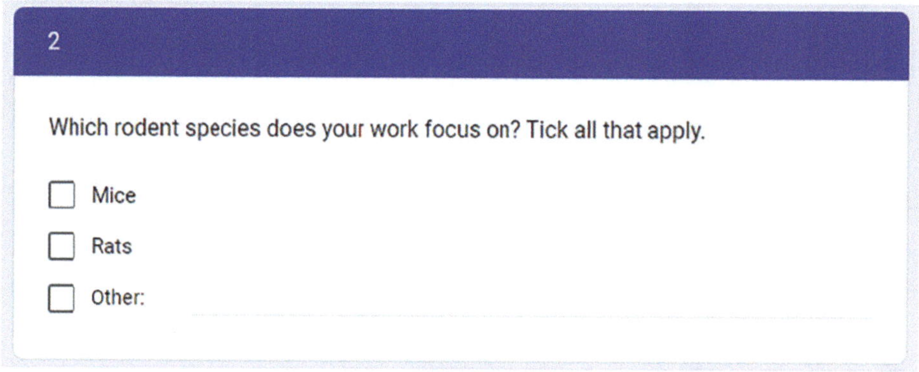
2

Which rodent species does your work focus on? Tick all that apply.

☐ Mice

☐ Rats

☐ Other:

Asked to all

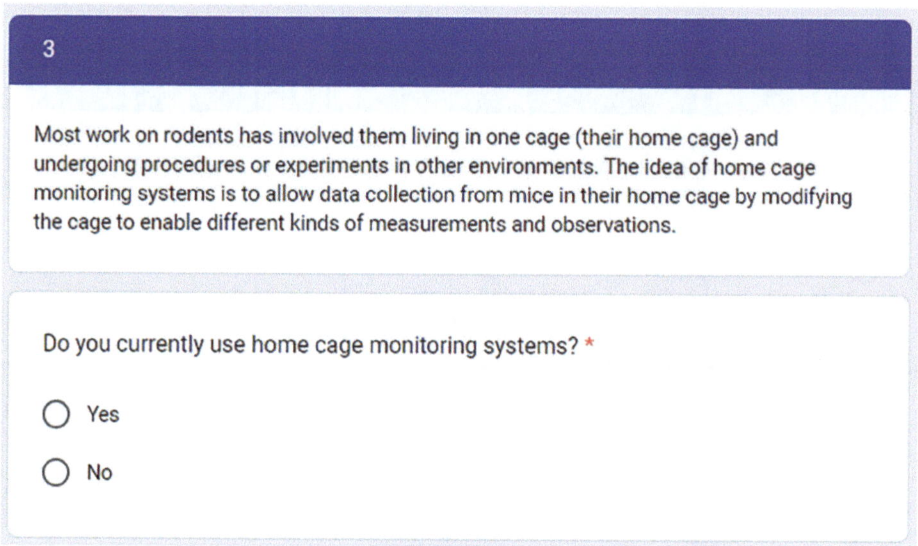
3

Most work on rodents has involved them living in one cage (their home cage) and undergoing procedures or experiments in other environments. The idea of home cage monitoring systems is to allow data collection from mice in their home cage by modifying the cage to enable different kinds of measurements and observations.

Do you currently use home cage monitoring systems? *

○ Yes

○ No

Asked to all

4

What do you mainly use for in vivo testing?

- ◯ Conventional outside home cage tests
- ◯ Home cage monitoring systems
- ◯ Both

Asked to those who answered "Yes" to Q3 (they currently use HCM)

5

In your opinion, what are the main benefits of home cage monitoring? Select up to 3.

- ☐ Reduced disturbance
- ☐ Recording different and novel experimental parameters
- ☐ Discovery of novel or subtle phenotypes
- ☐ Welfare insights
- ☐ Long-term continuous data that doesn't miss any part of the circadian cycle
- ☐ Other:

Asked to those who answered "Yes" to Q3 (they currently use HCM)

6

In your opinion, what are the main limitations of home cage monitoring? Select up to 3.

- [ ] Technical specification, e.g. limited range of parameters
- [ ] Technical reliability
- [ ] Technical support
- [ ] Data storage and back-up
- [ ] Data integration from different systems
- [ ] Single versus group-housed requirements
- [ ] Space
- [ ] Financial aspects
- [ ] Data analysis
- [ ] Maintenance and cleaning
- [ ] Types of caging required
- [ ] Using enrichment in the cage
- [ ] Other:

Asked to those who answered "Yes" to Q3 (they currently use HCM)

7

Do you predict a need to increase your use of home cage monitoring systems? *

○ Yes

○ No

Asked to those who answered "Yes" to Q3 (they currently use HCM)

8

Do you predict a need to continue your use of home cage monitoring systems? *

○ Yes

○ No

Asked to those who answered "No" to Q7 (they don't predict increase)

9

Not everything we do can currently be done with mice in their home cage. What procedures do you perform other than home cage monitoring?

☐ Additional handling (e.g. weight measurement)

☐ No other procedures

☐ Environmental perturbations

☐ Surgery, including device implantation

☐ Administration of drugs, gavage

☐ Behavioural testing

☐ Blood sampling

☐ Other: ______

Asked to those who answered "No" to Q7 (they don't predict increase)

10

Do you predict a need to start home cage monitoring?

◯ Yes

◯ No

Asked to those who answered "No" to Q3 (they don't currently use HCM)

11

Not everything we do can currently be done with mice in their home cage. What procedures do you perform outside of the home cage?

☐ Surgery, including device implantation

☐ Behavioural testing

☐ Environmental perturbations

☐ No special preparation

☐ Additional handling (e.g. weight measurement)

☐ Administration of drugs, gavage

☐ Blood sampling

☐ Other: ______

Asked to those who answered "No" to Q3 (they don't currently use HCM)

12

Do you currently see demand for 24/7 monitoring of animals in their home cage?

◯ Yes

◯ No

Asked to all

13

In your opinion, what are the main obstacles to adopting home cage monitoring technologies? Select up to 3.

- ☐ Technical and IT support/data management support
- ☐ Acceptance of new testing methods
- ☐ Awareness of capabilities
- ☐ Lack of qualified personnel
- ☐ Facility space
- ☐ Justification for use
- ☐ Legislation
- ☐ Cost of ownership
- ☐ Difficulty of choice due to the large number of different systems available
- ☐ IT infrastructure limitations
- ☐ Procurement processes
- ☐ Other:

Asked to all

14

What data are you mainly interested in?

- ○ Behaviour
- ○ Physiology
- ○ Both
- ○ None of the above
- ○ Other:

Asked to all

15

Many researchers use a mix of studies in the home cage and outside the home cage. We'd now like to ask about the out-of-cage methods you use.

For the following types of studies, how well do your current out-of-cage methods suit your needs? Please only complete for those you have experience or an interest in.

	1 - Very badly	2	3 - Moderately	4	5 - Very well	N/A
Understanding basic behaviour in animal models of disease	○	○	○	○	○	○
Regulatory testing/toxicology	○	○	○	○	○	○
Quality/validity translational data	○	○	○	○	○	○
Disease progression	○	○	○	○	○	○
Complex traits	○	○	○	○	○	○
Long-term data on treatment effects	○	○	○	○	○	○
Multi-morbidities	○	○	○	○	○	○
Complex traits	○	○	○	○	○	○
Long-term data on treatment effects	○	○	○	○	○	○
Multi-morbidities	○	○	○	○	○	○

Asked to all

16

What additional research data would you like to obtain that your current tests are missing?

- ☐ Continuous 24/7 data
- ☐ Social interactions
- ☐ Urine/faeces composition/quantity
- ☐ Data of individual mouse in social context
- ☐ Fine motor activity
- ☐ Water/food consumption
- ☐ Body posture, e.g. stretch-attend posture, rearing, grooming
- ☐ Body temperature
- ☐ Integrated parameters, e.g. ECG and motor activity
- ☐ Other: ____________

Asked to all

17

Where do you see a clear impact of home cage monitoring on welfare? Rank from most important to least important.

	1 - Most important impact	2	3 - Least important impact
Minimally intrusive	○	○	○
24/7 monitoring	○	○	○
Enabling group-housing	○	○	○

Asked to all

18

How do you think using home cage monitoring could add to animal welfare monitoring? Select up to 3.

- ☐ Comprehensive 24/7 monitoring
- ☐ Undisturbed by human presence
- ☐ Objective and quantitative data
- ☐ Early identification of humane end-points
- ☐ Maximising data collection and analysis
- ☐ Sharing data/dissemination of information
- ☐ Other: ______

Asked to all

How important is it that the following automatic real-time notifications are implemented in a home cage monitoring system to trigger timely response?

	1 - Very unimportant	2 - Unimportant	3 - Slightly unimportant	4 - Slightly important	5 - Important	6 - Very important
Pre-identified critical behaviours						
Technical issues, e.g. with food, water, flooding of cage						
Body temperature						
Birth						
Notification of humane end-points (e.g. BW<15%)						
Sudden death						

Asked to all

20

What else would you like a home cage monitoring system to provide with respect to animal welfare? Select the 3 most important to you.

- ☐ Monitor food and water intake
- ☐ Identify abnormal behaviour (e.g. stererotypical behaviour)
- ☐ Monitoring of reproduction (e.g. mating, birth, litters)
- ☐ Regular body weight recording
- ☐ Monitor social interaction and/or aggression
- ☐ Other:

Asked to all

21

Please rank the impact of the following points on animal welfare.

	1 - Highest impact	2	3	4 - Lowest impact
Non-enriched or suboptimal environment	○	○	○	○
Environmental stressors caused by the system (e.g. ultrasonic noise)	○	○	○	○
Single-housing	○	○	○	○
ID tagging	○	○	○	○

Asked to all

22

Are there additional welfare challenges?

Your answer

Asked to all

23

Please write any additional thoughts or comments.

Your answer

Asked to all

24

What country are you based in?

Your answer

Asked to all

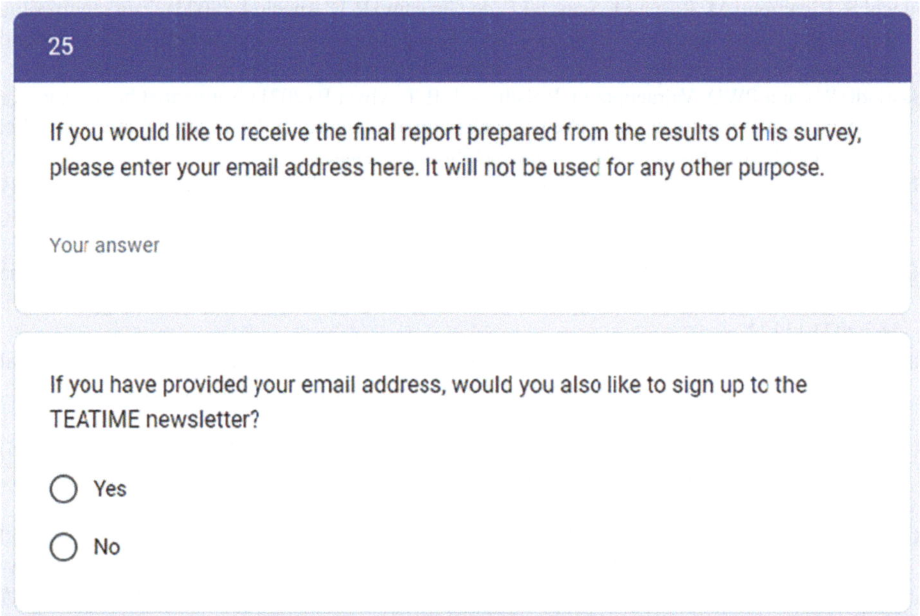

25

If you would like to receive the final report prepared from the results of this survey, please enter your email address here. It will not be used for any other purpose.

Your answer

If you have provided your email address, would you also like to sign up to the TEATIME newsletter?

○ Yes

○ No

Asked to all

References

Bains RS, Forrest H, Sillito RR, Armstrong JD, Stewart M, Nolan PM, Wells SE (2023) Longitudinal home-cage automated assessment of climbing behavior shows sexual dimorphism and aging-related decrease in C57BL/6J healthy mice and allows early detection of motor impairment in the N171-82Q mouse model of Huntington's disease. Front Behav Neurosci 17:1148172. https://doi.org/10.3389/fnbeh.2023.1148172

Balzani E, Falappa M, Balci F, Tucci V (2018) An approach to monitoring home-cage behavior in mice that facilitates data sharing. Nat Protoc 13(6):1331–1347. https://doi.org/10.1038/nprot.2018.031

Begley CG, Ioannidis JP (2015) Reproducibility in science: improving the standard for basic and preclinical research. Circ Res 116(1):116–126. https://doi.org/10.1161/CIRCRESAHA.114.303819

Bonasera SJ, Chaudoin TR, Goulding EH, Mittek M, Dunaevsky A (2017) Decreased home cage movement and oromotor impairments in adult Fmr1-KO mice. Genes Brain Behav 16(5):564–573. https://doi.org/10.1111/gbb.12374

Cobey KD, Ebrahimzadeh S, Page MJ, Thibault RT, Nguyen PY, Abu-Dalfa F, Moher D (2024) Biomedical researchers' perspectives on the reproducibility of research. PLoS Biol 22(11):e3002870. https://doi.org/10.1371/journal.pbio.3002870

Collins HM, Pinacho R, Tam SKE, Sharp T, Bannerman DM, Peirson SN (2023) Continuous home cage monitoring of activity and sleep in mice during repeated paroxetine treatment and discontinuation. Psychopharmacology 240(11):2403–2418. https://doi.org/10.1007/s00213-023-06442-3

Fuochi S, Rigamonti M, Raspa M, Scavizzi F, de Girolamo P, D'Angelo L (2023) Data repurposing from digital home cage monitoring enlightens new perspectives on mouse motor behaviour and reduction principle. Sci Rep 13(1):10851. https://doi.org/10.1038/s41598-023-37464-8

Hasriadi, Wasana PWD, Vajragupta O, Rojsitthisak P, Towiwat P (2021) Automated home-cage for the evaluation of innate non-reflexive pain behaviors in a mouse model of inflammatory pain. Sci Rep 11(1):12240. https://doi.org/10.1038/s41598-021-91444-4

Ho H, Kejzar N, Sasaguri H, Saito T, Saido TC, De Strooper B, Bauza M, Krupic J (2023) A fully automated home cage for long-term continuous phenotyping of mouse cognition and behavior. Cell Rep Methods 3(7):100532. https://doi.org/10.1016/j.crmeth.2023.100532

Hsieh CM, Hsu CH, Chen JK, Liao LD (2024) AI-powered home cage system for real-time tracking and analysis of rodent behavior. iScience 27(11):111223. https://doi.org/10.1016/j.isci.2024.111223

Jankovic MJ, Kapadia PP, Krishnan V (2019) Home-cage monitoring ascertains signatures of ictal and interictal behavior in mouse models of generalized seizures. PLoS One 14(11):e0224856. https://doi.org/10.1371/journal.pone.0224856

Kahnau P, Mieske P, Wilzopolski J, Kalliokoski O, Mandillo S, Hölter SM, Voikar V et al (2023) A systematic review of the development and application of home cage monitoring in laboratory mice and rats. BMC Biol 21(1):256. https://doi.org/10.1186/s12915-023-01751-7

Kohler J, Mei J, Banneke S, Winter Y, Endres M, Emmrich JV (2022) Assessing spatial learning and memory in mice: classic radial maze versus a new animal-friendly automated radial maze allowing free access and not requiring food deprivation. Front Behav Neurosci 16:1013624. https://doi.org/10.3389/fnbeh.2022.1013624

Moore JL, Brook EI (2022) Using home-cage monitoring to determine the impact of timed mating on male mouse welfare. Front Neurosci 16:786652. https://doi.org/10.3389/fnins.2022.786652

Murphy TH, Michelson NJ, Boyd JD, Fong T, Bolanos LA, Bierbrauer D, Siu T, Balbi M, Bolanos F, Vanni M, LeDue JM (2020) Automated task training and longitudinal monitoring of mouse mesoscale cortical circuits using home cages. elife 9:e55964. https://doi.org/10.7554/eLife.55964

Piilgaard L, Rose L, Justinussen JL, Hviid CG, Lemcke R, Wellendorph P, Kornum BR (2023) Non-invasive detection of narcolepsy type I phenotypical features and disease progression by continuous home-cage monitoring of activity in two mouse models: the HCRT-KO and DTA model. Sleep 46(9):zsad144. https://doi.org/10.1093/sleep/zsad144

Ruby JG, Di Francesco A, Ylagan P, Luo A, Keyser R, Williams O, Spock S, Li W, Vongtharangsy N, Chatterjee S, Sloan CA, Ledogar C, Kuiper V, Kite J, Cosino M, Cha P, Karlsson EM (2023) An automated, home-cage, video monitoring-based mouse frailty index detects age-associated morbidity in C57BL/6 and diversity outbred mice. J Gerontol A Biol Sci Med Sci 78(5):762–770. https://doi.org/10.1093/gerona/glad035

Salem G, Cope N, Garmendia M, Pu A, Somenhalli A, Krynitsky J, Cubert N, Jones T, Dold G, Fletcher A, Kravitz A, Pohida T, Dennis J (2024) MouseVUER: video based open-source system for laboratory mouse home-cage monitoring. Sci Rep 14(1):2662. https://doi.org/10.1038/s41598-024-52788-9

Singh S, Bermudez-Contreras E, Nazari M, Sutherland RJ, Mohajerani MH (2019) Low-cost solution for rodent home-cage behaviour monitoring. PLoS One 14(8):e0220751. https://doi.org/10.1371/journal.pone.0220751

Spivak DI, Kent RE (2012) Ologs: a categorical framework for knowledge representation. PLoS One 7(1):e24274. https://doi.org/10.1371/journal.pone.0024274

Steel LCE, Tir S, Tam SKE, Bussell JN, Spitschan M, Foster RG, Peirson SN (2022) Effects of cage position and light transmission on home cage activity and circadian entrainment in mice. Front Neurosci 15:832535. https://doi.org/10.3389/fnins.2021.832535

Tannenbaum J, Bennett BT (2015) Russell and Burch's 3Rs then and now: the need for clarity in definition and purpose. J Am Assoc Lab Anim Sci 54(2):120–132. https://pmc.ncbi.nlm.nih.gov/articles/PMC4382615/

Voikar V, Gaburro S (2020) Three pillars of automated home-cage phenotyping of mice: novel findings, refinement, and reproducibility based on literature and experience. Front Behav Neurosci 14:575434. https://doi.org/10.3389/fnbeh.2020.575434

Zentrich E, Talbot SR, Bleich A, Häger C (2021) Automated home-cage monitoring during acute experimental colitis in mice. Front Neurosci 15:760606. https://doi.org/10.3389/fnins.2021.760606

Optimizing Operations with Home Cage Monitoring in Animal Facilities

James Bussell, Jeetendra Eswaraka, Matthew Keller, Giorgio Rosati, and Catriene Thuring

Abstract

Operational efficiency is a critical determinant of success in laboratory animal facilities, shaping financial sustainability, research quality, and the well-being of both staff and animals. This chapter focuses on how home cage monitoring (HCM) systems can serve as a central driver of efficiency when integrated thoughtfully into daily operations. By enabling continuous, noninvasive data collection within the animals' primary environment, HCM systems support more strategic use of time, personnel, equipment, and funding, ultimately enhancing scientific output while reinforcing ethical animal care and improving workplace conditions.

When incorporated into routine workflows, HCM technologies help standardize procedures, reduce redundant tasks, and streamline the flow of information. These improvements lower operational costs, strengthen data integrity, and ease regulatory compliance. Moreover, the precision and automation offered by HCM reduce delays, minimize human error, and ensure consistent adherence to protocol requirements. Staff benefit as well: by offloading labor-intensive or repetitive tasks to automated

J. Bussell
University of Oxford, Oxford, UK

J. Eswaraka · M. Keller (✉)
Rutgers University, New Brunswick, NJ, USA
e-mail: mlkeller@research.rutgers.edu

G. Rosati
Tecniplast S.p.A., Buguggiate, VA, Italy

C. Thuring
University of Groningen, Groningen, The Netherlands

S. Gaburro, S. Mandillo (eds.), *Home Cage Monitoring in Rodents: A Global Effort*,
https://doi.org/10.1007/978-3-032-19781-8_2

home-cage systems, employees experience reduced stress and increased opportunities for professional development, including hands-on experience with advanced digital tools.

To provide practical guidance, this chapter highlights strategies for optimizing operations through HCM implementation, including the use of Six Sigma methodologies to refine processes, sustainable practices to reduce environmental impact, and automation technologies that simplify routine monitoring and husbandry tasks. It also outlines how HCM can relieve operational burdens on researchers, allowing them to devote more effort to scientific innovation and discovery. By integrating HCM with broader operational improvement strategies, laboratory animal research facilities can achieve a level of operational excellence that advances scientific progress, supports humane and minimally invasive animal care, and cultivates a resilient, motivated workforce.

This chapter explores strategies for enhancing operational efficiency in laboratory animal facilities by examining process-optimization methods such as Six Sigma, sustainability practices, and automation technologies like HCM to provide a comprehensive framework for improving workflow and reducing burdens on scientists.

Keywords

Operational efficiency · Animal welfare · Research quality · Cost management · Staff well-being

1 Introduction

1.1 Introduction: The Importance of Operational Efficiency in Laboratory Animal Research Facilities

Operational efficiency is fundamental to the success of laboratory animal research facilities, as it enables the effective and strategic use of key resources including time, personnel, equipment, and finances to support high-quality scientific outcomes. By streamlining workflows, standardizing procedures, and reducing redundancies, facilities can not only lower operational costs but also enhance the precision and reliability of research data. Moreover, an efficiently run facility fosters a supportive and less stressful work environment, which improves staff morale, job satisfaction, and retention. In contrast, operational inefficiencies can lead to resource waste, increased expenses, inconsistent animal care, and elevated stress levels among employees, all factors that can ultimately compromise both scientific integrity and the welfare of animals and staff. Therefore, investing in operational efficiency is not just a matter of cost control, but a strategic approach for sustaining excellence in research, animal care, and organizational health.

1.2 Financial Implications of Operational Efficiency

Efficient operations in animal research facilities lead to significant cost savings. By optimizing processes such as record-keeping, inventory management, and equipment maintenance, facilities can reduce unnecessary expenditures. For instance, implementing a comprehensive cost accounting system allows for accurate allocation of expenses to specific animal categories and services, enabling better financial planning and control.

Moreover, energy-efficient equipment and automation technologies can lower utility costs and labor expenses. Investing in such technologies may have upfront costs but often results in long-term savings and improved operational efficiency.

1.3 Enhancing Research Effectiveness Through Operational Excellence

Operational efficiency directly influences the quality and timeliness of research outcomes. Streamlined processes ensure that researchers can focus on experimental design and data analysis rather than administrative tasks. Efficient scheduling, resource allocation, and data management, reduces delays and errors, leading to more reliable and reproducible results.

Furthermore, adherence to standardized protocols and best practices enhances the credibility of research findings. Facilities that prioritize operational excellence are better positioned to meet regulatory requirements and achieve accreditation, which are essential for maintaining funding and institutional reputation.

1.4 Impact on Staff Job Satisfaction and Well-Being

A well-organized and efficient work environment contributes significantly to staff satisfaction and morale. When operations run smoothly, employees experience less stress and are more likely to find their work fulfilling. Efficient processes reduce the burden of repetitive or unnecessary tasks, allowing staff to engage more deeply with meaningful aspects of their roles.

Additionally, facilities that invest in staff training and development foster a culture of continuous improvement and professional growth. Such environments not only retain skilled personnel but also attract new talent, committed to high standards of animal care and research excellence.

1.5 Overview of Topics Covered

1. *Process Optimization and Six Sigma Methodologies*: This section discusses how applying Six Sigma principles can identify inefficiencies and implement data-driven solutions to enhance operational workflows.
2. *Sustainability Practices*: An exploration of eco-friendly initiatives, including energy conservation, waste reduction, and sustainable procurement, to minimize the environmental footprint of research facilities.
3. *Reducing the Burden on Scientists through Operational Improvements*: Strategies to alleviate administrative and operational pressures on researchers, enabling them to focus more on scientific inquiry and innovation.
4. *Automation and Technological Integration*: An examination of how HCM can align process optimizations, sustainability, and reduced administrative burdens to enhance the overall operation.

By addressing these key areas, the chapter provides a roadmap for laboratory animal facilities to achieve operational excellence, thereby enhancing research quality, ensuring animal welfare, and promoting staff well-being.

2 Process Optimization and Six Sigma Methodologies

While Six Sigma is well established in manufacturing and commercial operations, its application in laboratory and research animal facilities remains relatively novel. At its core, Six Sigma is a data-driven methodology aimed at reducing variation, minimizing errors, and enhancing operational efficiency. Built around a simple but powerful premise: by identifying and eliminating the causes of defects or inconsistencies in a process, we can improve the output quality and meet the expectations of stakeholders. The approach typically revolves around the DMAIC framework (Define, Measure, Analyze, Improve, Control), a structured problem-solving cycle that drives continuous improvement.

When applied thoughtfully, Six Sigma methodologies can support implementations of HCM solutions, where precision in data capture and timeliness in responses is critical (Schweikhart and Dembe 2009). Reducing variability in routine processes can lead to fewer errors, smoother operations, and more reliable outputs. In this context, the development of meaningful key performance indicators (KPIs) becomes a logical next step, helping to benchmark progress, identify drift, and guide ongoing refinement.

In sum, while laboratory operations, particularly in animal facilities, come with their own unique complexities, the underlying goals of Six Sigma resonate strongly. As we move into deeper process analysis and mapping, there is a real opportunity to adapt and apply its tools in a way that suits our environment without compromising the flexibility and responsiveness that often define our work.

2.1 Process Mapping and Analysis

Understanding how a facility operates at a process level is essential if you want to identify where improvements can be made. Process mapping is a powerful way to visualize the flow of work, communication, and decision-making. It helps to reveal not only what happens but also when, by whom, and most importantly, why. In animal facilities, where operations span from cage changes and health checks to data collection and equipment sterilization, mapping these processes offers visibility into complexity we often take for granted.

2.2 Identifying Current Processes

The first step is to document what is currently happening; not what should happen. This often reveals a gap between assumed and actual practices. For example, one might think cage change frequency is standardized, but a closer look could uncover variability tied to staffing levels, researcher requests, or individual preferences. Starting with a few key processes (e.g., cage changing, health checks, cage wash operations) and tracing them from start to finish allows for a more accurate view of operational flow.

Process walkthroughs with staff are especially helpful. Observing daily routines, asking clarifying questions, and sketching out the steps in real-time often brings hidden work and decision points to light, many of which are invisible on paper. Standard operating procedures (SOPs), or detailed, written instructions that outline the exact steps required to perform specific tasks or processes should be created and implemented to match expectations. Since SOPs are the guiding documentation in these operations, staff should be knowledgeable and trained to execute accordingly.

2.3 Techniques for Mapping Workflows

- *Basic Flowcharts*—These are great for outlining tasks, decision points, and the order in which activities occur. For example, a flowchart of the animal census process can reveal whether double counting is happening or if data are being missed.
- *Swimlane Diagrams*—Helpful when multiple teams (e.g., technicians, vets, admin) are involved. Swim lanes show who does what and when, highlighting potential overlaps or gaps in communication (See Fig. 1).
- *Value Stream Mapping*—A slightly more advanced tool that breaks down each step in terms of value to the "customer" (researchers, animals, regulators, etc.). It helps distinguish between value-adding steps and non-value-adding activities (like waiting or redundant recording).

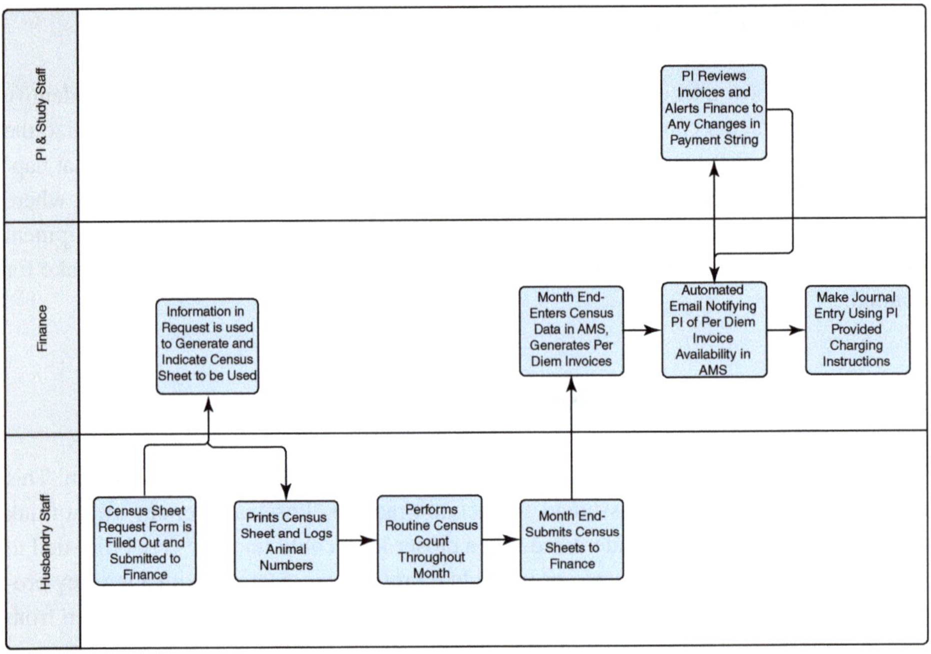

Fig. 1 Swimlane diagram showing an example of a census taking and billing procedure at an academic institution

2.4 Spotting Inefficiencies

Once the processes are mapped, it becomes much easier to begin spotting inefficiencies. These may not be dramatic individually but can add up. For example:

- *Time-consuming elements*—Are there steps that require significant time but offer little return (e.g., manual transcription and physical delivery of data versus entry into digital system)?
- *Critical path events*—What steps must happen before others can proceed? A delay here stalls the whole operation.
- *Redundancies*—Are multiple people checking the same thing? Are data being entered into two systems?
- *Bottlenecks*—Where do things tend to pile up (e.g., dirty cage backlog, waiting for approval, broken equipment)?
- *Rework*—How often are tasks redone because something was missed or incorrect?
- *Reorganization*—Identifying activity that may improve efficiency or save later activity if completed first.

These findings often point directly to areas for improvement, and importantly, they help move conversations from anecdotal complaints (“this takes forever”) to actionable insights (“this step delays every other task by 20 min”).

2.5 Tools Used

Even without specialized software, simple tools can be remarkably effective. Whiteboards and sticky notes can facilitate collaborative mapping sessions. In facilities where digital infrastructure is limited, using what is available and familiar to staff often works better than introducing something entirely new.

For more complex or cross-functional processes, value stream mapping can offer deeper insight. Though it originated in manufacturing, it is increasingly used in healthcare and research settings to capture the full scope of operations. It can be particularly useful when exploring processes like incoming animal shipments or emergency response protocols.

Process mapping, when done right, is not about documenting everything perfectly; it is about creating a shared understanding of how things really work. Once that clarity exists, it is far easier to apply frameworks like DMAIC to drive meaningful change. With visibility comes the opportunity to reduce errors, to optimize resource use, and to build better workflows that benefit both staff and animals.

2.6 Applying the DMAIC Framework

The DMAIC framework is a central pillar of Six Sigma. While traditionally associated with manufacturing, it translates well into operational environments like animal facilities, where consistency, quality, and efficiency are equally vital. Even if we do not formally label each step, the structure provides a practical roadmap for tackling inefficiencies and guiding change.

The following sections will describe each phase/step of DMAIC in detail:

2.6.1 Define

Every improvement project should begin with a clear understanding of what problem is being addressed and for whom. In our context, there are usually two "customers": researchers (who rely on accurate, timely data and well-maintained animals) and the animals themselves (whose welfare and environmental quality must be safeguarded).

Defining a project means answering a few key questions:

- What process or outcome needs improvement?
- Who is impacted by it?
- What would success look like?

For example, if we are addressing variability in health notification responses, the goal might be to reduce response time to alerts while ensuring data integrity is maintained. For this example, stakeholders could include technicians, researchers, veterinarians, and compliance officers.

A well-scoped project might sound like:

Reduce technician response time to automated welfare alerts by 20% over 3 months without increasing false positive rates.

2.6.2 Measure

With the goal defined, the next step is to understand the current state, which means collecting baseline data on performance. In a facility setting, useful metrics might include:

- Time taken from alert to resolution
- Number of false positives
- Error rates in manual data entry

Gathering these data often reveals unknown variability and assumptions. For instance, two technicians might interpret the same welfare alert differently, leading to inconsistency in documentation.

Reliable data do not have to be complex; they just need to be consistent and relevant. Even simple tallies or time logs can highlight trends when tracked over a few weeks.

2.6.3 Analyze

Once we understand how things are currently working, we can start asking *why*. Why does it take longer for some alerts to be addressed? Why is the animal census off by 5% each month?

Analysis aims to identify the root cause(s) or fundamental underlying reason(s) for an issue or problem to occur, rather than just the symptoms. Tools like the 5 Whys or Fishbone Diagrams (also known as the Ishikawa diagram) can help drill down into the drivers of inefficiency or error.

In one hypothetical scenario, a delay in response to health alerts might be traced to:

- Technicians do not see alerts quickly (lack of notification system)
- Confusion about who is responsible for addressing them
- Lack of proper triage or competing priorities

These kinds of insights allow for targeted, sustainable fixes.

2.6.4 Improve

With causes identified, it is time to develop and test solutions. This stage benefits from input across roles; those doing the work often have the clearest sense of what might help.

Improvements could be:

- Technological: Link alerts to handheld devices or dashboards with clear ownership tags
- Procedural: Standardize response protocols so all staff know what steps to take
- Operational: Adjust technician schedules and implement triage hierarchy

The key here is to pilot changes, monitor the impact, and refine as needed. Not every fix will work perfectly the first time. What matters is that changes are tracked and evaluated against the original goals.

2.6.5 Control

Finally, to make sure improvements stick, they need to be embedded into daily operations. This could include:

- Creating SOPs for new procedures
- Automating reminders or alert escalations
- Adding new KPIs to monthly reviews
- Training or refresher sessions for staff

Control is the most important and essential part of the DMAIC methodology, as without this control step, it is easy to slide back into old habits. The goal is not to add more bureaucracy, but to make improved ways of working the new default.

2.7 Case Studies of Successful Six Sigma Implementation

While the principles of Six Sigma may seem abstract at first, their impact becomes clear through real-world applications. In laboratory animal facilities, where even small inefficiencies can ripple out across teams and timelines, structured process improvement can deliver measurable benefits. The following case studies highlight how applying Six Sigma methods can improve both operational and data integrity outcomes, with potential takeaways for our own practices.

2.7.1 Case Study: Standardizing Bedding Type and Cage Fill Volume)

A mid-sized academic facility undertook a Six Sigma project to address inconsistencies in bedding type and quantity used for rodents across their various sites. Staff identified large variations in the different types and fill volumes of bedding across the sites, despite using similar style and size caging. The large variation in materials and standard operations made for a very inconsistent program of care and created difficulty with staff cross training and coverage. The project team began by collecting purchasing data, sampled bedding fill volumes across the sites and sourced testimonials from various staff to better understand the historical reasoning for why they used the material and/or corresponding fill volumes.

Using the DMAIC approach, they discovered several inefficiencies:

- Due to the large variety of bedding types utilized, the institution could not leverage its size and scale to receive preferential pricing.
- The large variety of materials utilized meant that a greater amount of storage space was needed to house the different products.
- A lack of standardized fill volumes created significant waste and even potential welfare issues:
  - Cages with too much bedding saw waste of the material and created an environment where wet spots could accumulate faster.
  - Cages with too little bedding saw cages that did not provide adequate liquid absorption and/or enough substrate for the animals to avoid walking on the cage bottom.

- Managing a large variety of bedding types also posed challenges when supply chain disruptions occur (e.g., COVID). Needing visibility into multiple suppliers to foresee potential disruptions and plan for contingencies made managing the operation extremely challenging.

  By analyzing the above measurements, the team was able to determine the following:
- Through discussions with staff and researchers, the project team determined that cellulose-based bedding was preferred. In addition, the staff liked this bedding type due to the lack of dust and the lighter weight per volume.
- Through literature review and internal testing, the team determined the optimal amount of bedding to fill a cage.
- By converging on a particular type of bedding (cellulose), the team evaluated potential options and ran tests to determine the best fit.
- Identifying a single bedding that met the above criteria enabled bulk discounts and easier supplier management, allowing for greater consistency and reduced administrative effort.

  Implementation involved the following:
- Internal marketing and selling the idea of a standardized bedding option to researchers.
- Procurement, deployment, and training of all staff on use of standardized scoops to ensure consistent bedding fill volumes across all sites.
- Planning and coordination of the shift in purchasing habits with the product distributor to ensure the institution received the best and most consistent pricing possible.

Due to the thoughtful approach to the changes, the selected product resonated well with the researchers, who readily bought into the option. Despite the product only making up 5% of the usage at the start, it quickly shifted to 85% + of the institution's usage over the next 6 months. In addition, this change saw a dramatic decrease in the overall amount of bedding used, due to the standardized fill volume. The financial savings from these changes were so staggering that once the change was implemented, it took 3 years of cost increases and a 20% increase in cage census to achieve the same level of total bedding spending that was seen before the switch.

2.8 Reflections and Insights

While each institution will have unique challenges and areas of focus, the principles of Six Sigma can be universally applied to all programs. By leveraging the DMAIC framework and other tools, programs can achieve the following objectives:

1. *Streamlined Operations*: Six Sigma tools help identify inefficiencies in daily routines, leading to more efficient workflows and better time management without compromising animal care.
2. *Improved Animal Welfare and Compliance*: Standardization reduces process variability and supports timely, consistent care. Six Sigma's data-driven approach enhances compliance with regulations and enables better adherence to SOPs.

3. *Improved Staff Engagement*: Involving animal care and other staff in problem-solving improves morale and encourages continuous improvement. Training in Six Sigma empowers employees to suggest practical and impactful changes.
4. *Data-Driven Decisions*: Switching from anecdotal to data-based decisions improves transparency, consistency, and collaboration across departments.

A thoughtful approach to the deployment of this methodology in an animal program is essential for the successful adoption and realization of the benefits. By engaging staff to evaluate the problems to help create and implement solutions, programs can best embody the teaching of Six Sigma and shift the culture to that of continuous improvement.

3 Addressing Labor Challenges and Enhancing Staff Well-Being

Laboratory animal caretakers play a vital and crucial role in the advancement of research by ensuring that animals are treated humanely and ethically. The key responsibilities of animal caretakers are to provide daily care, to monitor animal health and welfare, and to provide experimental support. All tasks should comply with regulations and ethical standards. Additional tasks may cover, e.g., transport of animals and carrying out breeding programs. The work requires a strong understanding of animal physiology and pathophysiology.

Laboratory animal caretakers face physical and mental burdens due to the nature of their work. The job involves physically strenuous activities such as lifting cages, crates of water bottles, and restraining animals. Caretakers often spend long hours standing, walking, and performing repetitive tasks. The mental burden, however, may even be more challenging. Caretakers must deal with the caring-killing paradox (King and Zohny 2022). This paradox describes the stress of nurturing animals while knowing they may be euthanized as part of the breeding strategy or experiments. This can lead to feelings of guilt, sadness, and moral distress (Murray et al. 2020).

Ultimately, the physical and mental stress experienced by caretakers may result over time in compassion fatigue. An employee suffering from compassion fatigue will not be able to contribute to the daily tasks that have to be carried out in a laboratory animal facility, either partially or fully. Reduced deployment comes with a risk: insufficient caretaking may lead to unnecessary discomfort for the animals. Full deployment increases the burden for the animal caretaking team and over time, this cycle of increased burden, reduced capacity, and escalating stress can contribute to high staff turnover, as caretakers facing compassion fatigue may feel unable to sustain the emotional and physical demands of their roles (Jianchun 2024).

A high turnover rate in a team of animal caretakers can have several disadvantages:

1. Loss of experience and knowledge: frequent turnover means losing experienced staff who have a lot of knowledge about the animals and the facility's operations. This can lead to a decline in the quality of care provided.

2. Training costs: Frequent hiring and training new employees is costly and time-consuming. New staff need time to become competent in their roles, which can temporarily reduce overall productivity.
3. Disruption of team dynamics: a high turnover rate can disrupt the cohesion and morale of the team. It can create an unstable work environment where remaining staff may feel overburdened and stressed.
4. Impact on animal welfare: consistency in care is important for maintaining the well-being of animals. High turnover can lead to inconsistencies in how animals are handled and cared for.
5. Increased workload for remaining staff: when positions are vacant, the remaining staff often must take on additional responsibilities, leading to a vicious circle: an even higher turnover rate.

It is the responsibility of the employer to minimize the risk factors for the onset of compassion fatigue by providing adequate support for the employees. This support should focus on two aspects:

1. Minimize physical strain by optimizing workflows and
2. Providing a Culture of Care: a positive work environment that supports animal welfare, human well-being, and quality in science.

3.1 Streamlining Workflows

In animal research facilities, streamlining workflows involves eliminating unnecessary steps to save time and effort. By analyzing each process, identifying redundancies, and removing them, facilities can enhance efficiency. An example of an unnecessary step is cleaning a rodent cage that technically does not yet need to be cleaned but is cleaned simply because other cages in the animal room are due for cleaning. Avoiding this step can significantly cut down on physical work, allowing animal caretaking staff to focus on more critical activities like monitoring animal health and welfare or carrying out experimental procedures.

Streamlining workflows may also be done through adopting data-driven decisions and consistent approaches. Collecting and analyzing data on KPIs such as number of pups weaned per breeding mouse may support the decision of continuation of a breeding pair. Developing and adhering to clear SOPs can streamline processes and ensure consistency.

3.2 Cross-Training Staff

Cross-training staff increases flexibility and coverage. Animal caretakers can, for example, be trained to work in both the breeding unit and the experimental unit. Or they can be deployed in both the rodent unit and the fish unit. This approach ensures that the workforce can adapt to varying demands and cover for absences without disrupting operations. This approach has advantages, but it also has a downside: Cross-training can lead to variability in performance. It is crucial to distinguish between straightforward tasks, which are less impacted by human variability (e.g., changing a bottle), and critical tasks that require minimal and clearly defined individuals to perform (e.g., body condition scoring or grimace scale scoring).

Operational resilience may enhance job satisfaction as employees gain diverse skill sets. If consistency is a requirement in tasks, the task should be assigned to a small group of specifically trained colleagues.

3.3 Achieving Staff Buy-In

Whatever steps are being taken to achieve efficiency in workflows, an essential aspect is to ensure that staff buy-in has been achieved. Implementing shifts and rotations that maximize productivity can significantly reduce labor demands. Versatile teams may play a significant role in achieving daily goals. However, removing a group's ability to determine how tasks are organized and the sequence in which they are performed can result in resistance. This effect may be even more pronounced in an academic environment where greater value is placed on autonomy in task structuring. Effective communication and involving staff in the preparatory phase of optimizing procedures can mitigate this issue. Highlighting the benefits, such as reduced workload and improved work-life balance, can help gain the support of the team.

3.4 Implementing Shifts and Rotations

Rotating staff through different tasks can prevent monotony and physical strain. It ensures that no single employee is overburdened with repetitive tasks, which can lead to fatigue and decreased productivity. In addition, rotation can help staff develop a broader skill set. By working in different areas of the facility, employees gain a better understanding of overall operations, which can improve teamwork and flexibility.

4 Reducing the Burden on Scientists Through Operational Improvements

Implementing HCM systems in laboratory animal research environments addresses several challenges faced by scientists, particularly in administrative tasks, data management, and research productivity. By automating data collection and enhancing information accessibility, HCM systems can significantly improve research efficiency and data quality.

4.1 Streamlining Data Collection and Management

4.1.1 Automated Data Acquisition

HCM systems utilize technologies such as RFID, sensors, and video tracking to continuously monitor animal behavior and physiological parameters within their home cages. For instance, implantable RFID chips allow researchers to track movement, location, and temperature of group-housed mice, providing real-time data without researcher interference.

4.1.2 Integration with Research Software

Modern HCM platforms are designed to integrate seamlessly with research software, facilitating the transfer of collected data to analysis tools and databases. This integration streamlines data management processes, reduces the need for manual data entry, and ensures that researchers have timely access to relevant information.

4.1.3 Reducing Errors

Automation minimizes human errors by standardizing data collection processes and eliminating manual transcription. Consistent data acquisition protocols enhance the reproducibility and reliability of research findings. Moreover, automated systems can flag anomalies in real-time, allowing for prompt corrective actions.

4.2 Enhancing Accessibility of Information

4.2.1 Real-Time Data Access

HCM systems provide researchers with the ability to monitor animal behavior and environmental conditions remotely, offering real-time insights into experimental subjects. This capability enables timely interventions and adjustments to experimental protocols as needed.

4.2.2 Customized Reporting

Advanced HCM platforms offer customizable reporting features, allowing researchers to generate reports tailored to specific research objectives. These reports can include detailed analyses of behavioral patterns, physiological changes, and environmental interactions, facilitating comprehensive data interpretation.

4.2.3 Collaborative Platforms

By centralizing data storage and providing secure access, HCM systems support collaborative research efforts. Multiple team members can access and analyze data concurrently, promoting interdisciplinary collaboration and accelerating research progress (Kos-Braun et al. 2022).

In summary, the adoption of HCM systems in laboratory animal research environments addresses key challenges related to administrative workload, data quality, and research productivity. By automating data collection, enhancing information accessibility, and supporting collaborative efforts, HCM systems contribute to more efficient and reliable scientific research.

5 Automated Animal and Cage Census Management

5.1 Importance of Accurate Census Data

5.1.1 Regulatory Compliance

Precise animal census data are fundamental in fulfilling both ethical guidelines and regulatory standards. Animal research facilities must comply with stringent regulations, including directives from institutions such as the Association for Assessment and Accreditation of Laboratory Animal Care International (AAALACi) and the Animal Welfare Act (AWA), as well as the Federation of European Laboratory Animal Science Associations (FELASA) under Directive 2010/63/EU. Accurate records of animal numbers, movements, and cage occupancy are necessary to demonstrate accountability and to ensure that research practices adhere strictly to ethical guidelines. Failure to maintain accurate census data can result in compliance violations, audits, fines, and significant reputational damage, which can severely impact research continuity and credibility.

5.1.2 Operational Efficiency

Reliable census data directly impacts the efficiency of research facility operations. Accurate and timely information about cage occupancy and animal counts is critical for optimizing resource allocation, including staffing, cage cleaning cycles, procurement of supplies (such as bedding, food, and enrichment items), and planning experimental schedules. Miscounted animals or inaccurately tracked cage occupancy data can lead to over- or under-utilization of resources, resulting in wasted effort, increased operational costs, or even disruption of experimental timelines. Thus, precise census management ensures smooth operational workflows, reduces unnecessary expenditures, and enhances overall facility performance.

5.1.3 Challenges of Manual Census

Traditionally, animal census management has relied heavily on manual counts and visual inspections performed by facility personnel. However, manual methods present significant challenges, notably their time-consuming nature and vulnerability to human error. Manual counts are often repetitive, tedious, and prone to inaccuracies arising from misidentification, fatigue, or oversight. Additionally, manual data entry can introduce transcription errors, causing discrepancies between recorded data and actual animal populations. These inaccuracies can lead to significant operational inefficiencies, potential regulatory noncompliance, and challenges in tracing animals accurately within the research environment.

5.2 Automated Census Systems

5.2.1 Technologies Employed

Automated systems for animal and cage census management utilize advanced technologies to overcome the limitations inherent in manual methods. Examples of current solutions include:

- *Barcode Systems*: Barcode labels affixed to cages enable rapid identification, simplifying cage occupancy tracking and status management. Personnel can efficiently scan cages, thereby can streamline inventory processes and reduce errors associated with manual data entry.
- *Radio Frequency Identification (RFID)*:
  - *Low Frequency (LF) RFID (134 kHz)—Animal Counting*: Utilizes microchip implants for accurate animal identification. This technology enables automatic tracking of individual animals as they enter or exit cages, move across facilities, or undergo specific procedures.
  - *Ultra-High Frequency (UHF) RFID (860–960 MHz)—Cage Counting*: UHF antennas integrated into labels or cage cardholders facilitate cage inventory through handheld devices or stationary antennas installed directly in animal rooms. This approach allows instant counting of all cages present within the designated area. However, it requires careful design of the reading areas to avoid capturing data from adjacent rooms.
  - *High Frequency (HF) RFID (13.56 MHz)—Real-time Cage Tracking*: Implemented via electronic boards within housing racks, HF RFID technology can automatically read cage tags upon insertion. This technology provides continuous, real-time cage tracking, offering enhanced operational insights beyond mere periodic census counts.

5.2.2 Benefits of Automation

Transitioning from manual to automated census systems brings substantial advantages:

- *Enhanced Accuracy*: Automation eliminates human counting errors, providing precise, reliable census data essential for compliance and operational effectiveness.
- *Time Savings*: Automated systems significantly reduce manual workloads, allowing personnel to focus on higher-value tasks, such as animal welfare, experimental support, and facility improvements.
- *Improved Traceability*: Continuous, accurate tracking enhances traceability, facilitating rapid audits and regulatory inspections. Improved data reliability supports robust documentation and accountability, strengthening institutional integrity.

5.3 Integration with Management Systems

5.3.1 Seamless Data Flow

Effective census management relies on the seamless integration of automated cage and animal census data with existing Laboratory Information Management Systems (LIMS), Animal Management Systems (AMS), and Enterprise Resource Planning (ERP) platforms. Integrated systems ensure that census data are automatically populated in centralized databases, streamlining information sharing across teams, departments, and management layers. This seamless data flow empowers facilities to achieve comprehensive operational visibility, supporting precise resource forecasting, experimental planning, and regulatory reporting.

5.3.2 Burdens of Non-Integrated Systems

Without integration between automated census systems and LIMS, AMS, and ERP, automated census solutions risk creating data silos. These isolated data repositories require manual intervention for data reconciliation and cross-referencing, resulting in inefficiencies, increased administrative workloads, and delayed decision-making. Non-integrated systems can also lead to discrepancies between different departments or management areas, complicating regulatory compliance, resource allocation, and traceability. Facility managers face significant challenges in coordinating accurate reports, often encountering duplications, inconsistencies, or incomplete data sets.

5.3.3 Case Study: Integration Resolving Facility Challenges

A mid-sized biomedical research facility previously relied on automated UHF RFID census systems without integration into their primary animal management system. Although cage counts were accurate, data resided in separate systems, requiring manual transfer and reconciliation. This resulted in inefficiencies, delays in reporting, and periodic compliance issues due to outdated or inconsistent records.

After implementing a full integration between the UHF RFID-based automated census system and their central LIMS, the facility observed substantial improvements. The seamless data exchange reduced administrative workload by approximately 4 h/week, eliminated reporting delays, and improved regulatory compliance scores. Real-time access to accurate census data streamlined experimental scheduling, improved animal welfare tracking, and significantly enhanced operational planning. This successful integration exemplified the critical importance of a unified, automated census management approach to achieve true operational excellence.

6 Sustainability and Reducing Environmental Impact

Implementing HCM systems in laboratory animal research not only enhances animal welfare and data quality but also offers significant opportunities to advance sustainability goals. This comprehensive overview explores strategies to reduce the environmental impact of research facilities through energy-efficient operations, waste reduction, and sustainable practices.

6.1 AI Driven Optimization of Facility Operations

6.1.1 HVAC

Heating, ventilation, and air conditioning (HVAC) systems are among the largest energy consumers in laboratory settings. Implementing AI-driven HVAC systems optimize air change rates and temperature settings based on real-time occupancy and environmental data. Air controls are aligned with actual needs of specific space, thereby greatly reducing the overall energy usage without compromising animal welfare or human safety (Carli et al. 2020).

6.1.2 Energy-Efficient Equipment

Newer HCM systems are designed with energy efficiency in mind, by integrating with existing housing equipment. For instance, mouse cages utilize Individually Ventilated Cage (IVC) technology that controls the animal environment at the cage level and modern HCM systems leverage and enhances this existing system. In this way, airflow, temperature, and humidity can be better managed at this level, which can differ from the macro/room level, while still allowing for continuous monitoring of the animals. This can greatly reduce the utilities needs to balance air rates for animal welfare, while ensuring that the macro environment is preserved for use by humans.

6.1.3 Minimizing Waste Generation

Reducing waste begins with evaluating and improving existing processes. Implementing HCM solutions that not only track animal activity but cage level parameters can be utilized to reduce unnecessary cage level activities. Tracking cage wetness or presence of ammonia can assist staff in implementing performance-based changes, thus only changing bedding when necessary. This implementation not only saves staff time, but reduces the amount of bedding, enrichment, cage wash chemicals, and other inputs needed to provision fresh caging for the animals.

6.2 Staffing and Business Continuity

HCM technologies enables a reevaluation of the roles and duties of staff that support research animal facilities. By leveraging the continuous monitoring of animals and cage parameters, staff will spend less time on the critical by mundane tasks of ensuring adequate food, bedding, and health condition of the animals under their care. This reduction in effort can be repurposed into developing and expanding other core responsibilities such as research support, breeding support, and provisioning of health care. Such tasks require an investment in the intellectual capital of the staff, leading to enhanced skill sets for a cutting-edge research environment.

By further developing staff for these new opportunities, laboratory animal programs can drive high level of engagement and overall staff retention, while providing enhanced services to help drive research activities.

Implementing HCM systems in laboratory animal facilities enhances animal welfare, data quality, and operational sustainability. By combining AI-driven HVAC optimization, energy-efficient equipment, and cage-level monitoring, HCM reduces energy use and waste without compromising care standards. Continuous monitoring also frees staff from routine tasks, allowing them to focus on higher-value responsibilities, develop skills, and improve engagement and retention. Overall, HCM advances efficient, sustainable, and ethically robust research operations.

7 Enhancing Operational Efficiency Through Integrated Systems

Implementing HCM systems in laboratory animal research facilities offers significant advancements in animal welfare, data accuracy, and operational efficiency. This comprehensive overview delves into two critical aspects of HCM implementation: Integrating HCM with facility management systems and leveraging real-time data analytics.

7.1 Integration of Home Cage Monitoring with Facility Management

7.1.1 Centralized Control Systems

Centralizing control systems in animal research facilities streamline operations by unifying various monitoring and management functions. By integrating HCM with centralized platforms, facilities can achieve:

- *Enhanced Operational Efficiency*: A centralized system logs maintenance requests, assigns tasks, and updates teams in real time, eliminating confusion and increasing accountability.

- *Improved Data Accessibility*: Centralized platforms facilitate the collection and analysis of data from various sources, enabling comprehensive monitoring of animal health and behavior.
- *Streamlined Maintenance and Resource Management*: Centralized systems can predict system failures, reduce downtime, and optimize resource allocation, leading to cost savings and improved facility operations.

7.1.2 Interoperability

Ensuring interoperability among different software and hardware systems is crucial for the seamless operation of HCM systems. Key considerations include:

- *Standardized Protocols*: Adopting open standards and protocols ensures that various devices and systems can communicate effectively, reducing integration challenges.
- *Modular System Design*: Modular HCM systems allow for flexibility in adding or upgrading components, facilitating customization and scalability.
- *Vendor Collaboration*: Working closely with vendors to ensure compatibility and support for integration can mitigate interoperability issues and enhance system performance.

7.2 Real-Time Data Analytics

7.2.1 KPIs

Identifying and monitoring KPIs is essential for assessing the effectiveness of HCM systems and facility operations. Important KPIs include:

- *Animal Health Metrics*: Continuous monitoring of vital signs and behavior provides early detection of health issues, improving animal welfare and research outcomes.
- *Environmental Conditions*: Tracking temperature, humidity, and other environmental factors ensures optimal living conditions for laboratory animals.
- *Operational Efficiency*: Metrics such as equipment utilization rates and maintenance response times help in evaluating and improving facility operations.

7.3 Data-Driven Decision Making

Leveraging analytics enables informed decision-making, leading to enhanced research quality and operational efficiency. Benefits include:

- *Predictive Maintenance*: Analyzing equipment performance data can predict failures, allowing for proactive maintenance and reducing downtime.
- *Resource Optimization*: Data insights assist in optimizing resource allocation, such as staffing and equipment usage, leading to cost savings.
- *Enhanced Research Design*: Real-time data allow researchers to adjust experimental protocols promptly, improving study accuracy and reliability.

7.4 Continuous Improvement

Continuous analysis of data collected through HCM systems fosters ongoing improvements in facility operations and research practices. Strategies include:

- *Feedback Loops*: Implementing systems that provide continuous feedback enables rapid identification and correction of issues.
- *Benchmarking*: Comparing performance metrics over time or against industry standards helps in setting goals and measuring progress.
- *Training and Development*: Data insights can identify areas where staff training is needed, promoting professional development and operational excellence.

In conclusion, integrating HCM systems with centralized facility management and leveraging real-time data analytics are pivotal in advancing laboratory animal research. These strategies not only enhance animal welfare and research quality but also drive operational efficiency and continuous improvement within research facilities.

8 Overcoming Operational Challenges with Process Optimization

8.1 Change Management and Staff Training

8.1.1 Engaging Stakeholders

Successful implementation of HCM systems requires the active involvement of stakeholders across all organizational levels. Engaging animal care technicians, researchers, veterinarians, and administrative personnel fosters a sense of ownership and facilitates smoother transitions. For instance, a facility addressed the issue of overfilling feed hoppers by involving technicians in identifying the root causes and collaboratively developing solutions. This participatory approach not only resolved the problem but also enhanced team cohesion and morale.

8.1.2 Training Programs

Comprehensive training is pivotal for the effective adoption of HCM technologies. Training programs should encompass both theoretical knowledge and practical skills, tailored to the specific roles of staff members. For example, initiatives like the TEATIME consortium (https://www.cost-teatime.org) have emphasized the importance of standardized training to improve reproducibility and robust experimentation. Such programs often include webinars, technology catalogues, and hands-on workshops to ensure that staff are well-equipped to utilize new systems effectively.

8.1.3 Communication Strategies

Transparent and continuous communication is essential during the transition to HCM systems. Regular updates, feedback sessions, and recognition of staff contributions can alleviate apprehensions and build trust. In the aforementioned facility, management maintained open lines of communication through team meetings and one-on-one interactions, providing positive reinforcement and addressing concerns promptly. This approach not only facilitated behavioral changes but also established a culture receptive to future innovations.

8.2 Cost-Benefit Analysis of Process Improvements

8.2.1 Evaluating Investments

Implementing HCM systems involves initial capital expenditures for equipment, software, and training. However, these investments can lead to significant long-term savings. For instance, transitioning to environmental health monitoring (EHM) methods, such as exhaust dust testing, has been shown to reduce annual costs by approximately 26% compared to traditional sentinel-based systems (Luchins et al. 2020). Savings stem from decreased animal purchasing, maintenance, and technician time.

8.2.2 Return on Investment (ROI)

Assessing ROI is crucial to justify the adoption of new technologies. Facilities that have implemented data-driven strategies, like optimizing cage utilization, have realized substantial financial benefits. Additionally, investments in automated systems, such as IVCs, have demonstrated labor cost reductions by extending cage-changing intervals, thereby increasing technician efficiency (Taylor et al. 2019).

8.2.3 Prioritizing Initiatives

To maximize impact, facilities should prioritize initiatives that offer the highest ROI and align with institutional goals. Implementing standardized digital forms and centralized data management systems can streamline operations, reduce errors, and enhance compliance.

8.3 Case Study: Performance Based Cage Change

Collins et al. (2025) evaluated the use of machine learning and predictive AI to determine cage change frequency for mice housed in IVCs. Traditional biweekly cage changes, often based on visual inspection, can be subjective and lead to unnecessary labor and resource use. The study developed an algorithm trained on human annotations of soiled bedding and the Bedding Status Index (BSI), a digital measure of cage wetness. The AI reliably identified soiled cages with >90% accuracy in standard-density cages and slightly lower accuracy in single-housed animals (76%). Using this approach, the researchers were able to extend cage change intervals, by implementing a system of visual indicators to perform spot changes (Jones et al. 2022). These actions were performed without compromising animal welfare, reduce labor, and improve vivarium operational efficiency, demonstrating how HCM systems can drive sustainable, data-driven management practices in research facilities.

Implementation of the AI algorithm resulted in a ~ 50% reduction in cage changes within the facility operations, saving significant labor and supplies. In addition, researchers were eager to adopt this practice, as it meant their research animals were less frequently disturbed and enjoyed a more stable caging environment.

In summary, the successful implementation of HCM solutions hinge on strategic change management, comprehensive staff training, and thorough cost-benefit analyses. By engaging stakeholders, providing targeted training, maintaining open communication, and carefully evaluating investments, research facilities can enhance animal welfare, improve data quality, and achieve operational efficiency.

9 Future Trends in Operational Management

1. Embracing Lean and Kaizen: A Fresh Approach to Daily Work
   Operational management in animal laboratory facilities is evolving. The need to work smarter, more flexible, and with greater accountability makes Six Sigma essential for cutting waste, simplifying processes, and fostering continuous improvement. Actively involving the entire team empowers everyone to enhance daily operations.
2. Integrated Digital Platforms: Building Blocks of Innovation
   At the heart of this transformation are digital platforms that link HCM with systems such as AMS, BMS, and LIMS. This centralized control and real-time insight support tech adoption even in existing setups, reducing barriers and protecting investments.
3. Data-Driven Decisions: From Information to Action
   Making informed decisions is more critical than ever. Advanced analytics, dashboards, and alerts help managers and technicians act early, preventing issues from escalating. Continuous monitoring of cage conditions, welfare, and resource utilization transforms data into actionable insights that enhance productivity and animal care (Fuochi et al. 2023).
4. Evolving Roles and Skills: The Workforce of Tomorrow
   The digital shift is redefining roles. Technicians and managers now require digital skills to interpret and utilize data effectively. Emerging roles, such as Digital Vivarium Managers and Automation Specialists, require ongoing training and internal champions to foster a culture that confidently embraces technology.
5. Sustainability and Environmental Responsibility
   Sustainability is becoming a priority, and HCM technologies support the identification of high-impact opportunities. Continuous monitoring reduces the use of supplies, utilities, and other consumables, cutting costs and minimizing environmental impact. These tools support institutional and governmental environmental goals and help progress toward carbon neutrality.

6. Smaller, Smarter Facilities with Ethical Commitment
   Digitally optimized facilities can function efficiently at any scale. Enhanced monitoring leads to better welfare and scientific outcomes, reducing the number of animals needed and upholding the 3Rs (Reduction, Refinement, Replacement).
7. Comprehensive Workflow Automation
   Automation now goes beyond cage monitoring. It supports broader workflow optimization, adjusting washing schedules by occupancy, tracking equipment with RFID or quick response (QR) codes, and using robots for transport and cleaning. This streamlines operations, reduces errors, and frees staff to focus on more skilled work.
8. Managing Change: Overcoming Challenges Together
   Reaching advanced standards requires managing change carefully. Digital transformation often meets resistance. Strong change management, thorough training, and trusted internal advocates are key to building confidence in new technologies.
9. Animal-Centered Operational Planning
   A shift toward animal-centered planning is underway. Using behavioral data to schedule tasks, such as cage changes or maintenance, improves welfare and resource efficiency.

10 Conclusion

The future of operational management in laboratory animal facilities lies in leveraging HCM systems to create a digital, connected, and sustainable research environment. By integrating continuous monitoring, automated data collection, and centralized platforms, HCM enhances operational efficiency by reducing errors, optimizing resource use, and freeing staff from repetitive tasks. These efficiencies allow personnel to focus on high-value activities, improving workflow and supporting professional development.

HCM monitoring directly contributes to overall sustainability of the operation, by not only lowering consumption of supplies and utilities, but through staff development and engagement. By providing avenues for growth and career opportunities, HCM systems enable staff to leverage their knowledge of these systems for future operational and research employment opportunities. At the same time, continuous, noninvasive monitoring improves animal welfare by providing more precise oversight of health and behavior, enabling early interventions, and responsible use of animals in accordance with the 3Rs (Replacement, Reduction, Refinement).

By combining smarter operations with ethical care, HCM systems strengthen research outcomes, ensuring more reliable, reproducible, and timely data while positioning facilities as leaders in efficiency, responsible innovation, and scientific excellence.

References

Carli R, Cavone G, Ben Othman S, Dotoli M (2020) IoT based architecture for model predictive control of HVAC systems in smart buildings. Sensors 20(3):781. https://doi.org/10.3390/s20030781. PMID: 32023965; PMCID: PMC7038446

Collins JM, Singh B, Zwick ME, Rosati G, Rigamonti M, Urdiales C, Eswaraka JR (2025) Using machine learning and predictive artificial intelligence to determine cage change frequency for mice housed in individually ventilated cages and drive vivarium operational efficiency. J Am Assoc Lab Anim Sci 64(4):1–14. https://doi.org/10.30802/AALAS-JAALAS-24-151. Epub ahead of print. PMID: 40683654; PMCID: PMC12379621

Fuochi S, Rigamonti M, Raspa M, Scavizzi F, de Girolamo P, D'Angelo L (2023) Data repurposing from digital home cage monitoring enlightens new perspectives on mouse motor behaviour and reduction principle. Sci Rep 13(1):10851. https://doi.org/10.1038/s41598-023-37464-8. PMID: 37407633; PMCID: PMC10322864

Jianchun Y (2024) employee job satisfaction through organizational climate and employee happiness at work: a mediated-moderated model. BMC Psychol 12(1):744. https://doi.org/10.1186/s40359-024-02269-5. PMID: 39696658; PMCID: PMC11657427

Jones T, Thaweethai T, Molk D, Ingram L, Palley LS, Jarrell D (2022) Evaluation and refinement of a spot-change-only cage management system for mice. J Am Assoc Lab Anim Sci 61(6):650–659. https://doi.org/10.30802/AALAS-JAALAS-22-000023. Epub 2022 Nov 1. Erratum in: J Am Assoc Lab Anim Sci. 2024;63(2):201. https://doi.org/10.30802/AALAS-JAALAS-24-000012. PMID: 36328418; PMCID: PMC9732769

King M, Zohny H (2022) Animal researchers shoulder a psychological burden that animal ethics committees ought to address. J Med Ethics 48(5):299–303. https://doi.org/10.1136/medethics-2020-106945. Epub 2021 Mar 31. PMID: 33789946; PMCID: PMC9046735

Kos-Braun IC, Gerlach B, Pitzer C (2022) Assessing and improving research quality in Core facilities. J Biomol Tech 33(1):3fc1f5fe.97057772. https://doi.org/10.7171/3fc1f5fe.97057772. PMID: 35837001; PMCID: PMC9258915

Luchins KR, Bowers CJ, Mailhiot D, Theriault BR, Langan GP (2020) Cost comparison of rodent soiled bedding sentinel and exhaust air dust health-monitoring programs. J Am Assoc Lab Anim Sci 59(5):508–511. https://doi.org/10.30802/AALAS-JAALAS-20-000003. Epub 2020 Jun 26. PMID: 32591028; PMCID: PMC7479769

Murray J, Bauer C, Vilminot N, Turner PV (2020) Strengthening workplace well-being in research animal facilities. Front Vet Sci 7:573106. https://doi.org/10.3389/fvets.2020.573106. PMID: 33330693; PMCID: PMC7673436

Schweikhart SA, Dembe AE (2009) The applicability of lean and six sigma techniques to clinical and translational research. J Investig Med 57(7):748–755. https://doi.org/10.2310/JIM.0b013e3181b91b3a. PMID: 19730130; PMCID: PMC2835466

Taylor JL, Noel P, Mickelsen M (2019) Evaluation of a 16-week change cycle for ventilated mouse cages. J Am Assoc Lab Anim Sci 58(4):443–449. https://doi.org/10.30802/AALAS-JAALAS-18-000070. Epub 2019 May 23. PMID: 31122312; PMCID: PMC6643086

Enhancing Animal Welfare Through Home Cage Monitoring Systems

Heidrun Potschka, Francisco Drusso Martinez-Garcia, Miriam van der Meulen, Jan Bas Prins, Özge Selin Çevik, and Oliver Stiedl

Abstract

Home cage monitoring (HCM) is increasingly being used in scientific studies but its application in the field of animal welfare is lagging. Advances in animal research are predominantly driven by scientific projects whose primary goal is increasing scientific knowledge but not animal welfare. Harnessing the potential of HCM to optimize animal welfare is clearly an ethical matter of Refinement, but it is also a prerequisite for improved quality and replicability in science and acceptance in society. HCM developments allow for uninterrupted recording of various parameters, and their analyses can be exploited for improved welfare monitoring. Here we provide an overview regarding animal welfare measures used in HCM studies and describe new developments in different research areas based on new methodological developments. We point at the importance of combining different readouts as integrative toolbox for an optimal

H. Potschka
Institute of Pharmacology, Toxicology, and Pharmacy, Ludwig-Maximilians-Universität, Munich, Germany

F. D. Martinez-Garcia · M. van der Meulen
Laboratory Animal Experts—Board of the University, University of Groningen, Groningen, The Netherlands

J. B. Prins
Leiden University Medical Centre, Leiden, The Netherlands

Ö. S. Çevik
Physiology Department, Faculty of Medicine, Mersin University, Mersin, Turkey

O. Stiedl (✉)
Animal Welfare Body, Amsterdam UMC and Vrije Universiteit, Amsterdam, The Netherlands
e-mail: o.stiedl@amsterdamumc.nl

S. Gaburro, S. Mandillo (eds.), *Home Cage Monitoring in Rodents: A Global Effort*,
https://doi.org/10.1007/978-3-032-19781-8_3

severity assessment regarding experimental and/or humane endpoints as refinement to reduce unnecessary and avoidable discomfort. Dynamical analyses are required because for example alterations of circadian activity (fragmented sleep-wake cycles) require discrimination of deviations during light and dark phase, e.g. hyperactivity during the light and hypoactivity during the dark phase. Finally, we must be careful about the changeover from physiology to pathology because basic knowledge about many measures in 24/7 HCM is not yet known. Most studies predominantly used young adult animals and provide data originating from short-term experiments performed outside the home cage. These cannot serve as gold-standard when it comes to animal welfare. Many factors such as age, sex, and (sub-)strain can all affect HCM measures and require further exploration to better understand the current physiology-pathology gap to support animal welfare assessment. Future perspectives of HCM technologies and their potential applications for animal welfare monitoring are discussed.

Keywords

Animal models · Animal welfare · Physiology · Pathology · Refinement · Discomfort assessment · Monitoring of breeding with discomfort

Abbreviations

AI	Artificial intelligence
BP	Blood pressure
CRF	Corticotropin-releasing factor
ECG	Electrocardiogram
EEG	Electroencephalogram
EEP	Experimental endpoint
HC	Home cage
HCM	Home cage monitoring
HEP	Humane endpoint
LPS	Lipopolysaccharide
ML	Machine learning
T_b	Body temperature

1 Introduction

“Happy animals make good science.” This statement was coined by Poole (1997). He concluded that “happy” animals are busy, confident, and behave normally. He went on to say that good, kind treatment and simple humane training are beneficial both in reducing stress and in producing confident, cooperative animals that are easily handled. Subsequently, these animals will also be the best subjects for scientific investigation. While the essence of his account is still appreciated today, his choice of words is not well-received nowadays due to its anthropomorphic nature and association with psychological well-being, whereas animal welfare encompasses physical health, emotional state (psychological state), and the chance to display natural behaviours in a proper environment. Ohl and Van Der Staay (2012) argued that the general concept of animal welfare recognizes that an animal's welfare status at any given time lies on a continuum between negative welfare, i.e. suffering, and positive welfare, i.e. well-being. This concept acknowledges that animals are active participants in their environment, and they have the ability to adapt. According to this concept, animal welfare is not threatened as long as an animal is able to meet (cope with) environmental challenges. However, an animal's welfare may be compromised if adverse internal or external factors (or their interaction) challenge its adaptability to the extent that it cannot adapt to the prevailing environmental circumstances to reach a state that it perceives as positive (or at least neutral). Positive welfare implies that the animal has the freedom and capacity to react appropriately (i.e. adaptively) to both positive and potentially harmful (negative) stimuli. Lewejohann et al. (2020) extended the welfare concept to include a more holistic, quality of life, approach focusing on good living rather than the mere avoidance of adverse conditions through, for example, environmental enrichment by toys and palatable food rewards for psychological well-being besides physical well-being (see Chap. 9). Consequently, the core unit of animal welfare is the subjective perception of an individual. This raises the important question of how to effectively assess animal welfare, not just for the sake of the animal, but also to ensure the quality and reliability of the scientific results obtained if sub-optimal welfare is not the topic under investigation but may impact on the readout measures of this investigation. Here longitudinal automated measures assessed in the home cage play a vital role as objective criteria of well-being (the physiology), compromised states of well-being, and its (gradual or more sudden) turnover to pathology.

In research facilities, rodents are kept in standard housing conditions comprising a "shoebox" cage containing bedding, food and water, nesting material, and some form of enrichment, such as a wooden block, cardboard house, or loft. In Europe (EU), the minimum standards are set out in Appendix A of the EU Convention for the protection of vertebrate animals used for experimental and other scientific purposes (ETS No. 123) and Annex III of the EU Directive 2010/63/EU. According to the EU Directive, animals must be provided with accommodation and an environment that is appropriate to their health and well-being. This includes food and water. The minimum standards regarding cage dimensions and provisions inside and outside the cage according to Appendix A of ETS No. 123 are a compromise between what is practically achievable and acceptable within the scientific context and what are considered appropriate housing conditions for the species. Compared to conspecifics living in the wild, captive animals exhibit restricted behavioural repertoires. However, it was shown with rats bred and kept in a laboratory setting for generations that they have not lost the capability for more "wild-like" behaviours if released in the wild (Berdoy 2002). In accordance with the welfare principles described earlier, laboratory rodents have adapted to the laboratory conditions and may have reached a state that is perceived as positive. That said, different strains of mice and rats exhibit different behavioural repertoires that may require different provisions in the cage (Tam and Cheung 2020; Dwinell et al. 2025) in line with article 33, 1 a. of the EU Directive 2010/63/EU requiring that *all animals are provided with accommodation, an environment, food, water, and care which are appropriate* and b. requiring that *any restrictions on the extent to which an animal can satisfy its physiological and ethological needs are kept to a minimum to their health and well-being. Daily checks of the environmental conditions in which animals are bred, kept, or used* are required by article 33, 1 c. of the EU Directive 2010/63/EU and *arrangements* should be *made to ensure that any defect or avoidable pain, suffering, distress, or lasting harm discovered is eliminated as quickly as possible* (2010/63/EU Art. 33, 1 d.).

Mice and rats are nocturnal animals, which generally sleep during the daytime when daily checks are performed. The prevailing view is that unnecessary disturbance of nocturnal animals does not contribute to their welfare. Therefore, it is not common practice to carry out thorough daily checks on each animal. Instead, each animal will typically undergo a physical check and be handled at least once a week, for example, during cage cleaning. However, the EU Commission's working document on a severity assessment framework sets out general considerations for a severity assessment (Severity assessment framework (2010/63/EU). Luxembourg: Publication office of the European Union; 2018. p. 76.) explains that it should be a continuous process. This process begins with the initial study design and continues through the day-to-day monitoring of animals during the project and the actual severity assessment upon completion of the study providing opportunities to identify further refinement options for future studies. The working document specifies the requirements for an effective severity assessment. Amongst these day-to-day severity assessment systems, those that are appropriately tailored to the species, strain, and project are listed. This includes informed and structured observations of animals at appropriate intervals and analysis of these observations to make an informed judgement on the nature and level of suffering.

Recognizing abnormalities requires a good knowledge and understanding of what is considered normal for the species, strain, and sex in question. Monitoring day-to-day behaviour of laboratory animals and comparing time budgets allocated to different behavioural domains is a feasible approach to analyse normal behaviour in laboratory rodents (Lewejohann et al. 2020). Similarly, pain-associated behaviours have been identified in rodent species (Roughan and Flecknell 2003; Leach et al. 2012; Wright-Williams et al. 2013). A comprehensive protocol for the welfare assessment of laboratory animals includes assessment of behaviours that are associated with animal suffering (Hawkins et al. 2011). However, detecting spontaneous behaviours in rodents that are associated with pain or distress is complicated because mice and rats are prey animals that attempt to elude the attention of predators, including humans, by concealing signs of weakness, injury, or pain (Arras et al. 2007). The inclusion of easily visible indicators of welfare albeit indirect, like the appearance of the cage, the condition of the nest and the bedding, and the organization and condition of the territory add to the validity of the welfare assessment. Since the cage area of animals in a positive state of welfare should be clearly structured with obvious areas for defecation and sleeping. In contrast, direct indicators, such as provoked behaviour assessment require direct interaction with the animal while body condition, and posture can only be assessed when the animal is visible. As is the assessment of the mouse or rat facial expressions according to the respective grimace scales (Langford et al. 2010). Physiologic parameters such as heart rate, blood pressure and body temperature can be recorded over longer periods but require implanted telemetric devices (Wright-Williams et al. 2013).

In a study aimed at identifying the most valid, reliable, and practical indicators of laboratory mouse welfare, participants in a Delphi consultation survey ranked 59 welfare indicators according to whether they were suitable for either a half-day (4 h) unit audit or a daily welfare assessment. For each scenario, they identified ten key indicators (Campos-Luna et al. 2019). For the daily welfare assessment, these were: (1) Hunched position; (2) Coat condition; (3) Bite wounds/marks; (4) Exhibition of abnormal behaviour; (5) Room temperature; (6) Wounds (other than bite wounds); (7) Exhibition of normal behaviour; (8) Usage of nesting material; (9) Pups outside the nest; (10) Alertness. Behavioural indicators were considered important with over 95% of the participants deeming the exhibition of both normal and abnormal behaviour to be valid. However, fewer than 75% of the participants assessed them as reliable, and around 80% as practical (Campos-Luna et al. 2019). This was in 2019, before Home Cage Monitoring (HCM) became more widespread (Kahnau et al. 2023). HCM allows the recording and real-time analysis of animal activity and behaviours 24/7 over extended periods by installing movement-sensitive plates under the cage, often in combination with one or more cameras and neural network data analysis. This enables the detection of activity and behaviours, as well as changes thereof, also at times when mice and rats are most active and humans are least likely to be present, and therefore, it went unnoticed until the introduction of HCM.

An animal's behavioural response depends on the context, its species-specific behavioural repertoire and its individual adaptability at any given moment (Ohl and van der Staay 2012). By observing changes in an individual's response to a given stimulus over time and recognizing behaviours and activity patterns that are indicative of reduced welfare, it is possible to assess an animal's state of welfare. HCM provides continuous monitoring of behaviours and activities that are among the top ten of welfare indicators, thereby achieving an unprecedented level of surveillance of laboratory rodents.

The main aim of this chapter is to provide an overview of the spectrum of measures that can serve as readouts for HC animal welfare assessment, current methodological developments applicable in HCM animal welfare monitoring as well as limitations and future needs for successful refinement of animal experiments.

2 The Importance of Knowledge of Physiology and Its Turnover to Pathology

In animal disease models, understandings of physiological systems provide the fundamental framework required to differentiate pathological processes. By knowing the range of values of physiological functions, scientists can detect and quantify deviating values that may be indicative of discomfort and/or disease. Understanding baseline physiological functions and how these are altered under pathological conditions is essential for interpreting experimental outcomes. This forms the basis to unravel systemic disruptions, their molecular basis, and evaluate therapeutic interventions. Preclinical researchers must therefore have a thorough knowledge of both normative biological processes and the compensatory responses that emerge when these processes are dysregulated, to accurately assess disease mechanisms and evaluate potential therapeutic interventions (van der Worp et al. 2010). By monitoring baseline biological processes, scientists can detect deviations indicative of disease, unravel molecular and systemic disruptions, and evaluate therapeutic interventions.

In this context, accurate knowledge of physiological values (ranges) under undisturbed conditions—such as within the home cage (HC)—is essential not only for detecting disease-related deviations but also for evaluating animal welfare. Home Cage Monitoring (HCM) systems offer a powerful, non-invasive means of continuously assessing spontaneous behaviours and physiological rhythms in rodents without the confounding effects of human handling or exposure to novel environments. These automated systems can detect objectively quantifiable parameters such as locomotor activity, circadian rhythm, feeding, drinking, and sleep patterns in real time, providing robust longitudinal data under minimally stressful conditions (Richardson 2015; Redfern et al. 2017). For instance, glucocorticoids—steroid hormones released in response to stress—exhibit a circadian rhythm and are tightly regulated under physiological conditions. Deviations from this baseline, such as prolonged or excessive glucocorticoid secretion, can profoundly disrupt homeostatic mechanisms and lead to long-term alterations in brain function and behaviour (McEwen 2007). In anxiety-related research, the hypothalamic-pituitary-adrenal (HPA) axis plays a central role in mediating stress responses through the release of glucocorticoids such as corticosterone in rodents. Home Cage Monitoring allows for the indirect assessment of HPA axis activity by tracking behavioural correlates of stress, such as changes in circadian locomotion or feeding suppression, while also reducing the confounding stress induced by traditional testing paradigms (Balci et al. 2013). Circadian rhythms regulate a wide range of physiological functions—including hormone secretion, immune activity, and drug metabolism—and their disruption or neglect in experimental design can lead to misleading efficacy profiles that fail to replicate in human trials (Perel et al. 2007; Dallmann et al. 2014). For instance, HCM of circadian activity of male C57BL/6J mice has been performed in the HC environments by different methods such as camera tracking (Hager et al. 2014; Loos et al. 2014), RFID sensors (Freund et al. 2013), movement detection (Lynch et al. 2011), or capacitance sensing technology (Pernold et al. 2019). In general, nocturnal rodent species show a relatively characteristic activity pattern that is altered depending on the group size, age, and sex of mice. Consequently, deviations from the circadian activity pattern can have different directions depending on the phase of the day. Deviations can be induced by mild stressors such as cage change or health checks leading to adrenergic activation (arousal) resulting in transient hyperactivity when commonly performed in the light phase by animal care personnel (Pernold et al. 2019). This leads to increased arousal that in the light (inactivity) phase leads to increased activity (e.g. novelty exploration after cage change). In turn, during the dark phase, when rats and mice are generally more active, emotional challenges such as shock exposure in aversive learning leads to a 2-h post-shock activity suppression in C57BL/6J and 6N mice as index of altered affect respectively increased anxiety (Hager et al. 2014). This effect can be explained by the bi-directional effects of corticotropin-releasing factor (CRF), an early neuropeptide signal in the hypothalamic-pituitary-adrenal cortex ("stress") axis activation cascade resulting in a transient corticosterone increase in rodents. Under habituated resting conditions in the home cage, CRF increases locomotor activity by increasing arousal, whereas under challenged conditions, CRF reduces locomotor activity (Stiedl et al. 2005).

Locomotor activity changes triggered by novelty are generally accompanied by corresponding heart rate, blood pressure and body temperature changes indicative of physiological support of behaviour as shown in rats (Beerling et al. 2011). When these changes are correlated with physical activity these changes reflect physiological functions and are adaptive changes in response to altered metabolic demands. The situation becomes different with emotional stressors that can elicit for example transiently tachycardia in the home cage to a conditioned fear stimulus in the absence of increased physical activity. Furthermore, the recovery (physiological readjustment) to baseline values may be prolonged/delayed after the offset of the stressor as shown for heart rate and blood pressure after conditioned auditory cue exposure (Tovote et al. 2005) and for rats long after social defeat with elevated heart rate despite low activity (Koolhaas et al. 2011). Even more pronounced is the delay of stressor-induced hyperthermia (Beerling et al. 2011). Thus, HCM with long-term recordings of physiological parameters is well suited to identify deviations from the physiological state and draw conclusions on pathological changes. However, interpretations about transient increases in physiological values due to physiological support of behaviour instead of potential pathological deviation must be taken care. Increased locomotor activity during the light phase and decreased locomotor activity in the dark phase are a starting point for more specific checks. An important issue here is the general state of the animals such as posture (arched back, rough coat, facial expression, body weight, etc.) as complementary indirect information about the general health status of animals. Short recordings may provide additional information. However, linear methods especially for cardiovascular measures of animals are inferior to assessment of heart rate dynamics by nonlinear methods to identify pathological states but requires high data quality (Hager et al. 2025). In case of heart rate measures, this can currently only be obtained in HCM by radiotelemetry, which has the disadvantage of being an invasive approach requiring considerable postsurgical recovery times (Stiedl et al. 2004). However, near-infrared imaging allows to measure heart rate non-invasively (Pereira et al. 2019; Mösch et al. 2023) besides providing additional valuable measures in HCM such as temperature and respiration rate as described below.

In mouse models of neurodegenerative disease such as Alzheimer's disease a fragmented circadian activity is indicative of a progressed pathological state (Sheehan and Musiek 2020). In general, HCM allows to especially detect activity changes faster than body weight changes as recently reported after SARS-CoV-2 virus exposure of mice (Gaburro et al. 2022; Kaufmann et al. 2022). This can be exploited to detect deviant states relatively fast so that decisions can be made about HEPs to limit the discomfort experienced by laboratory animals. This provides a basis for the implementation of early HEP decisions as important contribution to animal welfare refinement. When evaluating the outcome of Dementia- and Alzheimer-related pathology in animal models, it should be noted that normal aging process also can make some contribution to the cognitive decline. Care is required in discriminating between cognitive impairment from emotional effects such as increased anxiety on higher cognitive function (Diamond et al. 2007) with negative impact of adverse states on cognitive function as reported in mouse models of Alzheimer's disease such APPswe/PSEN1dE9-transgenice mice with elevated anxiety (Abdollahi Nejat et al. 2024). Consequently, HCM approaches improve animal welfare and scientific precision by reducing unspecific confounding stressors.

Environmental enrichment is widely recognized for its role in improving animal welfare. Enriched environments and long-lasting HCM approaches reveal individual differences (Freund et al. 2013; Hager et al. 2014) that remain suppressed under standard barren conditions (Würbel 2001). Essentially, enrichment is a form of experience-dependent adjustment of the individuals' response to any novel stimulus and avoids the general hyperresponsiveness of naïve unexperienced mice in many tests (Stiedl et al. 2004). Interindividual differences can emerge especially in emotional responsiveness due to different coping styles, which are associated with different stress-susceptibility and turnover from adaptive to maladaptive consequences. Higher vulnerability of proactive responders is associated with increased aggression, impaired decision-making and/or increased impulsivity (Koolhaas et al. 2017). Thus, environmental enrichment may increase the interindividual differences (individuality) resulting in increased data variation depending on the measures and the duration of behaviour tests. Variation in transfer latencies in passive avoidance latencies is lower in out-of-the cage tests compared to a HCM approach (Hager et al. 2014). However, rather than treating environmental enrichment as a confounding variable, it should be seen as an opportunity to increase ecological and translational validity. Importantly, HCM systems provide a powerful platform to assess the effects of environmental enrichment in real time and under minimally stressful conditions and to monitor its effects on animal welfare under these refined housing conditions (e.g. reduced stereotyped behaviour). By integrating environmental enrichment into HCM systems, researchers can systematically study how individual animals respond to complex and dynamic environments over time, offering insights into resilience, adaptability, and early behavioural markers of disease. We do not elaborate on environmental enrichment here in more detail since this topic is covered more specifically in Chap. 9.

Finally, understanding physiology and its turnover into pathology is especially important when considering the age of the animals used in preclinical research and its impact on animal welfare. Most of the available studies are performed in young adult animals, whereas the age-dependency of disease progression is frequently not investigated simply for financial reasons. Studies on biological aging of mice by longitudinal HCM underscore the importance of the investigations of sex- and age-related changes resulting in increased frailty (age-related functional decline with increased physical vulnerability) with ageing that is more pronounced in male than in female mice and accelerated by environmental conditions such as Western diet (Santin et al. 2021, 2024). These results demonstrate the impact of different factors such as age, sex, sub-strain, and added experimental and many environmental variables on animal welfare, highlighting the need to create internal standards due to unavoidable idiosyncratic differences between animal facilities (see also Chap. 13).

3 Identifying Reliable Clinical/Animal Welfare Symptoms Through Continuous HCM

The predominantly used current daily monitoring of animal well-being by brief visual inspection and its limitations (as mentioned in the Introduction) are a motivating factor to improve animal welfare as important refinement in laboratory animal facilities. As discussed above, clinical scores provide valuable information about the general state of the health status of laboratory animals. However, they only inform about obvious changes in behavioural and physiological measures that can reflect pronounced alterations of the affective state. By going beyond standard clinical scores and integrating more sensitive parameters into a HCM concept, the affective/emotional state of the animals can be assessed in more detail. This can take the continuous routine assessment of well-being and severity in individual animals to a substantially improved new level of sensitivity. On the other hand, such approaches provide a basis for a comparative assessment of severity, which enables the refinement of models and techniques based on animal welfare considerations and its comparative validation. In addition, HCM with multidimensional schemes can support the classification of new models including new genetically modified lines and their legal demands. Thereby, a better characterization of genetically modified lines for potential breeding with hampered phenotype (Zintzsch et al. 2017) is possible with a range of various candidate parameters described in more detail below. Therefore, HCM can improve or augment the phenotyping of GA lines to the benefit welfare (assessment) and science.

The dynamics of alterations in the readout parameters, as discussed above, needs to be taken into account when working with chronic models. Age can have a tremendous impact on the burden related to specific pathophysiological mechanisms and symptoms. This requires careful considerations with application of continuous monitoring concepts when assessing cumulative severity in models with progressive disease states, neurodevelopmental disorder models, or age-related disorder models.

3.1 Activity-Related Measures (General Locomotion, Rearing, Climbing, Nest Building, Burrowing, Grooming)

An obvious parameter that can be continuously assessed in an HCM system with automatic tracking of animals via different technical approaches is *locomotor activity*. Circadian rhythmicity needs to be considered in daily routine monitoring of the well-being of animals. Among other parameters locomotion and activity-related behavioural parameters show pronounced circadian patterns (Bermudez Contreras et al. 2022; Perry et al. 2025). While bursts of activity and periods of resting occur during the entire day, higher activity levels are characteristic for the dark phase and lower levels for the light phase. The long-lasting hyperactivity during the light phase disrupting the sleep phase by the weekly cage change and thorough health check is well documented (Pernold et al. 2019). Even more importantly alterations in circadian rhythmicity can constitute a valuable readout parameter. Post-surgical pain, tumour-related disease states, adverse effects of analgesic drugs, chronic disorders, and tethered recording techniques can result in a loss of pronounced circadian rhythms or an alteration of rhythms (Arras et al. 2007; Möller et al. 2019; Golini et al. 2020; Colwell 2021; Zhang et al. 2021b; Aulehner et al. 2022a). This does not only apply to locomotion and activity but also other parameters changing in parallel with activity such as heart rate and body temperature (Arras et al. 2007). The adaptability to cope with stressors has been shown by rats in a specific home cage (closed economy) experiment. Rats deliberately changed their feeding patterns from nocturnal to diurnal to avoid unpredictable foot shocks in the dark phase encountered in the area providing access to food and water. Thereby, the rats deliberately regained control resulting in shock avoidance (Pellman et al. 2015).

Hyperlocomotion has for instance been described in models of neurological or neuropsychiatric disorders in GluA1 receptor subunit-deficient mice (Reiber et al. 2022c), and in a series of genetic and induced epilepsy models (van Dijk et al. 2020; Reiber et al. 2022b). Hyperactivity can reflect an increased level of arousal or restlessness, which can be associated with a transient and/or chronic distress situation for the animals, as they might be more sensitive towards influencing factors such as cage changes or handling. *Hypolocomotion* may be directly related to model- or intervention-induced motor deficits, but more often to impaired general health and well-being, e.g. related to sickness behaviour, general distress, anxiety, and/or pain (e.g. in a colitis model (Zentrich et al. 2021)). In this context, wheel running behaviour has also been validated as a well-being- and severity-related readout parameter with alterations reported across different models and paradigms including a colitis model, a pancreatic cancer model, and a restraint stress paradigm (Häger et al. 2018; Weegh et al. 2020, 2021).

The analysis of *vertical activity* with *rearing, climbing,* and *cage lid hanging* can be of additional interest. Cage-lid hanging behaviour was the most interesting readout parameter in the HomeCageScan® automated behavioural scoring system with alterations linked to different types of pain and informative value confirmed by a response to analgesics in different pain states (Zhang et al. 2021a).

HCM monitoring allows a comprehensive collection of data for parameters related to innate behavioural patterns that are evolutionary determined but not necessarily essential for survival in a laboratory animal facility. A reduction or alteration in such behavioural patterns among others comprising *social interaction, nest building, burrowing, or grooming* can be a consequence of a compromised general well-being for instance related to disease symptoms, sickness behaviour or pain (Jirkof 2014; Turner et al. 2019; Aulehner et al. 2022b).

Nest building activity can be analysed by measurement of the time to handle or integrate nest material (Häger et al. 2015; Oliver et al. 2018). Moreover, the quality of the constructed nest can serve as an indirect measure of nest building (Schwabe et al. 2020). An impact of pain states and of sickness behaviour has been reported because of different surgical interventions and disease models (e.g. Arras et al. 2007; Jirkof et al. 2013; Jirkof 2014; Aulehner et al. 2022b). According to Schwabe et al. (2020), who reported a pronounced inter-facility variability, the impact of vendor, experience, exact animal strain information, sex, and local environmental influences needs to be considered when integrating this parameter in well-being and severity assessment schemes. However, this is also relevant for other parameters.

Burrowing was identified as indicator of postsurgical pain states in laboratory rodents based on a validation in mice (Jirkof et al. 2010). In this and subsequent studies by various groups, a reduction in burrowing activity was observed in response to pain states with a preventive effect of potent analgesics (e.g. Wodarski et al. 2016; reviewed by Turner et al. 2019; Aulehner et al. 2022b; Riedesel et al. 2023). Based on these findings the analysis of burrowing activity has more recently been validated in the context of general severity assessment in different disease models. A negative impact on burrowing activity has been reported in various disease models and following interventions by different groups (Koska et al. 2019; Seiffert et al. 2019; Boldt et al. 2021).

Along this line, a negative influence on *grooming* (*generally autogrooming*) activity has been described in response to exposure to anaesthesia/analgesia and surgical procedures (Oliver et al. 2018). Grooming can be analysed based on transfer of a fluorescent substance applied to the skin between the ears of mice (Grooming transfer test scoring, (Oliver et al. 2018)) or based on an analysis of movement patterns. Grooming can lead to stereotyped (obsessive-compulsive-like) behaviour resulting in skin irritations of self and/or cage mates (Feusner et al. 2009).

3.2 Posture and Gait

Changes in *posture and gait* are commonly analysed to detect and classify pain in laboratory animals. The alterations largely depend on the type (somatic, visceral, neuropathic; acute/chronic) and localization (body region and deep or superficial) of the pain. As an example, abdominal pain can be associated with arching of the back, writhing, and pressing of the abdomen to the cage floor. Thus, it is of particular interest to not only assess behavioural patterns but also monitor alterations in posture and gait of the animal. However, gait change as observed in lipopolysaccharide (LPS)-induced neuroinflammation models is commonly performed outside the HC (Carregosa et al. 2024).

3.3 Grimace Scale

Since the first intense evaluation in laboratory mice by Langford and colleagues (Langford et al. 2010), grimace scales have been intensely characterized and studied across different laboratory animal species and various pain states (for detailed reviews see Turner et al. 2019; Aulehner et al. 2022b; Onuma et al. 2024). While the grimace scales can also be affected by general sickness behaviour or by adverse effects of drugs such as anaesthetics and analgesics, they have been well validated in the context of the assessment of acute pain states (Onuma et al. 2024). Intense efforts have already been made to develop algorithms allowing automated analysis of facial expressions in the home cage setting (Andresen et al. 2020; Ernst et al. 2020a, b; McCoy et al. 2024).

3.4 Social Interaction and Vocalization

Among these parameters, social interaction is standing out as rodents are highly social animals, which seek contact with other animals. Associated with model- or intervention-associated distress or suboptimal husbandry conditions, animals might exhibit a reduction in social interaction or an increased level of aggressive behavioural patterns. In this context, the impact of sex and age requires consideration (Reiber et al. 2022a; Granza et al. 2023).

HCM toolkits include the recording and analysis of vocalizations through the installation of microphones in the cage. Vocalizations are important in the communication of mice and rats (Capas-Peneda et al. 2022; Agarwalla et al. 2023; Klaus et al. 2025) and will contribute to the refinement of welfare assessment.

Long-term monitoring of vocalization in the HC is expected to contribute to refined phenotypic characterization of social interactions in mice. Intraspecific communication signals from mating to aggression range from lower-frequent (10 kHz) up to the ultrasonic range (e.g. Hobson et al. 2020) and can also be picked up from mouse and rat pups after birth (Hofer et al. 2001).

3.5 Drinking, Feeding, and Body Weight

Drinking and feeding can be monitored by tracking in specific areas, including contact with food or water bottles. More accurate information about the actual *water or food intake* per unit of time requires measurement of remaining water or food at predefined intervals. Both parameters can be affected by distress, suffering, and pain of the animals. When interpreting the data, it must be carefully considered that thirst and hunger can also be influenced by direct or indirect effects on specific brain regions (e.g. related to neurostimulation or neuropathological alterations in a model of a neurological disorder or by metabolic diseases).

Anhedonia-associated behavioural patterns can be assessed based on measuring saccharin or sucrose preference with exposure to two bottles, one filled with water, and the other one with a sweet solution. A reduction in the preference for a sweet solution has been described in different disease models, following interventions or related to specific husbandry and housing conditions (e.g. Renner et al. 2016; Boldt et al. 2021; Kurogi et al. 2023). The lack of anticipatory behaviour in response to signalled palatable food reward (appetitive conditioning) is one of the prominent symptoms of motivational deficits and negative bias in a rat depression model (Von Frijtag et al. 2000).

In some HCM systems, a balance has been integrated to capture *body weight* information about group-housed mice tagged with RFID chips, whenever they enter a specific area such as a tunnel connecting two adjacent cages (Noorshams et al. 2017) or leading to the food dispenser (Ahloy-Dallaire et al. 2019).

Near infrared-imaging has also been applied to monitor wound healing based on temperature distribution profile in the wound area and to monitor inflammation-associated regional alterations of the temperature in specific disease models (Pereira et al. 2019).

3.6 Heart Rate, Respiratory Rate, and Body Temperature

An integration of near-infrared imaging techniques in a HCM system can allow continuous non-invasive assessment of *vital parameters including body temperature, heart rate, and its variability, and respiratory rate* (Pereira et al. 2019; Mösch et al. 2023). Depending on the model or intervention, these parameters are of relevance for health monitoring and for determination of early (HEPs) endpoints. Increase in heart rate and its concomitant decrease in heart rate variability occur in relation to arousal and various stressors due to altered autonomous nervous system function regulating the response of the cardiovascular system to demands (Stiedl et al. 2009; Koska et al. 2019; Buchecker et al. 2023; Hager et al. 2025). In general, stressors result in fast parasympathetic withdrawal and slower sympathetic activation to increase heart rate followed by a delayed recovery (return) to baseline values in both mice and rats (Tovote et al. 2005).

3.7 Selection of Parameters and Design of Multidimensional Schemes for Monitoring of Health, Well-Being, and Severity

Taken together a variety of parameters and candidate parameters exist, which can be integrated in HCM concepts aiming to continuously monitor the well-being of laboratory animals. It is emphasized that not all of these parameters have so far been assessed based on automated HCM with application in the context of animal welfare. Thus, further efforts are necessary to design more complex smart HC systems applying well validated algorithms to capture comprehensive information about an animal's health and affective state.

Agreement exists that there is no single parameter providing sufficient information about the level of pain or suffering of animals. A thorough assessment of the well-being of animals requires a selection and combination of parameters tailored to the species, strain, laboratory/husbandry conditions, model, and/or intervention. The design of composite multidimensional schemes for monitoring of animal-welfare related alterations has predominantly focused on the development of ethograms for different pain states in various laboratory animal species. As discussed above the alterations largely depend on the type and localization of pain. Examples of ethograms suitable for assessment of pain states have for instance been published (Roughan and Flecknell 2003; Leach et al. 2012; Oliver et al. 2018). Studies applying the HomeCageScan software tool for automated analysis of behaviours failed to clearly differentiate between groups of mice subjected to vasectomy with and without post-surgery analgesia, but they provided evidence for chronic non-evoked pain (Wright-Williams et al. 2013; Burand Jr. et al. 2023). These studies indicate that it is not sufficient to apply general behavioural scoring tools but underscore the need for a tailored design of the scoring schemes in combination with appropriate analgesic dose as animal welfare refinement to lower animal discomfort.

It has been repeatedly demonstrated that combining selected parameters as a basis for cluster analysis or ROC analysis can guide comparative severity assessment and can increase the sensitivity of the monitoring approaches (Häger et al. 2018; Abdelrahman et al. 2019; Tang et al. 2020; Wassermann et al. 2020; Mallien et al. 2022).

A bioinformatic workflow has been developed for the design of multidimensional composite scoring schemes (CMS) suitable for assessment of well-being and severity (van Dijk et al. 2020). An initial cross-correlation analysis identifies parameters with a high level of correlation allowing to exclude parameters providing redundant information. This pre-selection of parameters is followed by a principal component analysis allowing identification of the top parameters best distinguishing between experimental and control groups of animals. Applying data sets for these top parameters to *K*-means based cluster analysis allows a classification of individual animals to levels of severity and compromised well-being. The workflow has initially been applied to rat data sets from various epilepsy models. A more recent study validated the workflow by application to mouse models of neurodevelopmental, neuropsychiatric, and neurological disorders (Reiber et al. 2023). An online tool (R package) has been shared, which provides a ready-to-use application of the bioinformatic workflow FOR assessment of well-being and severity regardless of the models, interventions, and readout parameters (Reiber et al. 2023).

Another valuable tool has been developed by Talbot and colleagues (Talbot et al. 2022). The RELative Severity Assessment procedure (RELSA) is an algorithm-based weighted composite scoring system that can integrate information for various input variables. The RELSA approach has been successfully applied to different models and interventions resulting in a comparative severity grading in relation to predetermined reference data (Mallien et al. 2022; Talbot et al. 2022, 2023, 2024; Schreiber et al. 2024).

4 Examples of Animal Welfare Improvements by HCM Approaches

4.1 Early Detection of Compromised Welfare Through Mobility Monitoring

The more relevant the markers the better, but general locomotor activity tracking appears to be very informative by itself. Home-cage monitoring (HCM) systems enable continuous, non-invasive tracking of locomotor activity in laboratory mice, offering a powerful tool for early detection of compromised welfare. Immobility, particularly during the active (dark) phase, is a sensitive indicator of distress or illness. A study on dextran sodium sulphate (DSS)-induced colitis demonstrates that mice exposed to higher DSS concentrations exhibited significantly reduced activity and prolonged inactivity bouts, detectable before overt clinical signs emerged (Zentrich et al. 2021). Similarly, Huntington's disease (HD) models showed that climbing and cage-floor activity declined as early as 8 weeks of age, prior to visible motor deficits, highlighting immobility as an early behavioural marker of disease burden (Bains et al. 2023). In narcolepsy models using orexin/hypocretin (HCRT)-deficient mice exhibited fragmented activity patterns and an inability to sustain long activity bouts, which were detectable using HCM before full signs onset (Piilgaard et al. 2023). In an LPS inflammation model, climbing, locomotion, and rearing were significantly reduced along with increased immobility within hours of LPS administration. These changes were evident in both short-term (5-min) and long-term (24-h) assessments, particularly during the dark phase when mice are most active. The system also detected associated reductions in food and water intake and body weight, reinforcing its utility for early welfare surveillance. In a Streptozotocin (STZ)-induced pancreatic β-cell destruction type-1-like diabetes model, HCM monitoring corroborated the activity decline previously reported by standard methods. Contrastingly, Alzheimer's disease models showed increased nocturnal activity (Sun et al. 2024).

Even routine procedures, including handling, weighing, and particularly cage changes disrupted activity patterns, with effects lasting several hours among female mice, to days in male mice (Pernold et al. 2019). These findings underscore the sensitivity of HCM systems to both pathological and procedural stressors, making them valuable tools for early welfare assessment, enabling earlier intervention and refinement of care.

4.2 Continuous Monitoring for Disease Progression and Humane Endpoint Detection

The high-resolution temporal data provided by HCM allow for tracking disease progression in real time, facilitating the early identification of humane endpoints (HEPs). In oncology research, tumour bearing mice decreased their locomotor activity in the dark phase as tumour development progressed. Mice undergoing chemotherapy exhibited reduced nocturnal activity well before clinical signs were apparent (Terry et al. 2023). This behavioural activity decline, captured continuously, provides a more humane and objective basis for endpoint decisions than traditional daytime scoring.

In neurodegenerative models, such as amyotrophic lateral sclerosis (ALS) and HD, HCM detected progressive reductions in activity and increased rest fragmentation, correlating with disease advancement (Golini et al. 2020; Bains et al. 2023; Moore et al. 2024). Behavioural impairments persisted across both light and dark phases, with the most pronounced effects during the dark phase in the LPS model (Hasriadi et al. 2021). In narcolepsy models, HCRT-deficient mice exhibited fragmented activity patterns and an inability to sustain long activity bouts, which were detectable using HCM sub-clinically, i.e., before full clinical symptom onset (Piilgaard et al. 2023).

These findings support the use of HCM to monitor disease trajectory and refine endpoint criteria since changes were not only consistent across time but also aligned with known pathological milestones, supporting the use of activity data to refine endpoint criteria and reduce unnecessary suffering.

4.3 Objective Biomarkers for Disease Models

An advantage of HCM is its potential to identify biomarkers—quantifiable, objective indicators of disease state. Across multiple studies, specific activity metrics emerged as reliable proxies for disease burden. For instance, the "activity maintenance score," calculated as the ratio of long activity (≥32 min) versus short inactivity episodes (<8 min), was validated in narcolepsy models as a robust marker of severity (Piilgaard et al. 2023). Similarly, in HD models, the frequency and duration of climbing behaviour served as early indicators of motor impairment (Bains et al. 2023). In an LPS model, reductions in mobile behaviours (climbing, locomotion, rearing), average speed, and distance travelled were strongly correlated and inversely related to immobility. These metrics, captured in both short- and long-term assessments, provide a behavioural fingerprint of sickness and pain-like states. The authors also used ethograms and position distribution maps to visualize behavioural shifts, offering a rich data set for biomarker development (Hasriadi et al. 2021). In colitis models, a binary classifier was applied combining activity data and body weight to categorise animals into "burdened" and "non-burdened" states (Zentrich et al. 2021). This classifier mirrored the clinical course of colitis and outperformed traditional scoring in sensitivity and objectivity. These examples illustrate how HCM-derived measures can serve as early, reproducible biomarkers across diverse disease models, enhancing translational relevance and experimental rigour.

4.4 Predicting Optimal Timing for Humane and Experimental Endpoints

The ability to continuously monitor behaviour enables researchers to predict the optimal timing for HEPs and experimental endpoints (EEPs), thereby avoiding or reducing severe discomfort. A critical issue here is the detection of precisely defined pathological conditions in the continuum of often slowly progressive changes. Unfortunately, we generally have only limited empirical circadian data on what constitutes the normal physiological range and when the threshold for intervention has been reached. A narcolepsy study (Piilgaard et al. 2023) showed that activity fragmentation and loss of sustained wakefulness emerged within the first week of HCRT neuron degeneration, suggesting a narrow window for early intervention. In colitis models, activity reductions preceded clinical weight loss, allowing for earlier, more humane decisions regarding endpoint timing (Zentrich et al. 2021). In the LPS model, behavioural impairments emerged within 3 h of LPS administration and persisted for at least 24 h (Hasriadi et al. 2021). These early and sustained changes in activity (generally hypoactivity) could be a key signal about the timing of interventions and/or HEP decisions, particularly in acute inflammation models or in advanced stages of tumour growth in brain areas (brainstem, cerebellum) leading to impaired motor coordination, potentially replacing laborious motor tests by more complex HCM environments including climbing.

4.5 Monitoring Recovery and Refining Peri-Operative Analgesia

HCM also supports refinement of peri-operative care by enabling objective monitoring of post-intervention (surgery) recovery. In a study involving intracranial surgery, HCM detected reduced dark-phase activity and abnormal hyperactivity patterns in mice that later died unexpectedly—signals not captured by body weight alone (Pernold et al. 2019). This suggests that the system can serve as an early warning tool for post-operative complications.

Moreover, the ability to detect subtle changes in rest/activity cycles allows for the evaluation of analgesic efficacy. For instance, in models where analgesia was administered post-surgery, HCM could be used to assess whether normal activity patterns resumed, providing a non-invasive measure of pain relief and recovery quality. For example, surgery for brain infusion of viral vector solution leads to a long-lasting reduction of locomotor activity in the dark phase without affecting the overall circadian rhythm. Post-surgery hypoactivity is prevented by buprenorphine but not carprofen treatment (Abdollahi Nejat et al. 2024). However, buprenorphine is known to elicit hyperactivity by itself (Jirkof et al. 2015). In the LPS model, the system's sensitivity to pharmacological intervention by administering indomethacin, a non-steroidal anti-inflammatory drug was validated. Indomethacin significantly improved locomotor activity, reduced immobility, and restored food and water intake (Hasriadi et al. 2021). These effects were most pronounced during the dark phase, aligning with the drug's expected pharmacodynamics. This pharmacological validation supports the use of HCM for screening analgesic and anti-inflammatory compounds and determination of the necessary recovery period before actual experiments and/or subsequent interventions should be started.

5 Limitations of Home-Cage Monitoring for Animal Welfare Assessment

Despite its many advantages, HCM systems are not without limitations, particularly in the context of animal welfare monitoring.

5.1 Lack of Individual Resolution in Group-Housed Settings

Most systems, including the DVC® platform (Tecniplast), LABORAS (Metris), and LabMaster (TSE Systems), measure activity at the cage level. For optimal data quality, animals are often singly housed, which may negatively impact welfare by disrupting social behaviours. Although some studies have explored group-housing, the resulting data are less precise and more difficult to interpret (Golini et al. 2020). This limits the ability to assess individual animal welfare in group-housed settings, where the activity of multiple individuals may mask a dominant or sick animal's activity profile (Pernold et al. 2019; Zentrich et al. 2021; Bains et al. 2023; Sun et al. 2024).

While some studies have used RFID or video tracking to overcome this, these approaches require additional infrastructure and may introduce new variables. While HCM effectively captured sickness and pain-like behaviours in the LPS model, it could not distinguish between pain, fatigue, and motivational changes—all of which contribute to the sickness phenotype (Hasriadi et al. 2021). The authors recommended combining HCM with reflexive and other non-reflexive behavioural tests to improve specificity. Additionally, they cautioned that some analgesics may alter locomotor activity independent of pain relief, potentially confounding interpretation. For example, morphine may increase activity, while gabapentin may reduce it. Therefore, drug effects on motor coordination should be evaluated alongside HCM data to ensure accurate conclusions. This limitation is particularly relevant when interpreting inactivity, which may reflect rest, sleep, or illness (Piilgaard et al. 2023). Thus, HCM primarily captures gross locomotor activity and with basic monitoring (e.g. centre of gravity) cannot distinguish between specific behaviours such as grooming, eating, or quiet wakefulness. Unpublished DVC® data, from a breeding facility in the Netherlands, demonstrate contradictory activity patterns (hypoactivity vs hyperactivity) during breeding, once pups become active and leave the nest. Thus, complementary readouts are required together in combination with activity-based HCM to more reliably identify states of compromised animal welfare of an individual with a group.

5.2 Data Analysis

While the technical details of HCM are described specifically in Chaps. 7 and 9, we would like to point out some general aspects that are of high relevance for improving animal welfare through HCM systems.

Based on experience with customized systems for HCM of fear learning (Hager et al. 2014) and the Phenotyper® (Loos et al. 2014) with data analysis systems partly developed independently from the original vendor (Koopmans et al. 2017), it is obvious that quality control of HCM data analysis is an important issue. Scientifically, this requires absolute transparency on the raw data quality and editing, which are time-consuming and require full access to code used for analysis for reproducibility and replicability in science where "show me" must replace "trust me" (Kafkafi et al. 2018).

Video data are extremely valuable to assure proper quality control of automated HCM data. However, this may lead to huge amounts of data (in the order of tera- to petabytes) that must be stored and checked. Although algorithms, as for nest detection, can improve behavioural resolution, they remain proxies and require validation against gold-standard methods like EEG/EMG.

While HCM can detect fragmentation and immobility, it cannot reliably identify complex neurological states such as cataplexy or REM sleep unless when combined with additional specialized electrophysiological monitoring systems. Attempts to infer cataplexy-like episodes based on inactivity outside the nest found that these could not be distinguished from normal quiet behaviours (Piilgaard et al. 2023). This limits the utility of basic HCM system in models where such states are critical endpoints.

Finally, online data analysis is necessary to be able to act as soon as possible within certain time limits upon detection of compromised welfare. The worse the welfare state, the more urgent the required action. One consequence of more sensitive automatic 24/7 detection systems for welfare issues is that alerts are also received at night and at weekends. Timely follow-up of these alarms has implications for staff deployment and requires strategic choices to be made. However, as in clinical monitoring, fast online analysis is required to identify sudden activity drops that can emerge from unforeseen events to identify risks for fast action. Examples here may be bolus constriction by intraperitoneal ECG leads when using radiotelemetry implants or unexpected septic shock. Despite being a rare event, to avoid that mice die in a painful state with severe discomfort, fast action is required to apply a HEP as soon as possible after the detection of an expected (predefined) but also unexpected health issue. This is possible with the DVC® system and its automatic notification system. However, one should be aware of delays of automated emails by variable server settings that should be checked beforehand (e.g. emails sent 1x/hour). Additionally, new technical developments based on training of ML algorithms by experts can provide support as a basis for alarms, which would be easier to handle during nights/weekends.

5.3 Costs and Infrastructure

Lastly, the initial investment in HCM systems and the associated data infrastructure can be substantial. This may limit accessibility for smaller institutions or individual research groups (Pernold et al. 2019; Piilgaard et al. 2023). Additionally, the ongoing costs for analytical needs (personnel) and IT demands should not be underestimated (again see Chap. 7 for more details).

6 Conclusions and Perspective

In summary, HCM is a powerful, non-invasive approach for welfare assessment and disease monitoring providing data of a much higher quality than brief visual observations especially in the light phase. HCM and other assessment tools (see Sect. 3.1) contribute significantly to improvement of animal welfare and description of phenotypes. These augment research data by adding to research quality (replicability, etc.). However, HCM limitations must be carefully considered when focussing predominantly on activity-derived measures. Complementary readouts, based on video analysis, and physiological monitoring, remain essential for a comprehensive welfare assessment strategy. This is required to generate a reliable clinical score to apply early EEPs or HEPs to avoid experimental mortality with unnecessarily increased (up to severe) discomfort.

Besides performing experiments exclusively in a defined HC environment, the power to start experiments from a home-base and the option to visit attached environments to explore intrinsic deliberate motivation of novelty-seeking (Kas et al. 2011) cannot be underestimated especially in behavioural neuroscience. This will allow to better combine housing and testing needs, especially with the important refinement that unspecific stressors can be avoided by bringing an experiment to the animal and not vice versa that is important in view of the interaction between emotion and cognition, which has largely been ignored in animal research despite contributing to limited replicability in science.

While we are convinced that HCM quality will further develop and evolve (Wells and Members of the COST Action TEATIME CA20135 Welfare Group 2025), many aspects from improvements of animal welfare monitoring to better science in HCM are still in a relatively early developmental phase. Turnkey systems for all required options are not yet available, and customization of existing commercial systems is a complex and costly effort, limiting its wider use. For many readouts, their normal circadian range (physiology) and the threshold for identifying deviations (pathology) are yet to be determined. We need to bridge this *Physiology-to-Pathology gap* by considering many variables and influencing factors that play a role here, such as mouse and rat sub-strains, age, sex, food, housing conditions, microbiome, and many more. In the long term, HCM will further develop as (1) major contribution to refinement and (2) eventually is expected to contribute to a reduction in animal numbers used in experiments, and (3) in combination with improved data sharing (see Chap. 10) also a reduction in animal research. Since progress in animal research is predominantly driven by the funding of research projects rather than animal welfare improvements, it is essential to cooperatively merge these two areas for the ongoing improvement of animal welfare in science. Animal welfare and research quality go hand in hand.

Acknowledgements H.P., Ö.S.Ç. and O.S. have been members of the COST Action CA20135 TEATIME (http://www.cost-teatime.org/).

Funding H. P. received funding for the development of novel approaches (incl. Smart HCM) for evidence-based severity assessment and refinement by Deutsche Forschungsgemeinschaft (DFG FOR 2591 PO681/9-1, -2 and -3).

References

Abdelrahman A, Kumstel S, Zhang X, Liebig M, Wendt EHU, Eichberg J et al (2019) A novel multiparametric analysis of non-invasive methods to assess animal distress during chronic pancreatitis. Sci Rep 9:14084. https://doi.org/10.1038/s41598-019-50682-3

Abdollahi Nejat M, Stiedl O, Smit AB, van Kesteren RE (2024) Continuous locomotor activity monitoring to assess animal welfare following intracranial surgery in mice. Front Behav Neurosci 18:1457894. https://doi.org/10.3389/fnbeh.2024.1457894

Agarwalla S, De A, Bandyopadhyay S (2023) Predictive mouse ultrasonic vocalization sequences: uncovering behavioral significance, auditory cortex neuronal preferences, and social-experience-driven plasticity. J Neurosci 43:6141–6163. https://doi.org/10.1523/JNEUROSCI.2353-22.2023

Ahloy-Dallaire J, Klein JD, Davis JK, Garner JP (2019) Automated monitoring of mouse feeding and body weight for continuous health assessment. Lab Anim 53:342–351. https://doi.org/10.1177/0023677218797974

Andresen N, Wöllhaf M, Hohlbaum K, Lewejohann L, Hellwich O, Thöne-Reineke C et al (2020) Towards a fully automated surveillance of Well-being status in laboratory mice using deep learning: starting with facial expression analysis. PLoS One 15:e0228059. https://doi.org/10.1371/journal.pone.0228059

Arras M, Rettich A, Cinelli P, Kasermann HP, Burki K (2007) Assessment of post-laparotomy pain in laboratory mice by telemetric recording of heart rate and heart rate variability. BMC Vet Res 3:16. https://doi.org/10.1186/1746-6148-3-16

Aulehner K, Bray J, Koska I, Pace C, Palme R, Kreuzer M et al (2022a) The impact of tethered recording techniques on activity and sleep patterns in rats. Sci Rep 12:3179. https://doi.org/10.1038/s41598-022-06307-3

Aulehner K, Leenaars C, Buchecker V, Stirling H, Schönhoff K, King H et al (2022b) Grimace scale, burrowing, and nest building for the assessment of post-surgical pain in mice and rats—a systematic review. Front Vet Sci 9:930005. https://doi.org/10.3389/fvets.2022.930005

Bains RS, Forrest H, Sillito RR, Armstrong JD, Stewart M, Nolan PM et al (2023) Longitudinal home-cage automated assessment of climbing behavior shows sexual dimorphism and aging-related decrease in C57BL/6J healthy mice and allows early detection of motor impairment in the N171-82Q mouse model of Huntington's disease. Front Behav Neurosci 17:1148172. https://doi.org/10.3389/fnbeh.2023.1148172

Balci F, Shamy JL, El-Khodor BF, Filippov I, Mushlin R, Port R et al (2013) High-throughput automated phenotyping of two genetic mouse models of Huntington's disease. PLoS Curr. https://doi.org/10.1371/currents.hd.124aa0d16753f88215776fba102ceb29

Beerling W, Koolhaas JM, Ahnaou A, Bouwknecht JA, de Boer SF, Meerlo P et al (2011) Physiological and hormonal responses to novelty exposure in rats are mainly related to ongoing behavioral activity. Physiol Behav 103:412–420. https://doi.org/10.1016/j.physbeh.2011.03.014

Berdoy M (2002) The laboratory rat: a natural history. Oxford University. https://www.youtube.com/watch?v=giu5WjUt2GA

Bermudez Contreras E, Sutherland RJ, Mohajerani MH, Whishaw IQ (2022) Challenges of a small world analysis for the continuous monitoring of behavior in mice. Neurosci Biobehav Rev 136:104621. https://doi.org/10.1016/j.neubiorev.2022.104621

Boldt L, Koska I, Maarten van Dijk R, Talbot SR, Miljanovic N, Palme R et al (2021) Toward evidence-based severity assessment in mouse models with repeated seizures: I. Electrical kindling. Epilepsy Behav 115:107689. https://doi.org/10.1016/j.yebeh.2020.107689

Buchecker V, Koska I, Pace C, Talbot SR, Palme R, Bleich A et al (2023) Toward evidence-based severity assessment in mouse models with repeated seizures: (II.) impact of surgery and intrahippocampal kainate. Eur Surg Res 64:89–107. https://doi.org/10.1159/000522156

Burand AJ Jr, Waltz TB, Manis AD, Hodges MR, Stucky CL (2023) HomeCageScan analysis reveals ongoing pain in Fabry rats. Neurobiol Pain 13:100113. https://doi.org/10.1016/j.ynpai.2022.100113

Campos-Luna I, Miller A, Beard A, Leach M (2019) Validation of mouse welfare indicators: a Delphi consultation survey. Sci Rep 9:10249. https://doi.org/10.1038/s41598-019-45810-y

Capas-Peneda S, Saavedra Torres Y, Prins J-B, Olsson IAS (2022) From mating to milk access: a review of reproductive vocal communication in mice. Front Behav Neurosci 16:833168. https://doi.org/10.3389/fnbeh.2022.833168

Carregosa D, Loncarevic-Vasiljkovic N, Feliciano R, Moura-Louro D, Mendes CS, dos Santos CN (2024) Locomotor and gait changes in the LPS model of neuroinflammation are correlated with inflammatory cytokines in blood and brain. J Inflamm 21:39. https://doi.org/10.1186/s12950-024-00412-y

Colwell CS (2021) Defining circadian disruption in neurodegenerative disorders. J Clin Invest 131:e148288. https://doi.org/10.1172/JCI148288

Dallmann R, Brown SA, Gachon F (2014) Chronopharmacology: new insights and therapeutic implications. Annu Rev Pharmacol Toxicol 54:339–361. https://doi.org/10.1146/annurev-pharmtox-011613-135923

Diamond DM, Campbell AM, Park CR, Halonen J, Zoladz PR (2007) The temporal dynamics model of emotional memory processing: a synthesis on the neurobiological basis of stress-induced amnesia, flashbulb and traumatic memories, and the Yerkes-Dodson law. Neural Plast 2007:1–33. https://doi.org/10.1155/2007/60803

Dwinell MR, Takizawa A, Tutaj M, Malloy L, Schilling R, Endsley A et al (2025) Establishing the hybrid rat diversity program: a resource for dissecting complex traits. Mamm Genome 36:25–37. https://doi.org/10.1007/s00335-024-10102-y

Ernst L, Kopaczka M, Schulz M, Talbot SR, Struve B, Häger C et al (2020a) Semi-automated generation of pictures for the mouse grimace scale: a multi-laboratory analysis (part 2). Lab Anim 54:92–98. https://doi.org/10.1177/0023677219881664

Ernst L, Kopaczka M, Schulz M, Talbot SR, Zieglowski L, Meyer M et al (2020b) Improvement of the mouse grimace scale set-up for implementing a semi-automated mouse grimace scale scoring (part 1). Lab Anim 54:83–91. https://doi.org/10.1177/0023677219881655

Feusner JD, Hembacher E, Phillips KA (2009) The mouse who couldn't stop washing: pathologic grooming in animals and humans. CNS Spectr 14:503–513. https://doi.org/10.1017/S1092852900023567

Freund J, Brandmaier AM, Lewejohann L, Kirste I, Kritzler M, Krüger A et al (2013) Emergence of individuality in genetically identical mice. Science 340:756–759. https://doi.org/10.1126/science.1235294

Gaburro S, Winter Y, Loos M, Kim JJ, Stiedl O (2022) Editorial: home cage-based phenotyping in rodents: innovation, standardization, reproducibility and translational improvement. Front Neurosci 16:894193. https://doi.org/10.3389/fnins.2022.894193

Golini E, Rigamonti M, Iannello F, De Rosa C, Scavizzi F, Raspa M et al (2020) A non-invasive digital biomarker for the detection of rest disturbances in the SOD1G93A mouse model of ALS. Front Neurosci 14:896. https://doi.org/10.3389/fnins.2020.00896

Granza AE, Amaral IM, Monteiro DG, Salti A, Hofer A, El Rawas R (2023) Social interaction is less rewarding in adult female than in male mice. Brain Sci 13:1445. https://doi.org/10.3390/brainsci13101445

Hager T, Jansen RF, Pieneman AW, Manivannan SN, Golani I, van der Sluis S et al (2014) Display of individuality in avoidance behavior and risk assessment of inbred mice. Front Behav Neurosci 8. https://doi.org/10.3389/fnbeh.2014.00314

Häger C, Keubler LM, Biernot S, Dietrich J, Buchheister S, Buettner M et al (2015) Time to integrate to nest test evaluation in a mouse DSS-colitis model. PLoS One 10:e0143824. https://doi.org/10.1371/journal.pone.0143824

Häger C, Keubler LM, Talbot SR, Biernot S, Weegh N, Buchheister S et al (2018) Running in the wheel: defining individual severity levels in mice. PLoS Biol 16:e2006159. https://doi.org/10.1371/journal.pbio.2006159

Hager T, Agorastos A, Ögren SO, Stiedl O (2025) Identifying cardiovascular risk by nonlinear heart rate dynamics analysis: translational biomarker from mice to humans. Brain Sci 15:306. https://doi.org/10.3390/brainsci15030306

Hasriadi H, Dasuni Wasana PW, Vajragupta O, Rojsitthisak P, Towiwat P (eds) (2021) Automated home-cage monitoring as a potential measure of sickness behaviors and pain-like behaviors in LPS-treated mice. PLoS One 16:e0256706. https://doi.org/10.1371/journal.pone.0256706

Hawkins P, Morton DB, Burman O, Dennison N, Honess P, Jennings M et al (2011) A guide to defining and implementing protocols for the welfare assessment of laboratory animals: eleventh report of the BVAAWF/FRAME/RSPCA/UFAW Joint Working Group on Refinement. Lab Anim 45:1–13. https://doi.org/10.1258/la.2010.010031

Hobson L, Bains RS, Greenaway S, Wells S, Nolan PM (2020) Phenotyping in mice using continuous home cage monitoring and ultrasonic vocalization recordings. Curr Protoc Mouse Biol 10:e80. https://doi.org/10.1002/cpmo.80

Hofer MA, Shair HN, Brunelli SA (2001) Ultrasonic vocalizations in rat and mouse pups. Curr Protoc Neurosci 8:Unit 8.14. https://doi.org/10.1002/0471142301.ns0814s17

Jirkof P (2014) Burrowing and nest building behavior as indicators of well-being in mice. J Neurosci Methods 234:139–146. https://doi.org/10.1016/j.jneumeth.2014.02.001

Jirkof P, Cesarovic N, Rettich A, Nicholls F, Seifert B, Arras M (2010) Burrowing behavior as an indicator of post-laparotomy main in mice. Front Behav Neurosci 4:165. https://doi.org/10.3389/fnbeh.2010.00165

Jirkof P, Leucht K, Cesarovic N, Caj M, Nicholls F, Rogler G et al (2013) Burrowing is a sensitive behavioural assay for monitoring general wellbeing during dextran sulfate sodium colitis in laboratory mice. Lab Anim 47:274–283. https://doi.org/10.1177/0023677213493409

Jirkof P, Tourvieille A, Cinelli P, Arras M (2015) Buprenorphine for pain relief in mice: repeated injections vs sustained-release depot formulation. Lab Anim 49:177–187. https://doi.org/10.1177/0023677214562849

Kafkafi N, Agassi J, Chesler EJ, Crabbe JC, Crusio WE, Eilam D et al (2018) Reproducibility and replicability of rodent phenotyping in preclinical studies. Neurosci Biobehav Rev 87:218–232. https://doi.org/10.1016/j.neubiorev.2018.01.003

Kahnau P, Mieske P, Wilzopolski J, Kalliokoski O, Mandillo S, Hölter SM et al (2023) A systematic review of the development and application of home cage monitoring in laboratory mice and rats. BMC Biol 21:256. https://doi.org/10.1186/s12915-023-01751-7

Kas MJ, Golani I, Benjamini Y, Fonio E, Stiedl O (2011) Longitudinal assessment of deliberate mouse behavior in the home cage and attached environments: relevance to anxiety and mood disorders. NeuroMethods 63:1–20. https://doi.org/10.1007/978-1-61779-313-4_1

Kaufmann E, Khan N, Tran KA, Ulndreaj A, Pernet E, Fontes G et al (2022) BCG vaccination provides protection against IAV but not SARS-CoV-2. Cell Rep 38:110502. https://doi.org/10.1016/j.celrep.2022.110502

Klaus T, Wernisch B, Zala SM, Penn DJ (2025) Courtship vocalizations of wild house mice show highly dynamic changes and correlate with male copulatory success. Anim Behav 220:123024. https://doi.org/10.1016/j.anbehav.2024.11.002

Koolhaas JM, Bartolomucci A, Buwalda B, de Boer SF, Flügge G, Korte SM et al (2011) Stress revisited: a critical evaluation of the stress concept. Neurosci Biobehav Rev 35:1291–1301. https://doi.org/10.1016/j.neubiorev.2011.02.003

Koolhaas JM, de Boer SF, Buwalda B, Meerlo P (2017) Social stress models in rodents: towards enhanced validity. Neurobiol Stress 6:104–112. https://doi.org/10.1016/j.ynstr.2016.09.003

Koopmans B, Smit AB, Verhage M, Loos M (2017) AHCODA-DB: a data repository with web-based mining tools for the analysis of automated high-content mouse phenomics data. BMC Bioinform 18:200. https://doi.org/10.1186/s12859-017-1612-1

Koska I, van Dijk RM, Seiffert I, Di Liberto V, Möller C, Palme R et al (2019) Toward evidence-based severity assessment in rat models with repeated seizures: II. Chemical post–status epilepticus model. Epilepsia 60:2114–2127. https://doi.org/10.1111/epi.16330

Kurogi K, Taniguchi F, Matsuo R, Shinozuka M, Suzaki R, Yasuo S (2023) Increased depression-like behaviors with altered brain dopamine metabolisms in male mice housed in large cages are alleviated by bupropion. Eur J Pharmacol 960:176126. https://doi.org/10.1016/j.ejphar.2023.176126

Langford DJ, Bailey AL, Chanda ML, Clarke SE, Drummond TE, Echols S et al (2010) Coding of facial expressions of pain in the laboratory mouse. Nat Methods 7:447–449. https://doi.org/10.1038/nmeth.1455

Leach MC, Klaus K, Miller AL, Scotto di Perrotolo M, Sotocinal SG, Flecknell PA (2012) The assessment of post-vasectomy pain in mice using behaviour and the mouse grimace scale. PLoS One 7:e35656. https://doi.org/10.1371/journal.pone.0035656

Lewejohann L, Schwabe K, Häger C, Jirkof P (2020) Impulse for animal welfare outside the experiment. Lab Anim 54:150–158. https://doi.org/10.1177/0023677219891754

Loos M, Koopmans B, Aarts E, Maroteaux G, van der Sluis S, Verhage M et al (2014) Sheltering behavior and locomotor activity in 11 genetically diverse common inbred mouse strains using home-cage monitoring. PLoS One 9:e108563. https://doi.org/10.1371/journal.pone.0108563

Lynch JJ, Castagné V, Moser PC, Mittelstadt SW (2011) Comparison of methods for the assessment of locomotor activity in rodent safety pharmacology studies. J Pharmacol Toxicol Methods 64:74–80. https://doi.org/10.1016/j.vascn.2011.03.003

Mallien AS, Pfeiffer N, Brandwein C, Inta D, Sprengel R, Palme R et al (2022) Comparative severity assessment of genetic, stress-based, and pharmacological mouse models of depression. Front Behav Neurosci 16:908366. https://doi.org/10.3389/fnbeh.2022.908366

McCoy ES, Park SK, Patel RP, Ryan DF, Mullen ZJ, Nesbitt JJ et al (2024) Development of PainFace software to simplify, standardize, and scale up mouse grimace analyses. Pain 165:1793–1805. https://doi.org/10.1097/j.pain.0000000000003187

McEwen BS (2007) Physiology and neurobiology of stress and adaptation: central role of the brain. Physiol Rev 87:873–904. https://doi.org/10.1152/physrev.00041.2006

Möller C, van Dijk RM, Wolf F, Keck M, Schönhoff K, Bierling V et al (2019) Impact of repeated kindled seizures on heart rate rhythms, heart rate variability, and locomotor activity in rats. Epilepsy Behav 92:36–44. https://doi.org/10.1016/j.yebeh.2018.11.034

Moore JL, Kennedy J, Hassan A-A (2024) Automated home cage monitoring of an aging colony of mice—implications for welfare monitoring and experimentation. Front Neurosci 18. https://doi.org/10.3389/fnins.2024.1489308

Mösch L, Kunczik J, Breuer L, Merhof D, Gass P, Potschka H et al (2023) Towards substitution of invasive telemetry: an integrated home cage concept for unobstrusive monitoring of objective physiological parameters in rodents. bioRxiv. (preprint). https://doi.org/10.1101/2023.05.12.540546

Noorshams O, Boyd JD, Murphy TH (2017) Automating mouse weighing in group homecages with raspberry pi micro-computers. J Neurosci Methods 285:1–5. https://doi.org/10.1016/j.jneumeth.2017.05.002

Ohl F, van der Staay FJ (2012) Animal welfare: at the interface between science and society. Vet J 192:13–19. https://doi.org/10.1016/j.tvjl.2011.05.019

Oliver VL, Thurston SE, Lofgren JL (2018) Using cageside measures to evaluate analgesic efficacy in mice (Mus musculus) after surgery. J Am Assoc Lab Anim Sci 57:186–201

Onuma K, Watanabe M, Sasaki N (2024) The grimace scale: a useful tool for assessing pain in laboratory animals. Exp Anim 73:234–245. https://doi.org/10.1538/expanim.24-0010

Pellman BA, Kim E, Reilly M, Kashima J, Motch O, de la Iglesia HO et al (2015) Time-specific fear acts as a non-photic entraining stimulus of circadian rhythms in rats. Sci Rep 5:14916. https://doi.org/10.1038/srep14916

Pereira CB, Kunczik J, Bleich A, Haeger C, Kiessling F, Thum T et al (2019) Perspective review of optical imaging in welfare assessment in animal-based research. J Biomed Opt 24:1. https://doi.org/10.1117/1.JBO.24.7.070601

Perel P, Roberts I, Sena E, Wheble P, Briscoe C, Sandercock P et al (2007) Comparison of treatment effects between animal experiments and clinical trials: systematic review. BMJ 334:197. https://doi.org/10.1136/bmj.39048.407928.BE

Pernold K, Iannello F, Low BE, Rigamonti M, Rosati G, Scavizzi F et al (2019) Towards large scale automated cage monitoring—diurnal rhythm and impact of interventions on in-cage activity of C57BL/6J mice recorded 24/7 with a non-disrupting capacitive-based technique. PLoS One 14:e0211063. https://doi.org/10.1371/journal.pone.0211063

Perry LJ, Ratcliff GE, Mayo A, Perez BE, Rays Wahba L, Nikhil KL et al (2025) A circadian behavioral analysis suite for real-time classification of daily rhythms in complex behaviors. Cell Rep Methods 5:101050. https://doi.org/10.1016/j.crmeth.2025.101050

Piilgaard L, Rose L, Justinussen JL, Hviid CG, Lemcke R, Wellendorph P et al (2023) Non-invasive detection of narcolepsy type I phenotypical features and disease progression by continuous home-cage monitoring of activity in two mouse models: the HCRT-KO and DTA model. Sleep 46:zsad144. https://doi.org/10.1093/sleep/zsad144

Poole T (1997) Happy animals make good science. Lab Anim 31:116–124. https://doi.org/10.1258/002367797780600198

Redfern WS, Tse K, Grant C, Keerie A, Simpson DJ, Pedersen JC et al (2017) Automated recording of home cage activity and temperature of individual rats housed in social groups: the Rodent Big Brother project. PLoS One 12:e0181068. https://doi.org/10.1371/journal.pone.0181068

Reiber M, Koska I, Pace C, Schönhoff K, von Schumann L, Palme R et al (2022a) Development of behavioral patterns in young C57BL/6J mice: a home cage-based study. Sci Rep 12:2550. https://doi.org/10.1038/s41598-022-06395-1

Reiber M, Miljanovic N, Schönhoff K, Palme R, Potschka H (2022b) Behavioral phenotyping of young Scn1a haploinsufficient mice. Epilepsy Behav 136:108903. https://doi.org/10.1016/j.yebeh.2022.108903

Reiber M, Stirling H, Sprengel R, Gass P, Palme R, Potschka H (2022c) Phenotyping young GluA1 deficient mice—a behavioral characterization in a genetic loss-of-function model. Front Behav Neurosci 16:877094. https://doi.org/10.3389/fnbeh.2022.877094

Reiber M, von Schumann L, Buchecker V, Boldt L, Gass P, Bleich A et al (2023) Evidence-based comparative severity assessment in young and adult mice. PLoS One 18:e0285429. https://doi.org/10.1371/journal.pone.0285429

Renner M, Feng R, Springer D, Chen M-K, Ntamack A, Espina A et al (2016) A murine model of peripheral irradiation-induced fatigue. Behav Brain Res 307:218–226. https://doi.org/10.1016/j.bbr.2016.03.035

Richardson CA (2015) The power of automated behavioural homecage technologies in characterizing disease progression in laboratory mice: a review. Appl Anim Behav Sci 163:19–27. https://doi.org/10.1016/j.applanim.2014.11.018

Riedesel A-K, Helgers SOA, Abdulbaki A, Hatipoglu Majernik G, Alam M, Krauss JK et al (2023) Severity assessment of complex and repeated intracranial surgery in rats. Eur Surg Res 64:108–119. https://doi.org/10.1159/000520678

Roughan JV, Flecknell PA (2003) Evaluation of a short duration behaviour-based post-operative pain scoring system in rats. Eur J Pain 7:397–406. https://doi.org/10.1016/S1090-3801(02)00140-4

Santin Y, Lopez S, Ader I, Andrieu S, Blanchard N, Carrière A et al (2021) Towards a large-scale assessment of the relationship between biological and chronological aging: the Inspire mouse cohort. J Frailty Aging 10:121–131. https://doi.org/10.14283/jfa.2020.43

Santin Y, Chiesa M, Alfonso A, Doghri Y, Kang R, Haidar F et al (2024) Computational and digital analyses in the INSPIRE mouse cohort to define sex-specific functional determinants of biological aging. Sci Adv 10:eadt1670. https://doi.org/10.1126/sciadv.adt1670

Schreiber T, Koopmann I, Brandstetter J, Talbot SR, Goldstein L, Hoffmann L et al (2024) Evidence-based severity assessment of animal models for pancreatic cancer. Biomedicine 12:1494. https://doi.org/10.3390/biomedicines12071494

Schwabe K, Boldt L, Bleich A, van Dijk RM, Helgers SOA, Häger C et al (2020) Nest-building performance in rats: impact of vendor, experience, and sex. Lab Anim 54:17–25. https://doi.org/10.1177/0023677219862004

Seiffert I, van Dijk RM, Koska I, Di Liberto V, Möller C, Palme R et al (2019) Toward evidence-based severity assessment in rat models with repeated seizures: III. Electrical post-status epilepticus model. Epilepsia 60:1539–1551. https://doi.org/10.1111/epi.16095

Sheehan PW, Musiek ES (2020) Evaluating circadian dysfunction in mouse models of Alzheimer's disease: where do we stand? Front Neurosci 14. https://doi.org/10.3389/fnins.2020.00703

Stiedl O, Tovote P, Ögren SO, Meyer M (2004) Behavioral and autonomic dynamics during contextual fear conditioning in mice. Auton Neurosci 115:15–27. https://doi.org/10.1016/j.autneu.2004.07.006

Stiedl O, Meyer M, Jahn O, Ögren SO, Spiess J (2005) Corticotropin-releasing factor receptor 1 and central heart rate regulation in mice during expression of conditioned fear. J Pharmacol Exp Ther 312:905–916. https://doi.org/10.1124/jpet.104.075820

Stiedl O, Jansen RF, Pieneman AW, Ögren SO, Meyer M (2009) Assessing aversive emotional states through the heart in mice: implications for cardiovascular dysregulation in affective disorders. Neurosci Biobehav Rev 33:181–190. https://doi.org/10.1016/j.neubiorev.2008.08.015

Sun R, Gaerz M-C, Oeing C, Mai K, Brachs S (2024) Accurate locomotor activity profiles of group-housed mice derived from home cage monitoring data. Front Neurosci 18. https://doi.org/10.3389/fnins.2024.1456307

Talbot SR, Struve B, Wassermann L, Heider M, Weegh N, Knape T et al (2022) RELSA—a multidimensional procedure for the comparative assessment of well-being and the quantitative determination of severity in experimental procedures. Front Vet Sci 9:937711. https://doi.org/10.3389/fvets.2022.937711

Talbot SR, Kumstel S, Schulz B, Tang G, Abdelrahman A, Seume N et al (2023) Robustness of a multivariate composite score when evaluating distress of animal models for gastrointestinal diseases. Sci Rep 13:2605. https://doi.org/10.1038/s41598-023-29623-8

Talbot SR, Heider M, Wirth M, Jörns A, Naujok O (2024) Exploring dose–response variability and relative severity assessment in STZ-induced diabetes male NSG mice. Sci Rep 14:16559. https://doi.org/10.1038/s41598-024-67490-z

Tam WY, Cheung K-K (2020) Phenotypic characteristics of commonly used inbred mouse strains. J Mol Med 98:1215–1234. https://doi.org/10.1007/s00109-020-01953-4

Tang G, Seume N, Häger C, Kumstel S, Abshagen K, Bleich A et al (2020) Comparing distress of mouse models for liver damage. Sci Rep 10:19814. https://doi.org/10.1038/s41598-020-76391-w

Terry S, Gommet C, Kerangueven A-C, Leguet M, Thévenin V, Berthelot M et al (2023) Activity in group-housed home cages of mice as a novel preclinical biomarker in oncology studies. Cancers (Basel) 15:4798. https://doi.org/10.3390/cancers15194798

Tovote P, Meyer M, Ronnenberg A, Spiess J, Pilz PKD, Ögren SO et al (2005) Dissociation of temporal dynamics of heart rate and blood pressure responses elicited by conditioned fear but not acoustic startle. Behav Neurosci 119:55–65. https://doi.org/10.1037/0735-7044.119.1.55

Turner PV, Pang DS, Lofgren JL (2019) A review of pain assessment methods in laboratory rodents. Comp Med 69:451–467. https://doi.org/10.30802/AALAS-CM-19-000042

van der Worp HB, Howells DW, Sena ES, Porritt MJ, Rewell S, O'Collins V et al (2010) Can animal models of disease reliably inform human studies? PLoS Med 7:e1000245. https://doi.org/10.1371/journal.pmed.1000245

van Dijk RM, Koska I, Bleich A, Tolba R, Seiffert I, Möller C et al (2020) Design of composite measure schemes for comparative severity assessment in animal-based neuroscience research: a case study focussed on rat epilepsy models. PLoS One 15:e0230141. https://doi.org/10.1371/journal.pone.0230141

Von Frijtag JC, Reijmers LGJE, Van der Harst JE, Leus IE, Van den Bos R, Spruijt BM (2000) Defeat followed by individual housing results in long-term impaired reward- and cognition-related behaviours in rats. Behav Brain Res 117:137–146. https://doi.org/10.1016/S0166-4328(00)00300-4

Wassermann L, Helgers SOA, Riedesel A-K, Talbot SR, Bleich A, Schwabe K et al (2020) Monitoring of heart rate and activity using telemetry allows grading of experimental procedures used in neuroscientific rat models. Front Neurosci 14. https://doi.org/10.3389/fnins.2020.587760

Weegh N, Füner J, Janke O, Winter Y, Jung C, Struve B et al (2020) Wheel running behaviour in group-housed female mice indicates disturbed wellbeing due to DSS colitis. Lab Anim 54:63–72. https://doi.org/10.1177/0023677219879455

Weegh N, Zentrich E, Zechner D, Struve B, Wassermann L, Talbot SR et al (2021) Voluntary wheel running behaviour as a tool to assess the severity in a mouse pancreatic cancer model. PLoS One 16:e0261662. https://doi.org/10.1371/journal.pone.0261662
Wells S, Members of the COST Action TEATIME CA20135 Welfare Group (2025) Advocating for automation in animal research: using home cage monitoring to advance welfare, reproducibility and scientific openness. Dis Model Mech 18:dmm052669. https://doi.org/10.1242/dmm.052669
Wodarski R, Delaney A, Ultenius C, Morland R, Andrews N, Baastrup C et al (2016) Cross-Centre replication of suppressed burrowing behaviour as an ethologically relevant pain outcome measure in the rat: a prospective multicentre study. Pain 157:2350–2365. https://doi.org/10.1097/j.pain.0000000000000657
Wright-Williams S, Flecknell PA, Roughan JV (2013) Comparative effects of vasectomy surgery and buprenorphine treatment on faecal corticosterone concentrations and behaviour assessed by manual and automated analysis methods in C57 and C3H mice. PLoS One 8:e75948. https://doi.org/10.1371/journal.pone.0075948
Würbel H (2001) Ideal homes? Housing effects on rodent brain and behaviour. Trends Neurosci 24:207–211. https://doi.org/10.1016/S0166-2236(00)01718-5
Zentrich E, Talbot SR, Bleich A, Häger C (2021) Automated home-cage monitoring during acute experimental colitis in mice. Front Neurosci 15. https://doi.org/10.3389/fnins.2021.760606
Zhang H, Lecker I, Collymore C, Dokova A, Pham MC, Rosen SF et al (2021a) Cage-lid hanging behavior as a translationally relevant measure of pain in mice. Pain 162:1416–1425. https://doi.org/10.1097/j.pain.0000000000002127
Zhang X, Lin J, Spruyt K (2021b) Sleep problems in Rett syndrome animal models: a systematic review. J Neurosci Res 99:529–544. https://doi.org/10.1002/jnr.24730
Zintzsch A, Noe E, Reißmann M, Ullmann K, Krämer S, Jerchow B et al (2017) Guidelines on severity assessment and classification of genetically altered mouse and rat lines. Lab Anim 51:573–582. https://doi.org/10.1177/0023677217718863

Home Cage Monitoring in Practice in Core Labs: Training, Infrastructure, and Research Workflow

Philipp Villiger, Michael Tsoory, Silvia Mandillo, and Stefano Gaburro

Abstract

This chapter provides a practical, science-driven guidance for establishing and scaling HCM as a core facility service. We outline design choices that raise rigor and power: longitudinal baselines aligned to light–dark cycles, pre-planned event tagging for husbandry and interventions, and synchronization of brief arena assays to circadian peaks revealed by continuous cage readouts. We show how to translate raw streams into robust endpoints through standard metadata, FAIR-aligned storage, automated quality control, and analysis templates for rhythms, rare events, and effect-size estimation.

For operations, we define an intake and governance framework covering protocol suitability, welfare approvals, authorship and data rights, and a transparent fee model that balances access and sustainability. A competency pathway for staff and users is presented, with tiered training, skills checks, and reusable notebooks that lower the barrier to high-quality analyses. Performance is tracked with a concise metric set: utilization, repeat users, turnaround, data-loss rate, and scholarly output.

P. Villiger (✉)
Zurich Integrative Rodent Physiology (ZIRP), Department of Physiology, University of Zurich UZH, Zurich, Switzerland
e-mail: philipp.villiger@uzh.ch

M. Tsoory
Behavioral and Physiological Phenotyping Unit, Department of Veterinary Resources, Weizmann Institute of Science, Rehovot, Israel

S. Mandillo
Institute of Biochemistry and Cell Biology, National Research Council, Rome, Italy

S. Gaburro
Tecniplast Spa, Buguggiate, Italy

S. Gaburro, S. Mandillo (eds.), *Home Cage Monitoring in Rodents: A Global Effort*,
https://doi.org/10.1007/978-3-032-19781-8_4

Use cases from cognition, neurodegeneration, and pharmacology illustrate how HCM exposes early sleep and activity shifts, optimizes assay timing, and detects treatment effects that short tests miss, improving reproducibility and supporting 3Rs. We close with a forward look at closed-loop paradigms, multimodal integrations, and voluntary test add-ons, positioning core directors to deliver scalable, high-value behavioral phenotyping across disciplines.

Keywords

Core facilities · Circadian timing · Longitudinal phenotyping · Reproducibility · 3Rs

1 Introduction

Home cage monitoring (HCM) is a transformative method in animal behavioral research, allowing continuous observation of laboratory animals in their most familiar environment (i.e., home/housing cage). This technology reduces human–animal interference, captures naturally occurring behaviors in a longitudinal (24/7) manner, allowing analysis of circadian behavior under otherwise undisturbed conditions. HCM can address some of the limitations of conventional short-term (behavioral) tests. The adoption of automated HCM systems has surged in the last two decades; a review noted a ~ 26-fold increase in HCM--related publications from the 1970s to 2020 (Kahnau et al. 2023b). This reflects growing recognition of HCM's benefits for data quality, animal welfare, and reproducibility. HCM provides rich longitudinal data on activity, physiology, and behavior, previously inaccessible with episodic out-of-cage assays. Integrating HCM into experimental workflows is both an opportunity and a challenge for laboratory directors: enhancing behavioral studies while developing necessary infrastructure and training.

This chapter offers guidance for directors and users implementing HCM in (core) facilities. We discuss the principles of HCM-based phenotyping, strategies for combining HCM with behavioral tests, internal user training, and operational guidance on infrastructure, workflows, governance, cost recovery, and performance metrics. Real-world examples illustrate best practices from core facility managers and researchers. By setting prospective users' expectations and building HCM competency, facility directors/managers can guide scientists to leverage HCM for more productive and reproducible research.

2 Basic Principles of HCM Phenotyping

Traditional rodent phenotyping commonly depends on short behavioral assays that are conducted outside the home cage, such as the open field test or the elevated plus maze (EPM), which typically last only a few minutes. These assays are carried out in specifically designed experimental setups that require direct handling of the animals and often elicit neophobia and anxiety, even when habituation protocols are applied to minimize unspecific stressors (provide example or reference). A comparable issue arises when animals are exposed to new housing environments. For certain experimental procedures or measurements, laboratory mice must be transferred to a cage that differs from their home cage. In a recent study by Villiger et al. (2025), our group observed that mice did not exhibit a reduction in stress levels in response to the new housing conditions, even after undergoing a short-term intermittent habituation protocol. Standard tests for locomotion and anxiety-like behavior (such as open field exploration and elevated plus-maze open--arm time) leverage rodents' natural aversion from novel and exposed spaces. Still, their readouts may only capture a narrow snapshot of behavior. Brief, invasive tests often fail to reflect the full complexity of an animal's behavioral repertoire and internal state. Moreover, the short-term aspect of such tests renders them more susceptible to unrelated factors like the laboratory environment and handling methods that may confound the outcomes. Studies have shown that even genetically identical mice from the same vendor do behave differently across laboratories in identical test systems due to subtle environmental differences, undermining reproducibility (Crabbe et al. 1999). Moreover, the reproducibility of outcomes from short-out-of-the-cage tests is notoriously low when examined across experimenters or institutions. For example, one multi-lab study found that the results of anxiety tests varied significantly between facilities despite using the same protocols, highlighting systemic issues with replicability in such "classical" assays (Grieco et al. 2021; Kafkafi et al. 2018).

HCM directly addresses these challenges by flipping the experimental paradigm: instead of bringing the animal to the test, HCM brings the test to the animal. In HCM systems, rodents are monitored continuously in their home environment, often over days or weeks, using sensors and automation to collect behavioral and/or physiological data. This approach minimizes human intervention and novelty to the bare minimum, thereby reducing unspecific stressor-related confounding effects. Even measurements that traditionally required animal restraint, such as core body temperature or heart rate, can be made via implanted or remote sensors in the home cage, avoiding acute stress hyperthermia caused by handling. By capturing behavior 24/7, including during the animals' nocturnal active phase, HCM allows to record intrinsically motivated behavior patterns, which cannot be provided by commonly used short daytime out-of-the-cage tests. Mice are far more active during the dark phase of their cycle than in light hours, a circadian effect that influences performance in open field tests. HCM experiments indicate deliberate exploration of a test compartment starting out from a home cage compartment almost exclusively during the dark phase (Hager 2014). Even if short episodic tests have revealed some behavioral traits, e.g., challenging experimental conditions will not capture the full behavioral repertoire, continuous monitoring also enables the detection of subtle or sporadic phenomena (e.g., micro-movements, sleep disturbances, early signs of disease, stereotyped behavior) that would likely go unnoticed in short-term observation. Ahloy-Dallaire et al. (2019) demonstrated that automated home cage tracking of mouse feeding and weight can detect health status changes sensitively. This allows continuous health assessment without removing the animals from their cage. Since HCM provides a far richer and unbiased behavioral dataset, it improves the signal-to-noise ratio and increases the chance of identifying actual relevant (more important than significant!) phenotypic differences (as opposed to chance findings based on high data variability in short-term datasets).

From a core facility perspective, the fundamental advantages of HCM may enhance rigor and reproducibility. Data gathered in the home cage tend to have higher within-group consistency because animals are less perturbed. However, inter-individual differences cannot be addressed (cage effect, Townsend et al. 2025) since many HCM systems work on the group level as experimental units. Automated HCM indicates reliable strain differences in behavior across multiple labs, illustrating improved reproducibility through automation (Krackow et al. 2010). Additionally, HCM expands the scope of measurable endpoints beyond what is feasible in brief tests, encompassing circadian activity patterns, social interactions (still an emerging field), and physiological readouts continuously over time (Horii et al. 2017; Kim et al. 2019). This comprehensive approach aligns with parts of the principles of the 3Rs (Replacement, Reduction, Refinement) by refining how behavioral data are collected and potentially reducing the number of animals needed (since each animal yields more data over time). However, capitalizing on these strengths requires careful experimental design and user training and competence. Researchers must understand the functional meaning (biological relevance) of longitudinal data and how these home cage metrics relate to classical human or experimental endpoints. The following sections delve into how HCM can be integrated with traditional assays and how core managers/directors may facilitate this.

3 Integrating HCM with Classical Behavioral Assays

While HCM offers a powerful alternative to conventional tests, it is often complementary rather than a wholesale replacement of conventional/classical screening/phenotyping approaches. Many researchers will wish to integrate HCM with established out-of-cage behavioral assays, such as novel object recognition or rotarod, to enrich their phenotypic assessments. Therefore, the following section discusses synchronizing HCM with classical tests, merging data streams for a holistic analysis and interpreting the findings comparatively. In a later section, possibilities of cage add-ons (to optimally exploit the animals' motivational states based on deliberate choice) will be explored.

Experimental Synchronization Planning is essential when incorporating continuous HCM and discrete behavioral tests in the same study. One key consideration is timing. Because rodents have circadian variations in behavior and physiology, the schedule of out--of-cage tests should be chosen with the animals' activity cycle in mind. To capture their peak performance, tests should be carried out in their active phase (dark phase). On the other hand, some tests intentionally occur in the light (when mice are naturally less active) to provoke anxiety-like behavior, as in the case of light–dark (or better dark–light) box tests, elevated plus maze or open field exploration. To leverage HCM effectively, researchers can use it to establish each animal's baseline activity pattern and then schedule the classical test at a meaningful time relative to that baseline. Importantly, the use of HCM systems does not replace commonly used phenotyping baselines; rather, it should be viewed as a complementary approach within an already established comprehensive phenotyping battery. For example, a behavioral core facility worked with a neuroscience research group to investigate a novel anxiolytic drug. The researchers used HCM to monitor locomotor activity and sleep disruptions of mice for 1 week, establishing baseline behavior for each animal before drug administration. HCM data during drug administration showed that the drug resulted in slightly higher activity during the early dark phase compared to baseline/controls. The scientists then conducted an elevated plus maze test at the onset of the dark phase, when differences were expected to be maximal, rather than during the day. This synchronized timing enabled a data-based interpretation of the drug's effects. Aligning test timing according to home cage activity insights may improve the detection of experimental effects and provide potential explanations for their lack because of an incorrectly selected time window of drug action and when to perform the tests. In addition, the commonly used serial testing may increase inter-individual variation due to differences in the exact time of testing within the circadian pattern. Individually housed C57BL/6 J mice particularly show a high activity level in the beginning and at the end of the dark phase. Another synchronization strategy is to use HCM as a pre-screen or post-test observation period. For instance, animals might be continuously tracked in the home cage before and after a specific (intermittent) behavioral challenge. This design allows researchers to see how a brief test or challenge (e.g., a stressor such as a foot shock or social defeat) impacts subsequent home cage behavior (recovery time, sleep patterns, etc.), or conversely, whether pre-test home cage metrics can predict performance in the test. In HCM, shock exposure during contextual avoidance training results in profound post-shock activity suppression in the dark phase (Hager 2014).

Moreover, automated HCM systems can also deliver stimuli or tasks parallel to classical assays into their home cage. Some advanced setups include gated connections between the home cage and a test apparatus, allowing animals to voluntarily enter a testing arena from their home enclosure. This "brings the test to the animal" approach preserves the home cage as a safe zone and may yield more ethologically relevant responses, particularly because it is easier to start a new test in a novel environment that has the full attention of the animals. With such a setup, human interaction can be kept to a minimum. Core facilities that can implement such hybrid setups (for example, an automated gate allowing a mouse to move from its home cage into an adjacent open field arena) can offer scientists a novel way to conduct behavioral tests (Hager 2014).

Comparative Interpretation Integrating HCM with traditional assays requires careful interpretation, as the two approaches might not always yield congruent results, the question arises as to what we consider as the gold standard testing method. Core scientists should guide users in understanding why an animal's standard behavior (out-of-the-cage) test may differ from its behavior determined by HCM. For example, a mouse may exhibit high anxiety in an open field test (rearing along the walls, reduced center exploration) but appear quite active and exploratory in the familiarity of its home cage during nocturnal periods. Rather than viewing these outcomes as contradictions, researchers are encouraged to interpret them as complementary facets of the phenotype, e.g., the fear of novelty, neophobia, is not induced by pure basal increased locomotion. The discrepancy may illustrate context-dependent behavior: the classical test measures the animal's acute reaction to novelty-induced arousal due to many additional unspecific stressors, such as cage transfer and handling, whereas HCM measures its behavior by avoiding these unspecific stressors. Notably, continuous home cage data can help distinguish between a consistent low-activity phenotype and a context-specific suppression of activity, e.g., reduced exploration of a novel area that may be related to increased anxiety. Suppose experimental treatment (or genetic modification) yields no change in open-field exploration, but HCM detects increased voluntary running-wheel activity at night. In this case, one should infer that the treatment (or genetic modification) effect emerges only in a familiar environment. Conversely, HCM may reveal subtle but longer-lasting small differences with larger statistical power that traditional tests cannot detect. Core unit managers/directors should educate users to consider factors like habituation, unspecific stressors, and intrinsic motivational differences when comparing HCM data that relies on voluntary behaviors and data that reflects the animal responses to the assay's setup. It can be helpful to perform habituation trials or repeated testing, if feasible, to gauge how quickly animals adapt to novel tests, and to use HCM to evaluate if their home cage behavior changes after the test (indicating residual stress or learning). The integration of these approaches ultimately strengthens the overall conclusions: convergent findings build confidence in a result's robustness and replicability, while divergent findings spur deeper investigation into underlying mechanisms and/or contributing factors depending on different experimental variables. Data Integration Strategies A practical challenge in combined studies is integrating the disparate data streams—continuous time-series data from HCM and point-in-time measurements from behavioral tests. Core facilities should establish data management and analysis pipelines that allow these datasets to be merged or compared on common timelines. One approach is to mark events from classical tests on the continuous time-series: for example, timestamp the exact period when an animal was removed for testing and when it was returned to the home cage. Moreover, most HCM systems include built-in surveillance, enabling continuous monitoring of the cage environment and facilitating the collection of information on potential confounders, such as planned or unexpected events (e.g., cage changes, routine procedures, injections, apparatus inspections, fluctuations in light or temperature, construction noise, and more). Although generally undesired, these events cannot be avoided. This enables retrospective analyses of home cage activity immediately before and after the test or the interruption. Researchers can then quantify the stressor-induced deviation in home cage activity combined with other indicators of confounding events occurring during the performance of any test. Another approach is to derive summary metrics from HCM data analogous to experimental endpoints in classical tests (without temporal constraints such as short test duration). For instance, "time spent in center vs periphery" is an open field measure of anxiety; similarly, one could use video-based home cage tracking to calculate how often a mouse ventures into an open area of an enriched home cage or how it distributes time across zones. Although the home cage lacks the aversive properties (novelty, high light intensity) of an open field test arena, creative analyses can yield comparable metrics for anxiety or exploration measured in the home environment, e.g., by analyzing the dynamic changes in the cage exploration after introducing the animal to the new home cage or latencies to enter and explore an attached test compartment. Core data scientists might also assist users with multivariate analyses incorporating both data types. Techniques like principal component analysis or machine learning models can combine features from HCM (e.g., circadian activity amplitude, bout duration of activity, feeding frequency and timing, social interaction counts) with classical outcomes (e.g., maze latency, distance traveled) to identify underlying factors or predict phenotypic classifications or even inter-individual variation. For example, a machine learning model could be trained to predict whether a mouse is in a high-anxiety or control group based on a combination of its home cage metrics and open field test results, potentially improving sensitivity over either measure alone. By guiding such data integration, core facilities help researchers maximize the insight gained from each experiment and thereby may support the reduction of mice needed for the experiment, e.g., when longitudinal data can identify larger effect sizes.

Case example (scientist's perspective): A neuroscientist is studying a transgenic mouse model of Alzheimer's disease. With assistance from the behavior core, she designs a study where each mouse undergoes periodic, repetitive cognitive out-of-the-cage testing while being continuously monitored in the home cage for general activity and sleep. HCM data reveal subtle sleep disruptions and nighttime hyperactivity emerging in the transgenic mice months before any cognitive deficit is detected in the object recognition test (Martin et al. 2024). When cognitive impairments finally appear, the neuroscientist integrates the two datasets and discovers that the extent of early sleep fragmentation (from HCM) precedes the emerging memory deficits (from cognitive testing). This combined approach strengthens her findings by linking an early phenotype to a later outcome, something neither method alone would have uncovered.

In summary, integrating HCM with classical behavioral assays can provide a more comprehensive picture of an animal's phenotype than either approach alone. The core facility should serve as an interface/integrator between these methodologies, helping to synchronize experimental timing, teaching users how to interpret context-dependent behavior, and providing guidance with tools to merge and analyze complex datasets. When executed thoughtfully, this integration enables scientists to draw nuanced conclusions about behavior, yielding both robust results in controlled tests and longitudinal circadian (home cage) activity data of high scientific value.

4 Strategic Integration Pathways for Core Facilities

Successfully adopting HCM in an animal facility requires more than just buying new equipment—it demands a strategic plan that aligns technology implementation with the needs of diverse stakeholders. Core directors must navigate questions of which systems to adopt, how to incorporate HCM into existing workflows, and how to build user support and creativity for new possibilities. This section outlines strategic pathways for integrating HCM into core phenotyping workflows, focusing on stakeholder engagement, workflow compatibility, data interoperability, and resource sharing.

Stakeholder Alignment and Needs Assessment Early in the integration process, core directors should engage with the stakeholders of the core facility—principal investigators (PIs), research staff, veterinarians, and institutional leadership—to assess the demand and requirements for home cage monitoring. Understanding the scientific use cases researchers are most interested in, it will guide system selection and protocol development tailored to the needs of the core facility and its users. For example, some groups may be interested in HCM for high-throughput screening of locomotor activity or circadian rhythms. In contrast, others might focus on specific behaviors like social interactions, learning tests, or physiological functions. A collaborative requirement-gathering exercise ensures that the chosen HCM platform and its configuration meet the broadest possible range of needs. Animal welfare bodies are frequently interested in improved surgical recovery and monitoring of new mouse lines with potential discomfort. In practice, this might involve surveys or workshops where potential users discuss what features (e.g., video tracking, RFID individual identification, operant task capability) are most important. An example framework is the "PhenoKey" concept, an informal strategy emphasizing cross-departmental input in core design: by bringing together neuroscientists, pharmacologists, ethologists, and data analysts, the core director can create a roadmap that addresses everyday research needs and identifies any technical gaps. This proactive engagement builds a sense of community ownership of the new HCM system and helps manage user expectations (e.g., clarifying what HCM can and cannot measure reliably). Moreover, involving institutional animal care committees or welfare officers at this stage ensures that any HCM protocols align with animal welfare standards and regulatory guidelines. Initiatives at national and international levels are also paving strategic pathways that cores can follow. For instance, the COST Action "TEATIME" consortium in Europe has explicitly focused on improving biomedical research by automated HCM, bringing together experts across academia and industry. Through TEATIME, best-practice guidelines and standardized definitions of what constitute an HCM system have been developed (e.g., an online catalog of HCM technologies and an ontology of home cage (COST-Action, TEATIME 2025). Core directors can leverage such resources to make informed decisions to shape their strategy, adopting internationally recognized standards. Another example is the UK's NC3Rs-sponsored CRACK IT Challenges, which have funded multidisciplinary projects to develop or validate new automated monitoring technologies. By aligning with these broader efforts, a core facility gains credibility and plugs into a network of expertise for troubleshooting and future upgrades.

Workflow Compatibility and Implementation Integrating HCM should be done to complement and improve existing core services, rather than disrupt them. A thorough workflow compatibility analysis helps identify which traditional assays can be augmented or replaced by HCM. A more detailed breakdown of the system can be found in Chapters "Technologies for Home Cage Monitoring in Preclinical Research" and "Study Design and Data Analysis in Home Cage Monitoring Experiments". For example, if the core routinely offers conventional telemetry for recording vital signs, integrating telemetry into an HCM system can streamline those studies. A valuable example is indirect calorimetry systems such as Sable Systems Promethion Core System, which, combined with radiotelemetry, enables quantification of metabolic rate and, depending on the transmitters used, measurement of additional parameters such as blood glucose levels, heart and respiratory rate, or temperature. If the core conducts many nighttime behavior tests (e.g. running wheel monitoring or metabolic assays), transitioning those into automated HCM systems might increase throughput and consistency. Another example is RFID-based group housed solutions, exemplifies the type of platform that can integrate into phenotyping workflows. One example is the IntelliCage, which automatically allows group-housed mice to be assessed for various behaviors (activity, drinking, learning tasks) within their home cage via RFID-tagged individuals and computer-controlled operant corners. It was developed to measure complex behaviors such as spatial learning and reversal learning in a fully automated fashion. For instance, Urbach et al. (2014) demonstrated automated phenotyping in a Huntington's disease mouse model using the IntelliCage by capturing cognitive and motor readouts continuously without human intervention. Such longitudinal data sets can help to determine early markers of diseases etiology and progression helping to identify optimal intervention timepoints. By examining such cases, core directors can judge how an HCM system can be used to perform assays that are originally performed manually out-of-the-cage. It may emerge that some tests (like simple locomotor activity or preference tests) can be transferred entirely into HCM setups, whereas others (like fine motor coordination on a rotarod or specific motor coordination test [e.g., catwalk]) may still require separate equipment and experimenter support. In the latter case, the core might still use HCM to monitor animals before/after the rotarod to enrich the data, as discussed earlier. In this case, HCM systems such as the DVC system are highly valuable because they function as typical IVC cage racks while also providing continuous monitoring of the housed mice. Unlike many other HCM systems, this system can be seamlessly integrated into daily laboratory and husbandry workflows due to its strong similarities to the widely used IVC cage racks. Therefore, it can be seen as an HCM system, which truly complements a classical phenotyping battery since it offers the same standard cage environment widely used in research. In addition, this approach allows to observe longitudinally to determine age-related alterations, such as changes in activity in combination with potential disease etiology and progression. The goal is to weave HCM into the fabric of the core workflow so that it adds value seamlessly. Piloting the new workflow with a small project or an internal test run is an advisable strategy. This allows the involved team to optimize settings, data handling, and animal acclimation procedures and prepare for data analysis before advertising the service widely to users. During implementation, flexibility is key: the core might start with offering a limited set of HCM-based assays and gradually expand as staff and users become more comfortable.

Data Interoperability and Standards A significant aspect of strategic integration is ensuring that the data generated by HCM systems can interface with the core's data pipelines and the researchers' analysis tools. Different HCM technologies produce diverse data types: RFID-based systems log timestamps and IDs for each interaction, video-tracking systems output position coordinates and images. At the same time, pressure or capacitance sensors generate continuous analog activity signals. Without a plan for harmonizing these formats, the core (and the end-users) may struggle with data overload or incompatibility. Adopting data standards and interoperability practices is therefore a priority. Wherever possible, core directors should utilize or develop software that can import and convert HCM data into standard formats (CSV, HDF5, EDF, etc.) and integrate it with existing databases. The principles of FAIR data management—making data Findable, Accessible, Interoperable, and Reusable—are highly relevant in this context. For example, a core might require that all HCM study data be accompanied by metadata in a standard schema (describing animal IDs, timestamps, variables recorded, etc.), which enables future re-analysis or multi-study comparisons. Collaborative groups like the TEATIME consortium work on bioinformatics tools for large-scale HCM data analysis, which core facilities can adopt or contribute to. In practice, a core director may set up a centralized data storage server for HCM outputs and provide users with analysis notebooks or pipelines (potentially using cloud-based platforms for heavier computational tasks). Standardizing on a limited number of HCM platforms in the facility also helps reduce complexity. If all data comes from one or two systems with known data structures, it is easier to develop robust analysis workflows and cross-compare results. Interoperability extends beyond data formats and includes experimental protocols as well: cores should promote standardized protocols for standard HCM assays. If both labs want to use HCM to test circadian activity under a drug treatment, the core can recommend a standard experimental design and data reporting format. This makes life easier for scientists and builds a repository of comparable datasets over time, enhancing the core's scientific impact and comparability with available data to better discriminate normal variation from real pathological changes, e.g., as observed in a specific mouse line. Resource Pooling and Shared Infrastructure HCM systems, especially high-end commercial ones, can be expensive and have considerable long-lasting costs from IT (e.g., server capacity) to online software packages from vendors (e.g., analysis software). A strategic approach for a core is to use a shared equipment model to maximize utilization and cost-effectiveness. This model entails centralizing HCM equipment within the core and making it available to all investigators on a schedule, rather than individual labs purchasing their own systems that might sit idle. Some institutions have pioneered this approach; for instance, a cardiovascular research core at Stanford incorporated an HCM-based telemetry system as a shared resource, supporting multiple studies on cardiac function in rodents (Bernstein 2003). By pooling resources, the core facility ensures that the costly equipment serves many projects, improving the return on investment. It also allows the core staff to maintain and troubleshoot the system, rather than each lab struggling independently. When planning a shared HCM resource, core directors should perform a cost–benefit analysis that includes maintenance costs, throughput (how many cages can be run and how often), and the user pricing model. Often, supplementary funding (via equipment grants or institutional support) is needed to acquire the system, with the expectation that user fees will cover operating costs over time. Transparent communication of the cost-recovery plan to users will help manage expectations—researchers should understand, for example, whether they will be charged per cage per monitoring day or experiment, and what technical support is included. Resource sharing also opens collaboration opportunities: the core might encourage two labs interested in similar HCM applications to run a joint experiment, thereby sharing data and costs. Such cooperative use is beneficial when demand is still growing in early adoption phases. Furthermore, the core can organize user groups or monthly meetings for HCM users to share tips and experiences, effectively pooling knowledge in addition to equipment. This community-building fosters a culture where HCM is seen not as a black-box service but as a collaborative scientific endeavor, increasing its acceptance and successful integration. In summary, strategic integration of HCM into a core facility revolves around careful planning and stakeholder collaboration. By aligning HCM capabilities with user needs—ensuring compatibility and standardization in workflows and high data quality (replicability)—and leveraging shared resource models, core directors can embed HCM as a sustainable and valued component of their services. This strategic groundwork sets the stage for the practical operational steps—infrastructure setup, training, and governance—discussed in subsequent sections.

5 Infrastructure and Data Ecosystem Development

Implementing HCM in core facilities requires building a robust infrastructure and data ecosystem to support continuous, high-volume data collection. This involves selecting appropriate hardware configurations for housing and monitoring animals, establishing computational architecture for data handling, and employing software tools to analyze and share results. In this section, we outline key considerations for infrastructure development, drawing on current technologies and case studies of successful HCM implementations.

Modular Hardware Configurations Modern HCM systems have various hardware configurations, each suited to different experimental needs. Broadly, we can classify these as single-housing modules, social housing arrays, and hybrid environments. In single-housing modules, one animal per cage is monitored in isolation. This setup is proper when individual data without social interference is needed—for example, precise tracking of an individual's metabolism (Promethion Core), vital parameters (DSI radiotelemetry implants), food intake (FED3) and water intake, or phenotyping of traits where social interactions could be confounding (like measuring fine-grained locomotor patterns or sleep in a single mouse). Single housing can also be advantageous in pharmacological studies to avoid drugged animals affecting others. However, because many research questions and welfare guidelines favor group-housing, HCM vendors have designed systems that accommodate small groups of animals together. Social housing arrays allow group-housed rodents (often 4–5 per cage for mice, or 2–3 for rats, depending on the sizes of animals and cage) to be continuously monitored while living together, thereby preserving natural social behavior. These monitoring systems must solve the challenge of attributing observed behaviors to the correct individual in a group. In some systems, this issue is managed by defining the cage (group) rather than the individual mouse as the experimental unit. Tecniplast's DVC system, for example, can still detect differences between groups if only one mouse is affected by disease or shows welfare impairment in a group of 3–4 mice, but it cannot identify the specific individual. Other companies, such as Olden Labs, use cameras instead of electromagnetic fields and, with the help of color codes, can differentiate individual animals within a group. Moreover, individual baselines can be established. Another solution is to include RFID transponders implanted in each animal, antennae or detectors at interaction sites (feeding stations, wheels, etc.). RFID-based HCM systems, such as the Home Cage Analyzer, mouse matrix, and IntelliCage, can identify specific animals as they nose-poke a sensor or visit a corner, linking each data point to an individual ID. This technology allows group housing with the resolution of individual animal performance. Social housing is critical for studies of social hierarchy, dominance, and collective behaviors, and simply increases throughput by monitoring several animals at once. Some systems even enable competitive or collaborative tasks within the home cage (e.g., two mice competing in an operant task for a reward) to study social aspects of cognition. Hybrid environments combine features of home cage comfort with the scale of an arena or specialized testing environment. One example is an enlarged home cage enclosure that provides more complex space (sometimes called an "arena cage", Mieske et al. 2021). These hybrids allow animals to move and explore much more than a standard cage still as controlled environment. Another form of hybridization is connecting home cages to external devices via tunnels or gates (as mentioned earlier, Kahnau et al. 2023a). For example, an automated gate can allow a mouse to leave its home compartment to enter a testing chamber (like a puzzle box or maze) deliberately, effectively making the animal a voluntary participant in assays. In terms of hardware, implementing these hybrid setups may require modifying rack systems or purchasing specialized enclosures that fit into standard racks while providing extra capabilities (running wheels, maze compartments, etc.). Core directors should consider whether their facility space can accommodate the footprint of larger or custom cages and whether their vivarium husbandry practices (bedding changes, sanitation schedules) can adapt to more complex cage structures and sensitive sensors such as cameras, microphones, and others.

Computational Architecture and Edge Computing The data infrastructure is paramount alongside the physical hardware. HCM systems continuously generate large volumes of data—video recordings, sensor logs, and more—which can demand considerable computational resources if not managed well. A practical approach is to use edge computing, where initial data processing occurs on devices at the "edge" of the network (i.e., near the data source) rather than sending everything to a central server as raw data. Many contemporary HCM platforms include on-board processors or local computers that handle tasks like tracking an animal's position from video in real-time, or summing beam break counts in 1-min bins, thereby reducing the raw data stream to manageable features. For example, Iannello (2019) describe a HCM cage rack using electrical capacitance sensors that detect mouse movements through cage flooring; this system's electronics compute activity indices on the fly, dramatically cutting down the data that needs to be stored centrally. By implementing edge processing, cores can avoid network bottlenecks and only record salient processed data (with raw data optionally saved in a buffer if needed for later re-analysis). Nonetheless, for specific applications like behavior sequencing or novel behavior detection, saving raw video or high-resolution data may be necessary (e.g. for validation or analysis refinements), in which case a robust storage and transfer setup is required (e.g., a dedicated high-speed network-attached storage for the core). The core's computational architecture should include adequate data storage, backup, and processing power. Continuous monitoring can produce terabytes of data in weeks, especially with high-resolution video or ultrasound recordings. Establishing an automated pipeline where data from HCM experiments are regularly offloaded from the acquisition PCs onto a central server is advisable. Depending on the acquired data volume, this could be scheduled daily or weekly to avoid data loss and free up acquisition system space. Data backup strategies (to protect against disk failures) are essential, given the irreplaceable nature of experimental data; RAIDs or cloud-based backup solutions can be employed. On the processing side, having a local analysis workstation or a server with substantial CPU/GPU resources will aid in running computationally intensive tasks like video analysis or machine learning on behavior data. Suppose the institute has a high-performance computing cluster. In that case, integrating core data with that resource can accelerate analysis (for example, training a DeepLabCut; Mathis et al. 2018) neural network for pose estimation might be done on a GPU cluster rather than on the core director's laptop). A trend in recent years is also to utilize cloud-based collaboration platforms for data sharing and analysis such as CalR

(Mina et al. 2018). Core facilities might set up a secure cloud repository where users can log in to view their HCM data, perform analysis via hosted Jupyter notebooks, and even integrate their data with external datasets. This approach can be convenient for multi-center collaborations or PIs who want to access data remotely. The computational architecture, whether local or cloud, should also be designed with data security and privacy in mind, especially if any video data could show identifying features of animal caretakers or contain sensitive experimental details.

Software and Data Analysis Tools The full potential of HCM is realized only when the data is translated into biologically meaningful results. Thus, part of the infrastructure investment must include software tools and analysis pipelines. Many HCM systems come with proprietary software. For example, the Promethion Core system includes the Macro Interpreter and CalR-compatible outputs, enabling the use of an open-source analysis pipeline that allows the same type of data analysis as with a TSE system. Another example is the DVC system, which can be used with DVC Analytics, a powerful tool that translates artificial readouts from electrodes into meaningful activity or even behavioral patterns. Similarly, DSI implants generate data that can be analyzed with Data Insights, and IntelliCage provides IntelliCage Plus software for experiment configuration and basic analysis of nose-poke data. Regardless of the manufacturer or software, core staff should be well trained and continuously updated in these packages to effectively support users. However, often the built-in software has limitations in analysis sophistication and/or flexibility. Thus, complementary customized tools are frequently needed. Open-source software has flourished in this domain. For instance, DeepLabCut is a popular open-source tool that uses deep learning to track user-defined body points in videos, enabling detailed behavior and posture analysis from home cage video data. A core can set up DLC and even provide training data or pre-trained networks for common lab mouse behaviors, simplifying life for scientists who want to classify behaviors from video. DLC has been successfully used to reduce human scoring variability in behavioral analysis and can reach human-level accuracy in posture tracking with minimal effort (Mathis et al. 2018). Other tools include motion-detection and circadian analysis programs, machine learning pipelines for unsupervised behavior classification (such as Motion Sequencing or MoSeq for identifying movement motifs), and data visualization dashboards. The core's data scientist or informatician might create standardized scripts (in R, Python, or MATLAB) to generate reports for each experiment, for example, automatically plotting each animal's activity over time, average daily rhythms, correlation between metrics, etc. By providing these as templates, users can quickly gain insights without needing advanced coding skills. A commitment to interoperability also means ensuring that outputs from one system can feed into others; if a user exports timestamps of certain events from the HCM software, the core could have a script ready to integrate that with corresponding video files or external sensor data (like synchronized EEG or metabolic data, if any). This cohesive data ecosystem should be documented clearly so that users know what to expect: e.g., "At experiment end, you will receive a dataset with X, Y, Z metrics and a set of graphs; raw data is stored at location Q and is accessible for further analysis for up to N months". The inclusion of case studies and technical exemplars can be helpful; for instance, the SCORHE system (System for Continuous Observation of Rodents in Home cage Environment) is a case study highlighting how a simple hardware setup (a dual-camera unit mounted on a standard cage rack) combined with intelligent software can yield valuable activity and behavior data. Salem et al. (2015) described SCORHE as a low-cost, scalable solution that required minimal cage modification and produced automated readouts of mouse activity patterns. Learning from such examples, core facilities can adapt off-the-shelf tools or develop custom ones to fit their needs. In conclusion, establishing an HCM infrastructure in a core facility is a multidimensional task covering physical equipment, IT resources, and analytical software. By choosing flexible modular hardware, ensuring strong data handling capabilities (edge processing, storage, backup), and equipping the core with state-of-the-art analysis tools, a core director creates the foundation for successful HCM-based research. The next step is ensuring that people—both staff and users—are competent to use this infrastructure effectively, which we address in the following sections on training and operational processes.

6 Operational Guidance for HCM Core Management

Deploying HCM as a core service involves scientific and technical aspects as well as operational management to ensure the platform's success and sustainability. This section guides several key operational areas: project intake and workflow management, governance and ethics oversight, cost recovery and funding, and performance metrics for continuous improvement. A core director can run the HCM platform efficiently while meeting users' needs and institutional requirements by setting up clear processes in these areas.

Project Intake and Workflow Management Introducing HCM into a core's portfolio will likely generate interest from core users and new users with no prior experience in automated behavioral monitoring. It is crucial to have a structured project intake process that handles initial inquiries through to study completion. Typically, this begins with a consultation phase where the core team assesses the project's feasibility, design needs, and resource requirements. The core can then advise on experimental design, suggesting modifications if necessary (for example, recommending appropriate habituation time in the HCM system or including control groups monitored in parallel). Once a project is approved, an experimental plan (study plan or work protocol) is formalized, often as a service agreement or protocol document, and as required legal animal research documentation. This should outline the responsibilities of the core (equipment setup, data collection, preliminary analysis) and of the user (animal preparation, experimental treatments, final data interpretation), along with a timeline. Clear communication at this stage sets the tone for the project; users should know what data they will receive and when, while core staff should know the critical experimental events to coordinate, i.e., events that affect the

HMC, such as experimental manipulations, welfare assessments, and "out-of-the-cage" assays. During the execution of the project, standard operating procedures (SOPs) are vital. For instance, the core might have an SOP for habituating animals to the HCM system. Another SOP might cover how often to check on the animals and system (since HCM usually runs unattended overnight, clear instructions for daily animal welfare checks and system status checks must be in place). Maintaining a project log or notebook for each HCM system/study is advisable, noting any events such as system errors, animal removals, or anomalies (e.g., "Day 3: animal #5 found chew damage to sensor, replaced sensor pad"). Next to a project log, some HCM systems offer an environmental monitoring unit, which automatically tracks the environment for sound, light, and other emissions. This and personal documentation are essential for troubleshooting and transparency if results need to be interpreted in light of a technical issue.

Governance and Ethical Compliance Operating an HCM core intersects with institutional governance, including animal welfare regulations, data governance, and compliance with cost accounting rules (for billing). First and foremost, any use of HCM in live animals must be covered by appropriate ethical approvals (Institutional Animal Welfare Body or Animal Care and Use Committee, IACUC, in the United States or equivalent). Fortunately, HCM aligns well with the refinement tenet of the 3Rs, as it is generally less stressful than traditional testing, which committees often view favorably. Nevertheless, considerations such as maximal monitoring duration, ensuring provision of food/water if automated dispensers are used, and contingency plans for equipment failure affecting animal welfare need to be spelled out. Furthermore, some systems might require single housing, and depending on the authorities, this could limit the system. Additionally, core staff must be trained in animal care within the HCM context, for example, recognizing signs of distress in animals that might not be disturbed daily due to automated monitoring, or knowing when it is necessary to remove an animal from an experiment early for humane or experimental reasons. Data governance is another facet of oversight. The core should define who owns the data generated by the HCM experiments and how data sharing is handled. Typically, the researcher owns their experimental data, but if the core stores it centrally, policies must ensure confidentiality and integrity of that data. Multi-user systems might inadvertently allow one user to glimpse another's ongoing experiment data if not properly access-controlled. Thus, IT measures should include data protection as needed. If video recording is part of the monitoring and if any facility staff appear in those videos (even peripherally during cage maintenance), privacy issues might arise—cores may decide to position cameras or schedule personnel duties to avoid recording humans, or to redact/blur any such instances if videos are to be shared. Regarding intellectual contribution, if core staff significantly contribute to experimental design or analysis, authorship or acknowledgments in publications should follow institutional core guidelines to ensure proper credit, a governance aspect that core directors should communicate to users upfront.

Financial compliance and governance are crucial for cost recovery, but broadly, the core must operate in accordance with institutional policies for service centers. This often includes undergoing periodic rate reviews or audits to ensure that billing rates align with actual costs and do not generate undue profit (for federally funded institutions, for example, this is mandated). In summary, governance in an HCM core context means staying compliant with animal ethics, protecting data and privacy, and following administrative policies, all foundational to running a trustworthy and accountable core service.

Cost Recovery and Sustainability With their advanced hardware and software, HCM systems represent a significant investment for a core facility. To sustain operations, core directors typically implement a cost recovery model whereby users are charged fees for the services. Designing a fair and practical pricing model requires understanding the direct costs (equipment depreciation, maintenance contracts, consumables like RFID tags or bedding, staff time for setup and analysis) and indirect costs (facility space, utilities, administrative support). One approach is a per-cage-per-day charge, which directly ties to the capacity usage of the system. Alternatively, some cores may offer experiment-based package pricing. Package pricing can be simpler for users to budget. However, the core must pay attention to not underestimating required efforts and to be cost-neutral. Another model is tiered pricing depending on the level of service—for example, a lower rate if the user handles more of the work versus a higher rate if full service with core personnel doing analysis is provided. In the initial stages, full cost recovery might not be immediately feasible if user adoption is slow. However, surveys have shown that many academic cores operate at 80–90% cost recovery, with some exceptional cores achieving near 100% through high volume and efficiency (Turpen et al. 2016). The core director should strive for a sustainable balance: underpricing might attract users but could lead to budget shortfalls, whereas overpricing could deter usage and result in idle equipment (which is equally unsustainable). Regular review of finances is necessary—tracking metrics like utilization rate, number of distinct user groups served, and revenue vs expenses. If utilization is low, targeted outreach or workshops might be needed to drum up interest (often, investigators are unaware of what HCM can do until they see examples). On the expense side, careful maintenance is important; unexpected downtime due to equipment failure can be costly in terms of lost revenue and credibility. Therefore, service contracts with vendors or stocking of critical spare parts are usually justified for minimizing downtime of the HCM systems.

To bolster sustainability, core directors can explore supplementary funding avenues. For example, adding an HCM component might make the core eligible for equipment grants or instrumentation supplements from funding agencies. Collaboration with users on grant proposals (where they budget for core service costs or even write the core into the methods) ensures future income if those grants succeed. A fully sustainable HCM core is one where the inflow of projects and funding covers the operational costs and allows for maintenance and eventual upgrades; achieving this may take a few years of growth and adjustment. However, this is a long-term goal and therefore strongly depends on the size of the core, the scientific directions of the core, and the researcher turnover at the core.

Performance Metrics and Continuous Improvement To guide the success of a core facility, it is essential to define and track performance metrics and to use those metrics for continuous improvement. A 2016 analysis by Turpen et al. outlined categories for core facility performance evaluation, including financial health, user satisfaction, efficiency, and scientific impact. Applying these to an HCM core, key metrics might include: utilization rate, number of users and repeat users, turnaround time, publications, external funding, data quality/error rates, user satisfaction and training outcomes. By regularly reviewing these metrics, the core team can identify areas for improvement. Importantly, a culture of continuous improvement also means staying current with technological advances and user needs. The core director should maintain awareness of new HCM technologies (through literature, conferences, vendor demos). For instance, if a novel sensor could expand the core's capabilities (like HCM with EEG integration), it might be worth planning for. Regularly soliciting user input on desired features can guide future development; maybe users express interest in monitoring a specific behavior (e.g., ultrasonic vocalizations) that the core does not yet support, this feedback could direct investment in new modules or collaborations with developers. In essence, running an HCM core is an evolving process. Setting clear operational guidelines and metrics ensures that day-to-day activities align with larger scientific excellence and service quality goals. By paying attention to project management, governance, finances, and performance indicators, a core director can adapt and refine the core's operations, thereby maintaining a high level of service for researchers and sustaining the core's value to the institution.

7 Training and User Adoption Strategies

The successful integration of HCM into a research environment depends as much on people as technology. Both core staff and scientific users must develop new skills and understanding to make the most out of HCM systems. This section focuses on building internal training frameworks, setting user expectations, and cultivating a culture that embraces automated monitoring. We will cover competency-based training programs, data literacy initiatives (especially around handling the large datasets and novel analysis methods HCM produces), and strategies to encourage adoption through collaboration and communication.

Competency-Based Training for Core Staff and Users Introducing HCM often means that even experienced animal technicians or behavioral scientists must learn new methods. Competency-based training ensures individuals attain specific skills and knowledge milestones before operating the system independently. For core staff (technicians, technologists, or junior scientists in the facility), training might involve vendor-provided HCM hardware/software courses, followed by hands-on practice with dummy experiments. To conduct dummy experiments an animal experiment license is needed, which might be hard to get and training animals may be applied for in the ordinary experimental license (depending on the country and the current legislation). Further, core staff should be proficient in system setup, troubleshooting common issues, and basic data retrieval/analysis. Cross-training among staff is valuable so that HCM expertise is not siloed—multiple people should know how to maintain and run the system to cover absences and provide depth of support (redundancy). For scientific users, training is equally important. Many may be unfamiliar with continuous monitoring, or how to design experiments without the traditional "control vs test in a 5-min trial" mindset. The core should offer a tiered training program: introductory seminars for broad awareness, followed by practical workshops for those who intend to use the system, and one-on-one mentoring for initial projects. A notable initiative is the European TEATIME Training Schools, which provided instruction on home cage technologies including experimental design, operant task setup, and data analysis for complex behaviors (details can be found in the chapter on Education and Training). Inspired by such models, a core facility could host annual or semi-annual training courses covering HCM theory and practice. For example, a two-day workshop might include modules on: Day 1—theory (capabilities of HCM, examples of studies, limitations, and considerations like circadian factors); Day 2—hands-on (setting up a cage, configuring the software for a simple task, and a demo of analyzing the output). Participants could receive a certificate or simply be noted as "trained users" of the core. Impressing upon users the importance of proper training is part of managing expectations—they need to know that HCM is not a push-button magic box or "ready to use turnkey system". Experimental rigor and understanding of the system are still required for success.

Data Literacy and Analysis Skills HCM flips the data paradigm from sparse to rich, meaning scientists must be prepared to handle and interpret large datasets. Many users may initially not have the computational skills to fully analyze, for example, minute-by-minute activity data over several weeks for dozens of animals. A core facility should thus consider data literacy as part of its educational mission. This can range from basic training in how to use analysis software provided by the system manufacturer, to more advanced workshops on topics like statistical analysis of time-series data, machine learning for behavior classification, or integrating HCM data with other data types. In recent years, there has been a push to improve data skills in biology in general, often through workshops or online courses in coding and analysis. The core can partner with bioinformatics or biostatistics colleagues to offer tailored sessions (for example, a short course on "Analyzing Behavioral Time Series in R/Python"). Alternatively, if resources allow, the core might develop user-friendly analysis templates. Imagine providing a Jupyter Notebook that a user can run by simply pointing it to their dataset, and it will generate common analyses and visualizations—this empowers those who are not coding experts to still glean insights from HCM data. One particular area where data literacy is crucial is the application of machine learning for behavior analysis. Video-based HCM yields particularly complex data (often requiring behavior to be classified from footage). Tools like DeepLabCut have made it feasible for non-experts to apply deep learning to track animal movements. However, using these tools still demands understanding concepts like training a network, overfitting, and validating results. The core can help by pre-training some networks on typical behaviors, maintaining them for users to apply, and teaching the underlying principles at a high level. Hence, users trust and verify the outputs. For example, an interested lab might want to track rearing behavior in the home cage. The core could provide a baseline DLC model for mouse posture and show the lab how to refine it with a few annotated video frames of rearing vs non-rearing, then use that model to process their entire dataset. By doing so with guidance, the user gets their immediate result and learns the workflow for future analyses, achieving competency that they carry forward.

Another facet of data literacy is ensuring users know how to interpret HCM outputs biologically and meaningfully. As mentioned earlier, not every blip or change in an activity plot equates to a significant behavioral event. The core should counsel researchers on appropriate statistical analyses (for example, methods for repeated fluctuating measures over time, circadian rhythm analyses like Fourier or Cosinor analysis, or more adequately advanced nonlinear analyses with higher sensitivity and translational power (Hager et al. 2025). There may be cases where core analysts directly assist in higher-order analysis for a fee or collaboration, akin to a bioinformatics support model.

Promoting Acceptance Through Collaboration and Success Stories No matter how advanced the technology, a core will only thrive if researchers are motivated and convinced to use HCM. Cultural adoption can be encouraged by showcasing the success stories and promoting collaborative publication. When early adopter labs achieve compelling results with HCM, the core should work with them to disseminate these outcomes through seminars, internal newsletters, or conference presentations. Providing concrete examples of HCM leading to important scientific results providing scientific results. For instance, if one lab could detect subtle early signs of neurodegenerative disease in mice via HCM of disturbed circadian patterns, that story can be highlighted as a breakthrough that would not be possible with conventional methods. It is effectively an advertisement for the added value of HCM. Collaboration is a powerful incentive. Core directors can identify common interests among users and propose multi-group studies where the core might coordinate a larger project. Multi-disciplinary projects (like pairing a behavioral neuroscientist with a data scientist to do an HCM-based behavioral phenomics study) could produce more impactful results which cannot ge generated by single labs. In terms of publication, it helps to ensure core involvement is credited, either through co-authorship or at least acknowledgment, as this encourages core staff to invest deeply in projects and signals to the community the scientific contributions of the core. Some early HCM studies have been collaboration between technology providers and biologists, leading to cross-disciplinary publications. These papers also demonstrate how to report HCM data, setting precedents in the literature (Golini et al. 2020, 2023).

User expectations should also be managed by transparently discussing the capabilities and the current limitations of HCM. For example, while HCM can capture "more natural" behavior and reduce experimenter-induced variance, it is not inherently better at all types of assessments. A frank discussion might explain that for certain questions (like precise cognitive task performance), extensive training and particular hardware are needed, and even then, classical tests might still complement the findings. By setting realistic expectations on various available techniques, users will approach HCM projects with proper planning and avoid discouragement from initial hurdles. It is helpful to emphasize a growth mindset: automated monitoring may require a learning curve and some trial-and-error in experimental setup. However, the outcome can be gratifying regarding data richness and animal welfare improvement.

Role-Specific Example To ground the training and adoption strategies, consider two perspectives—the core director and the research scientist—in hypothetical case studies: Core Director's perspective: As a director of a behavioral phenotyping core that just acquired a HCM system he promotes adoption, and organizes an open house demonstration. They set up the HCM system with a few mice and project real-time data plots on a screen, inviting researchers to drop by. Seeing live activity and even video of mice behaving naturally generates a wider interest in the behavioral repertoire of the attending researchers. A pharmacologist also shares a case study where the core staff partnered with him to investigate a new anxiolytic drug: they ran a controlled study showing the drug increased nocturnal activity while reducing anxiety-like behavior bursts, a nuanced finding published in a high-tier journal. Following this, the director notices a surge in inquiries. He established a mentorship program where his staff will closely assist the following two labs to design and run HCM studies, in exchange for co-authorship and permission to present the outcomes in institutional forums. Within a year, several labs have integrated HCM into their grant proposals, citing the core's capabilities as strengths.

Research Scientist's perspective: A young investigator is intrigued by HCM but unsure how it fits her research on metabolic syndrome in rats. After attending the core workshop, she realizes HCM could continuously monitor feeding behavior, activity, and even body temperature of her rat model, providing an integrated picture of metabolism and behavior. Collaborating with the core's data expert, she sets up a study where rats are fed either a high-fat or control diet and are monitored 24/7 for 2 weeks using an automated system that logs each feeding event and locomotor activity, along with periodic telemetry for temperature. The young investigator may be initially concerned about data overload. Luckily, the core provides her with processed summaries showing clear patterns: high-fat diet rats have more fragmented feeding across the circadian cycle, reduced overall activity, and a slight elevation in nocturnal body temperature—indications of metabolic disturbance. These data strengthen her hypothesis and are included in a successful grant renewal.

Through such examples, it becomes evident that training, supportive collaboration, and communication of successes drive the adoption of HCM systems. Over time, as more scientists become proficient and share their experiences, HCM evolves from a "novel" to a mainstream, even indispensable, part of the behavioral research toolkit.

8 Future Directions and Emerging Technologies in HCM

As HCM systems are increasingly established in laboratories, the horizon continues to expand with emerging technologies and experimental paradigms promising to further revolutionize behavioral phenotyping. Core directors and researchers should be aware of these developments to future-proof their strategies and remain at the cutting edge. In this section, we discuss several exciting directions: closed-loop experimentation, integration of HCM with multi-omics and physiological data streams, and the fusion of virtual reality with home cage systems to create enriched cognitive testing environments. These innovations, some already in early use and others on the cusp, illustrate the concept of "cognitive laboratories" of the future, where automated systems observe and interact with subjects in real time.

Closed-Loop Experimentation Traditional experiments are mostly open-loop—we observe the animal and later adjust conditions. Closed-loop experimentation, by contrast, involves real-time modulation of experimental conditions based on the animal's behavior or physiology at that moment. HCM is ideal for closed-loop systems because it continuously collects data and can be connected to actuators that deliver stimuli or interventions. For example, imagine a setup that automatically triggers a stimulus like a mild tone, an electric brain stimulation, or drug infusion to prevent a behavioral pattern (e.g., prolonged inactivity that might indicate a seizure, stereotyped behavior, or the prevention of drug-seeking). Such systems could aid in the prevention of compromised animal welfare or enforce experimental conditions precisely (like delivering a stimulus exactly when a specific sleep stage is detected to prove its precise role in memory consolidation. Early versions of closed-loop HCM are being explored in pain and epilepsy research, where feedback loops adjust stimuli in real time (e.g., the trigger of seizure activity is removed or completely stopped once a critical (e.g., induction) threshold is reached). One practical implementation could be in operant learning. If an animal reaches a criterion in a self-training task at 2 AM, the system could immediately advance the task difficulty without human intervention, thus using the animal's timing and motivation to drive the experiment forward. Even though they are not completely new from the technological perspective, closed-loop approaches can reduce human-induced variability further and enhance the depth of data and precision of conclusions, but they require robust detection algorithms and fail-safes (Ho et al. 2023; Remmelink et al. 2017). As reported by some pilot studies, these setups significantly reduce the need for experimenter intervention, which further minimizes unspecific stressors and yields more reliable data (Richter 2020). However, they also highlight a challenge: sophisticated closed-loop platforms can be technologically complex and expensive, putting them out of reach for many labs. Core facilities may play a key role in popularizing closed-loop experimentation by hosting such advanced systems and making them available as a shared resource. Multi-omics and Physiological Integration While HCM primarily focuses on behavior, the next frontier is to link continuous behavioral data with underlying biological changes. Integrating multi-omics data (genomic, transcriptomic, proteomic, metabolomic) with behavior is highly attractive for understanding complex disorders. For instance, consider an experiment where mice are monitored for behavior around the clock. At the same time, intermittent sampling or sensors provide data on hormone levels, or where tissue samples (or blood microsamples) are taken at key behavioral inflection points for transcriptomic analysis. Already, some studies have combined telemetry (for electrophysiological signals such as EEG or ECG) with HCM of activity, generating combined datasets of brain activity and behavior over long periods (Coborn et al. 2019). Soon, we might see cages equipped with non-invasive biochemical sensors—for example, to detect cortisol metabolites in urine or infrared spectrometers to gauge CO_2/O_2 exchange for metabolic readings—synchronized with behavioral outputs. Multi-omics integration might also occur at the data analysis stage: behavioral phenotypes identified via HCM can be correlated with gene expression profiles or genomic variants. With large enough datasets, machine learning could predict an animal's molecular phenotype from its behavior or vice versa. Such comprehensive phenotyping would contribute to better understand the mechanisms behind observed behaviors, moving the field toward a systems biology-focused approach. Core facilities venturing into this area must collaborate closely with genomics/proteomics cores or have cross-disciplinary staff. The data management challenge also grows, ensuring that timestamps align across modalities and that analyses account for the multiple comparisons inherent in multi-omics data. Nonetheless, the payoff is significant: a holistic view of an organism's biology. In a sense, HCM coupled with—omics could help realize the idea of an in vivo phenotypic screen where behavior is another readout like a gene expression pattern, broadening the phenotype definition in preclinical studies, successfully demonstrated by the Mouse Phenotyping Consortium (Brown et al. 2018; Groza et al. 2023). Virtual Reality and Augmented Environments One of the more futuristic developments is using virtual reality (VR) setups for rodents in combination with home cage living. VR for animals typically involves devices like head-mounted displays or projection systems around the cage, and sometimes treadmills or ball platforms that allow a mouse to navigate a virtual space. Researchers have begun to merge these with home cage contexts so that the animal can seamlessly transition between a real home cage and a virtual environment. For example, a system might allow a mouse to voluntarily climb onto a spherical treadmill (the Servoball is one such device) placed adjacent to its home cage; once on the ball, motion sensors and computer graphics create the illusion that the mouse is running in a boundless virtual corridor or maze. If the mouse can return to its home cage deliberately, the setup qualifies as a home cage setup. Kaupert et al. (2017) demonstrated an approach where mice in a home cage extension experienced a virtual spatial navigation task with minimal unspecific stressor exposure, as they were neither handled nor restrained. Another approach by Kislin et al. (2014) involved a flat-floored air-lifted platform (essentially a virtual reality arena) that allowed freely moving rodents to experience virtual stimuli while still moving naturally, bridging classical experiments and HCM settings. These hybrid VR-HCM systems enable complex cognitive testing (like navigational memory, decision-making in mazes, etc.), which typically requires placing the animal in a specialized out-of-the-cage setup. The implication for core facilities is significant: if VR systems become more accessible, a core facility could theoretically host a "cognitive VR arena" where animals from different studies rotate in. At the same time, their behavior is monitored in VR and their home cage behavior is tracked before/after the voluntary behavioral test. If such systems are used on multiple home cages and additionally 24/7 on a voluntary basis (e.g., combined with a reward) this can save time and costs compared to the classical serial testing. Nevertheless, there are challenges to overcome, such as ensuring VR does not induce unintended stress (some argue that head-fixing mice for VR, as is sometimes done, is not ethologically friendly, but newer free-moving VR addresses that). Also, not all animals will spontaneously engage with a VR interface; some training or habituation is needed but this can be facilitated by increased motivation (e.g., by highly palatable food rewards after testing). Nonetheless, VR offers a way to present stimuli and environments that are otherwise impossible, greatly expanding what can be tested. As a concrete example, a mouse could be tested on a complex foraging task in a VR forest environment, then immediately be back in its home cage to eat and rest, effectively experiencing a "world" far larger than any physical lab apparatus could provide, with all data logged.

Toward the "Cognitive Laboratory" of the Future When combining all these emerging trends—closed-loop control, multi-omics integration, VR, and advanced sensing, we foresee a future cognitive laboratory largely automated, immersive, and data-rich beyond current imagination. In such a lab, an animal might live in a smart home cage rig for an extended period, during which it encounters various scenarios (some real, some virtual), perhaps experiences automated challenges (like a sudden temperature drop to mimic environmental challenges, or a puzzle to obtain a food reward), while an array of sensors captures everything from behavior to physiology to molecular signals. The system could adapt protocols on the fly (closed-loop), ensuring the animal is always appropriately challenged but not overloaded, resulting in reduced motivation. Data analytics, likely AI-driven, would parse this firehose of data to detect phenotypic signatures or changes. For the researchers, this means deeper and more exploratory experiments—instead of testing one hypothesis with one assay, they could gather data to test numerous hypotheses concurrently (behavioral, metabolic, neurological, etc.). The role of the scientist shifts somewhat from hands-on data collection to experimental design upfront and data interpretation afterwards, guided by sophisticated HCM systems. However, it is essential to remember that the remaining hands-on work and interaction with the animals are becoming increasingly important, both for the experiment itself and for early-career researchers to gain a full understanding of how an animal experiment is conducted. From a core facility perspective, the cognitive laboratory vision underscores the importance of keeping an eye on new technologies and thinking holistically. Core directors may eventually oversee integrated platforms that cut across what are today separate core areas (behavior, physiology, genomics). Early adoption of modular upgrades can pave the way, for instance, by adding a metabolic monitoring capability (like indirect calorimetry) to existing HCM cages or incorporating a few "VR-ready" cages into the standard rack for those who would benefit from this technology in their experimental assays. Collaboration with engineers and software developers might become a regular aspect of core operations to customize solutions.

Ethically, these advancements also push us to consider the welfare impact: an automated system that can intervene in an animal's environment must be carefully validated to truly benefit the animal and not inadvertently cause harm or serve as an intermittent stressor due to, e.g., false alarms. Fortunately, many of these innovations are being developed with animal welfare as a priority (the idea of reducing human handling and providing enrichment through VR, for instance, aligns with refinement goals).

To sum up, the future of HCM is poised to integrate cutting-edge technology to create an environment where laboratory animals can be studied more humanely, comprehensively, and rigorously. Core facilities will be instrumental in bringing these advances to the broader scientific community, acting as incubators for new methods and providing access to complex setups that individual labs might not manage alone. By staying informed and adaptable, core directors can ensure that their playbook evolves in step with these emerging opportunities, guiding scientists through the next era of behavioral research.

9 Conclusion

HCM has moved from a niche innovation to a central component of modern behavioral phenotyping, and its successful implementation requires a synergistic approach between technology, people, and required processes. For core laboratory directors, establishing an HCM platform is a technical acquisition and a strategic enhancement of their facility's capabilities. This chapter has provided a comprehensive overview for guiding scientists in this journey, from understanding fundamental benefits of HCM to integrating it with classical tests, setting up the necessary infrastructure, training users, managing operations, and looking ahead to future developments leading to a reduction of classical out-of-the-cage assays.

In summary, HCM systems offer continuous real-time monitoring, which complements traditional methods by capturing nuanced behavioral patterns and physiological parameters that episodic tests cannot provide. This strength leads to improved reproducibility and data richness in studies, as demonstrated by numerous examples where automated home cage data revealed phenotypes or drug effects that were missed by conventional assays (Sun et al. 2025; Theologidis et al. 2025). The core director's role is pivotal in translating these advantages into routine practice. By carefully planning integration pathways—aligning stakeholders, ensuring workflows and data streams are compatible, and pooling resources for efficiency—core animal facilities can embed HCM into their service lineup in a sustainable manner. Robust infrastructure, including modular hardware and advanced data management pipelines, forms the foundation that core staff must maintain and continuously improve.

Equally important are the human factors: through competency-based training programs and data literacy initiatives, core facilities equip researchers with the skills to optimally design insightful experiments and interpret the complex data that are generated. Managing user expectations and fostering a collaborative culture help in overcoming initial adoption barriers. The chapter's operational guidance highlights that clear project management, governance compliance, and financial planning are essential to running HCM as a reliable, highly valuable core service. Tracking performance metrics and iterating on processes ensures the core remains responsive to users' needs and accountable to its institution.

Real-world case studies illustrate how core directors and scientists can partner effectively—the core providing expertise and support, and the scientists bringing domain-specific questions to achieve results that push boundaries of scientific progress. As HCM technology continues to evolve, incorporating closed-loop interactions, multi-modal data integration, and even virtual reality, core facilities will likely be at the forefront of these innovations. Embracing new tools and maintaining flexibility will allow core directors to continue guiding their scientific users through increasingly sophisticated experimental paradigms.

Finally, the "core director's playbook" for HCM is one of integration—integrating new technology with existing methods, integrating rich datasets with biological insight, and integrating the efforts of core staff with the ambitions of researchers. When executed well, the outcome is a robust platform that enhances both experimental outcomes and animal welfare. This development educates and empowers a new generation of scientists in quantitative, systems-level behavioral research. HCM stands as a testament to how methodology can drive discovery in combination with animal welfare improvements. With knowledgeable core facilities leading the way, its full potential can be realized across disciplines ranging from neuroscience and pharmacology to physiology and beyond.

References

Ahloy-Dallaire J, Klein JD, Davis JK, Garner JP (2019) Automated monitoring of mouse feeding and body weight for continuous health assessment. Lab Anim 53(4):342–351

Bernstein D (2003) Exercise assessment of transgenic models of human cardiovascular disease. Physiol Genomics 13(3):217–226. https://doi.org/10.1152/physiolgenomics.00188.2002

Brown SDM, Holmes CC, Mallon A-M, Meehan TF, Smedley D, Wells S (2018) High-throughput mouse phenomics for characterizing mammalian gene function. Nat Rev Genet 19(6):357–370. https://doi.org/10.1038/s41576-018-0005-2

Coborn JE, Lessie RE, Sinton CM, Rance NE, Perez-Leighton CE, Teske JA (2019) Noise-induced sleep disruption increases weight gain and decreases energy metabolism in female rats. Int J Obes 43(9):1759–1768. https://doi.org/10.1038/s41366-018-0293-9

COST-Action, TEATIME (2025) About the TEATIME action. COST teatime. https://www.cost--teatime.org/about/

Crabbe JC, Wahlsten D, Dudek BC (1999) Genetics of mouse behavior: interactions with laboratory environment. Science 284(5420):1670–1672. https://doi.org/10.1126/science.284.5420.1670

Golini E, Rigamonti M, Iannello F, De Rosa C, Scavizzi F, Raspa M, Mandillo S (2020) A non-invasive digital biomarker for the detection of rest disturbances in the SOD1G93A mouse model of ALS. Front Neurosci 14:896

Golini E, Rigamonti M, Raspa M, Scavizzi F, Falcone G, Gourdon G, Mandillo S (2023) Excessive rest time during active phase is reliably detected in a mouse model of myotonic dystrophy type 1 using home cage monitoring. Front Behav Neurosci 17:1130055

Grieco F, Bernstein BJ, Biemans B, Bikovski L, Burnett CJ, Cushman JD, Van Dam EA et al (2021) Measuring behavior in the home cage: study design, applications, challenges, and perspectives. Front Behav Neurosci 15:735387

Groza T, Gomez FL, Mashhadi HH, Muñoz-Fuentes V, Gunes O, Wilson R, Cacheiro P et al (2023) The international mouse phenotyping consortium: comprehensive knockout phenotyping underpinning the study of human disease. Nucleic Acids Res 51(D1):D1038–D1045. https://doi.org/10.1093/nar/gkac972

Hager T, Jansen RÃ©F, Pieneman AW, Manivannan SN, Golani I, Van Der Sluis S, Smit AB, Verhage M, Stiedl O (2014) Display of individuality in avoidance behavior and risk assessment of inbred mice. Front Behav Neurosci 8:314. https://doi.org/10.3389/fnbeh.2014.00314

Hager T, Agorastos A, Ögren SO, Stiedl O (2025) Identifying cardiovascular risk by nonlinear heart rate dynamics analysis: translational biomarker from mice to humans. Brain Sci 15(3):306. https://doi.org/10.3390/brainsci15030306

Ho H, Kejzar N, Sasaguri H, Saito T, Saido TC, De Strooper B, Bauza M, Krupic J (2023) A fully automated home cage for long-term continuous phenotyping of mouse cognition and behavior. Cell Rep Methods 3(7):100532. https://doi.org/10.1016/j.crmeth.2023.100532

Horii Y, Nagasawa T, Sakakibara H, Takahashi A, Tanave A, Matsumoto Y, Nagayama H et al (2017) Hierarchy in the home cage affects behaviour and gene expression in group-housed C57BL/6 male mice. Sci Rep 7(1):6991. https://doi.org/10.1038/s41598-017-07233-5

Iannello F (2019) Non-intrusive high throughput automated data collection from the home cage. Heliyon 5(4):e01454

Kafkafi N, Agassi J, Chesler EJ, Crabbe JC, Crusio WE, Eilam D, Gerlai R et al (2018) Reproducibility and replicability of rodent phenotyping in preclinical studies. Neurosci Biobehav Rev 87:218–232

Kahnau P, Jaap A, Urmersbach B, Diederich K, Lewejohann L (2023a) Development of an IntelliCage-based cognitive bias test for mice. Open Res Eur 2:128

Kahnau P, Mieske P, Wilzopolski J, Kalliokoski O, Mandillo S, Hölter SM, Voikar V et al (2023b) A systematic review of the development and application of home cage monitoring in laboratory mice and rats. BMC Biol 21(1):256. https://doi.org/10.1186/s12915-023-01751-7

Kaupert U, Thurley K, Frei K, Bagorda F, Schatz A, Tocker G, Rapoport S, Derdikman D, Winter Y (2017) Spatial cognition in a virtual reality home-cage extension for freely moving rodents. J Neurophysiol 117(4):1736–1748

Kim DG, Gonzales EL, Kim S, Kim Y, Adil KJ, Jeon SJ, Cho KS, Kwon KJ, Shin CY (2019) Social interaction test in home cage as a novel and ethological measure of social behavior in mice. Exp Neurobiol 28(2):247–260. https://doi.org/10.5607/en.2019.28.2.247

Kislin M, Mugantseva E, Molotkov D, Kulesskaya N, Khirug S, Kirilkin I, Pryazhnikov E et al (2014) Flat-floored air-lifted platform: a new method for combining behavior with microscopy or electrophysiology on awake freely moving rodents. J Vis Exp JoVE 88:51869

Krackow S, Vannoni E, Codita A, Mohammed AH, Cirulli F, Branchi I, Alleva E et al (2010) Consistent behavioral phenotype differences between inbred mouse strains in the IntelliCage. Genes Brain Behav 9(7):722–731. https://doi.org/10.1111/j.1601-183x.2010.00606.x

Martin SC, Joyce KK, Lord JS, Harper KM, Nikolova VD, Cohen TJ, Moy SS, Diering GH (2024) Sleep disruption precedes forebrain synaptic tau burden and contributes to cognitive decline in a sex-dependent manner in the P301S Tau transgenic mouse model. eNeuro 11(6):ENEURO.0004-24.2024. https://doi.org/10.1523/ENEURO.0004-24.2024

Mathis A, Mamidanna P, Cury KM, Abe T, Murthy VN, Mathis MW, Bethge M (2018) DeepLabCut: markerless pose estimation of user-defined body parts with deep learning. Nat Neurosci 21(9):1281–1289. https://doi.org/10.1038/s41593-018-0209-y

Mieske P, Diederich K, Lewejohann L (2021) Roaming in a land of Milk and honey: life trajectories and metabolic rate of female inbred mice living in a semi naturalistic environment. Animals 11(10):3002. https://doi.org/10.3390/ani11103002

Mina AI, LeClair RA, LeClair KB, Cohen DE, Lantier L, Banks AS (2018) CalR: a web-based analysis tool for indirect calorimetry experiments. Cell Metab 28(4):656–666.e1. https://doi.org/10.1016/j.cmet.2018.06.019

Remmelink E, Chau U, Smit AB, Verhage M, Loos M (2017) A one-week 5-choice serial reaction time task to measure impulsivity and attention in adult and adolescent mice. Sci Rep 7(1):42519. https://doi.org/10.1038/srep42519

Richter SH (2020) Automated home-cage testing as a tool to improve reproducibility of behavioral research? Front Neurosci 14:383. https://doi.org/10.3389/fnins.2020.00383

Salem GH, Dennis JU, Krynitsky J, Garmendia-Cedillos M, Swaroop K, Malley JD, Pajevic S et al (2015) SCORHE: a novel and practical approach to video monitoring of laboratory mice housed in vivarium cage racks. Behav Res Methods 47:235–250

Sun R, Zimbalski L-K, Schreyer S, Baidoe-Ansah D, Harutyunyan A, Heuser A, Lippert RN et al (2025) Sex-specific changes in energy demand during the Preplaque stage in a transgenic Alzheimer's mouse model. Biol Sex Differ 16(1):54. https://doi.org/10.1186/s13293-025-00737-0

Theologidis V, Ferreira SA, Jensen NM, Moreira DG, Ahlgreen OA, Hansen MW, Rosenberg ED et al (2025) Bradykinesia and postural instability in a model of prodromal synucleinopathy with α-synuclein aggregation initiated in the gigantocellular nuclei. Acta Neuropathol Commun 13(1):32. https://doi.org/10.1186/s40478-025-01948-7

Townsend HGG, Osterrieder K, Jelinski MD, Morck DW, Waldner CL, Cox WR, Gerdts V et al (2025) A call to action to address critical flaws and bias in laboratory animal experiments and preclinical research. Sci Rep 15(1):30745. https://doi.org/10.1038/s41598-025-15935-4

Turpen PB, Hockberger PE, Meyn SM, Nicklin C, Tabarini D, Auger JA (2016) Metrics for success: strategies for enabling core facility performance and assessing outcomes. J Biomol Tech 27(1):25

Urbach YK, Raber KA, Canneva F, Plank A-C, Andreasson T, Ponten H, Kullingsjö J et al (2014) Automated phenotyping and advanced data mining exemplified in rats transgenic for Huntington's disease. J Neurosci Methods 234:38–53

Villiger P, Calvet C, Pastor-Arroyo EM, Wagner CA, Seebeck P (2025) Thermoneutral environment improves mouse welfare and reduces stress in metabolic cages. Lab Anim 54(11):303–312. https://doi.org/10.1038/s41684-025-01618-0

Home Cage Monitoring in Pharmaceutical Industries and Contract Research Organizations

Gommet Céline, Marcel M. van Gaalen, and Scorrano Fabrizio

Abstract

Home cage monitoring (HCM) systems enable continuous, automated observation of laboratory animals in their standard environment without human interference and are aligned with the 3Rs principle (reduction, refinement, replacement). They provide a variety of metrics, including locomotor activity, circadian patterns, feeding and drinking behaviors, which can support the development of new drugs by early detecting drug-related effects and potential toxicity.

In the context of harmonized and standardized drug development, digital measures generated by HCM systems must undergo a process of validation, evaluating if they can be used as surrogates to biomarkers or additional, enhanced, early metrics. This chapter focuses on the relevance of HCM in preclinical studies in drug development, based not only on literature but also on real-case studies.

The increased integration of HCM on a regular basis is expected in the following years with the emergence of more examples highlighting its inputs and maybe a consensus on how to use HCM technologies.

G. Céline (✉)
Sanofi, Vitry-sur-Seine, France
e-mail: celine.gommet@sanofi.com

M. M. van Gaalen
Evotec, Göttingen, Germany

S. Fabrizio
Novartis, Basel, Switzerland

S. Gaburro, S. Mandillo (eds.), *Home Cage Monitoring in Rodents: A Global Effort*,
https://doi.org/10.1007/978-3-032-19781-8_5

Keywords

Home cage monitoring · Research and development · Preclinical studies · Safety · Toxicology · Digital biomarkers

1 Introduction and Context

In the evolving landscape of healthcare and biomedical research, terms like biomarker, digital biomarker, and digital measure are frequently used. However, their overlapping usage can lead to confusion. Understanding their distinct definitions is crucial for accurate communication and application in clinical and preclinical research settings.

A *biomarker* is a measurable indicator of a biological state or condition. It is objectively measured and evaluated as an indicator of normal biological processes, pathogenic processes, or responses to therapeutic interventions. Examples include blood pressure, cholesterol levels, and specific genetic mutations (Califf 2018). A *digital biomarker* refers to objective, quantifiable physiological or behavioral data collected and measured by means of digital devices such as portables, wearables, implantables, or digestibles. These biomarkers are used to explain, influence, and/or predict health-related outcomes (Motahari-Nezhad et al. 2021). The term *digital measure* encompasses health-related data collected through digital devices, including smartphones, wearables, or sensors. These measures can include metrics like step count, heart rate, or sleep patterns. They offer objective insights into an individual's health status and can be used for monitoring and assessing health outcomes (Coravos et al. 2019). These definitions are very applicable to clinical research. Recently, Baran et al. (2025) provided definitions that can be more applicable to preclinical research. Digital measures are defined as quantitative data continuously collected from unrestrained and uninstrumented animals using digital in vivo technologies, such as sensors embedded in the animal's cage or environment. When a digital measure demonstrates objective, quantifiable responses to disease progression or therapeutic intervention, it may be considered a digital biomarker. If it further bridges preclinical and clinical contexts, it may be classified as a translational digital biomarker.

In vivo science remains a crucial step in drug discovery. In our discipline, we strive to adhere to the 3Rs principle: reduction, refinement, and replacement, as first articulated by Russell and Burch in 1953 and repeatedly revised (e.g., Louis-Maerten et al. 2024). Implementing Home Cage Monitoring (HCM) has the potential to reduce the size of animal experiment groups, thereby decreasing the number of animals used. Additionally, automatic observations without human interference in a home cage setting reduce stress for the animals, thus improving refinement. This is not only specific to applied in vivo science in the industry but is equally important for academic research. In vivo science in the industry is part of preclinical research and development (R&D) in drug discovery. It plays a role in pharmacokinetic, pharmacodynamic, and efficacy studies during the research stages. The latter two are particularly applicable for combining studies in this area with

HCM. Obviously, in vivo studies are also required for toxicological and safety assessments in the preclinical developmental stage. Although HCM certainly has the potential to add value during the drug discovery stage, employing these techniques under Good Laboratory Practice (GLP) may present challenges (see later in this chapter).

Although observing research animals in their natural living environment is not new, recent advancements have significantly enhanced these observations. First, more affordable hardware solutions have made HCM systems scalable and integrable with standard caging, potentially enabling the transition to digital vivariums where each animal cage is digitally monitored. Secondly, Artificial Intelligence- (AI) and Machine Learning-based (ML) algorithms now allow for swift and advanced analysis of the data generated by these new technologies. Consequently, HCM systems have become commercially available in recent years, and open-source solutions have also emerged, making these technologies appealing to in vivo scientists across academic institutions, contract research organizations (CROs), biotech firms, and large pharmaceutical companies. Additionally, HCM systems can improve the quality and efficiency of animal care.

Preclinical R&D is followed by the clinical phase. Overall, the cost of drug R&D and clinical development is continuously increasing. On average, to bring a new drug to the US market, the cost of non-clinical R&D is estimated to be $11.8 million. Clinical trials are significantly more expensive, ranging from $7.1 million (Phase I) to $21 million (Phase II) and $89.3 million (Phase III). This brings the total average cost, including FDA approval, to $131.5 million (Sertkaya et al. 2024). The probability of success (PoS) for clinical candidate drugs to achieve market approval varies significantly across therapeutic areas. Vaccines and ophthalmology have relatively high success rates (33% and 32%, respectively), whereas Central Nervous System (CNS) drugs (15%) and oncology drugs (3.4%) are at the lower end of the success spectrum (Wong et al. 2019), based on data from trials conducted between 2000 and 2015. When accounting for failures and the median capitalized research and development investment required to bring a new drug to market, the average cost was estimated at $1141.7 million (Wouters et al. 2020).

Interestingly, Wong et al. (2019) also calculated the difference in PoS between clinical trials that included biomarkers and those that did not, based on data from 2005 to 2015. In oncology, trials from this period had a PoS of 1.6% when no biomarkers were included, whereas the PoS was 10.7% in trials that did include biomarkers. During the same period, CNS trials had a PoS of 6.2% without biomarkers, compared to a PoS of 8.3% in trials with biomarkers. Given that HCM has the potential to reveal and validate digital biomarkers that can be translated to clinical settings (using wearables, smartphone applications, etc.), the implementation of HCM technology has the potential to improve PoS in clinical trials.

Over the last decade, many findings in preclinical animal research published in high-profile journals have been deemed unreliable and irreproducible, leading to a so-called reproducibility crisis. This crisis is attributed to poor scientific practices and neglect of rigorous methods. Contributing factors include flaws in experimental design, execution, statistical analysis, and reporting (Voehringer and Nicholson 2020). One of the execution factors has been demonstrated by Crabbe et al. (1999), who studied possible confounding influences of the laboratory environment. In their multi-lab study, apparatus, test protocols, and many environmental variables were rigorously equated. Despite standardization, the outcomes differed markedly in all behaviors. One of the factors contributing to these differences is likely the human experimenter, given that this human factor is hard to standardize. HCM does not rely on a human experimenter and, therefore, may result in more reproducible results. This will contribute to increased trust in in vivo results and thereby optimize the R&D processes and PoS in clinical development.

This chapter focuses on the use of HCM systems in R&D in pharmaceutical industries and CROs, from the evaluation of these systems to their implementation and use of the data obtained with these technologies.

2 Validation of HCM

2.1 Importance of Validating HCM-Derived Endpoints Against Pharmacological and Behavioral Benchmarks

To standardize drug R&D, the International Council for Harmonisation of Technical Requirements for Pharmaceuticals for Human Use (ICH 2025) issued guidelines on drug development, including scientific and technical aspects. In the set of safety guidelines, the organ systems that should be investigated and some associated biomarkers are even listed. Regulatory guidelines, such as the one issued by the European Medicines Agency (EMEA 2017), rely on ICH's guidelines for the evaluation of drug candidates and their transition to first-in-human or early clinical trials. For preclinical studies, most ICH guidelines focus on safety.

The ICH S7A guideline on pharmacology studies mentions that "data from unrestrained animals that may be chronically instrumented for telemetry, other suitable instrumentation methods for conscious animals, or animals conditioned to the laboratory environment are preferable to data from restrained or unconditioned animals". In the use of unanesthetized animals, the avoidance of discomfort or pain is a foremost consideration. As HCM systems collect data from unanesthetized and unrestrained animals, they perfectly fit with the guidelines on the test systems. However, as the studies are part of the development of drugs meant for human use and can be included in market authorization, the digital measures collected by HCM systems need to be proven dependable. Therefore, it is crucial to challenge and validate HCM systems' data through a consensual framework (Baran et al. 2025). In studies supporting regulatory submissions, data quality and integrity should be compliant with the principles of GLP to computerized systems (OECD 1995).

The validation process for HCM systems typically encompasses the following steps:

- Verification with reference compounds or models: assessing whether the system accurately detects anticipated effects when challenged with established reference drugs or validated models.

- Comparative analysis against standard methodologies: evaluating alignment with data obtained through conventional reference methods and determining relative sensitivity between approaches.
- Assessment of added value: determining the practical benefits and scientific advantages of integrating HCM systems into study designs.

2.2 Experimental Designs: Parallel Testing with Conventional Assays

In the validation process, HCM data are compared to reference methods. It is usually done by detecting expected effects of reference drugs (Tse et al. 2018; Robinson and Riedel 2014; Petersen et al. 2023; Piilgaard et al. 2023). According to Kahnau et al. (2023) in their review on HCM systems used in laboratory mice and rats, the main measures collected were locomotor activity, feeding, social behaviors, heart rate, and electrocardiography.

Depending on the study design, it may be necessary to reconsider or refine the time of drug administration, especially for studies with a limited observation/sampling window. However, this should not impair the other measured biomarkers. Drug administration is usually done in the morning, which enables close monitoring of the drug effect and repeated samplings. If we follow up the locomotor activity of rodents with our HCM system, a drug-induced hyperactivity will be well detected during the light phase, as rodents are resting during the daytime. But a drug-induced hypoactivity may not be detected if the effect lasts a couple of hours (see Fig. 1). Then, an administration at dusk would give a better insight into the hypoactive effect, but may not be compatible with non-automated sample collection.

This is a consideration that must be taken into account for acute monitoring in particular.

2.3 Strategies for Aligning HCM Data with Known Biomarkers and Endpoints

HCM data must align with the parameters monitored during the study, which include:

- The choice of biomarkers, related to the organ systems that must be evaluated during the study.
- The endpoints, which are pre-specified according to general ethical criteria and the potential specificity of the model.

The evaluation of biomarkers and endpoints represents a picture of what's happening at a specific time and can be repeated. HCM data, on the other hand, are quantitative data collected continuously. Even if we look at the same metric, manual data and HCM data may not refer to the exact same thing.

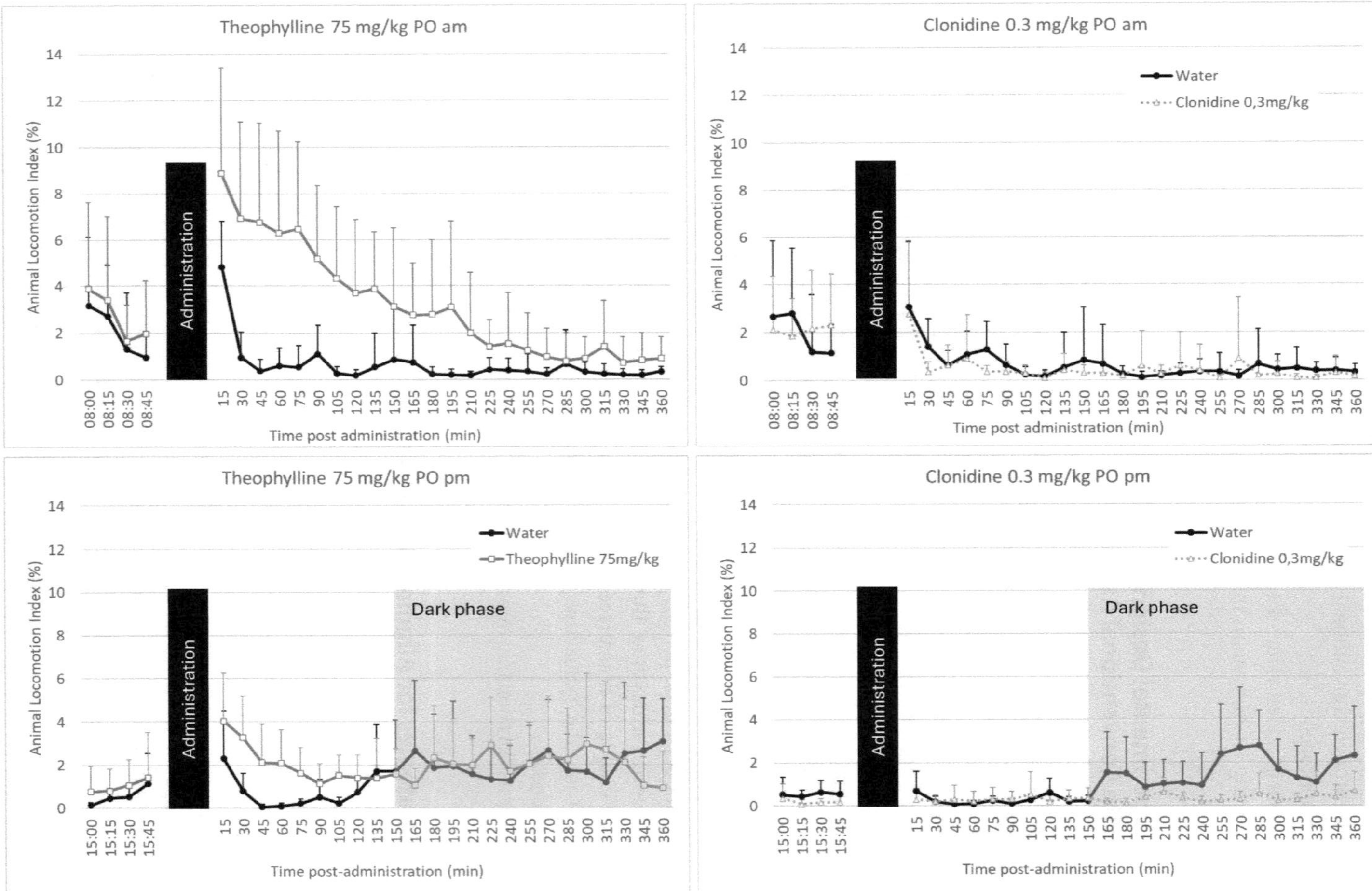

Fig. 1 Example of locomotor activity detected by the DVC® system after oral administration of theophylline or clonidine in the morning and in the afternoon (Sanofi's data)

If we take the example of the evaluation of water consumption, one reference method is to periodically weigh the bottle. Several HCM systems allow the evaluation of drinking behavior. Some continuously register the water consumption due to a weight transducer like the PhenoMaster. In this case, HCM data are comparable to the conventional measure and even add the circadian rhythm of water consumption. Other HCM systems will evaluate the water consumption not by weighing the water bottle but by counting when and how long the animal is drinking. It is another way to evaluate drinking behavior (Robinson and Riedel 2014; Petersen et al. 2023). Whether digital measures can replace or complement conventional data depends on their application and its correlation with the reference method.

The COST TEATIME Action has compiled the current HCM technologies as well as their associated metrics (TEATIME Action 2025). This compilation is a major help for choosing the more relevant HCM system according to the needs identified.

2.4 Data Quality and Relevance

Evans already discussed in 1989 the importance of using home cage behaviors to detect chemical toxicity in laboratory animals and the relevance of their inclusion in toxicity screening (Evans 1989). One huge benefit of using HCM systems is to automatically collect digital measures which could complement and/or replace already established biomarkers, such as behavioral tests.

Among the benefits pinpointed for HCM data are automated, non-biased, enabling the monitoring of the entire circadian rhythm, and can be applied to long-term studies. HCM data may also be useful in the early detection of health degradation (Baran et al. 2020; Vagima et al. 2020).

For rodents in vivo studies, HCM 24/7 gives access to the nocturnal activity patterns, which are more sensitive than the diurnal activity patterns, as mice and rats are nocturnal animals. With continuous data, HCM allows the confirmation or the unveiling of the timing of drug effects, the maximum effect but also potential delayed or rebound effects which could not be detected during time-limited observations (Tse et al. 2018).

However, not all HCM systems provide the identification of individual animals. With the refinement of the studies and the reduction of the number of animals used, this is a challenge that needs to be addressed as group-housing is the standard. The ability to identify individual animals in group housed cage is a key feature to consider when purchasing an HCM system.

3 Key Performance Indicators (KPIs) and Metrics

3.1 Common Automated Behavioral Metrics and Linked KPIs

HCM systems automatically record a wide array of animal behaviors continuously in the animals' home environment, minimizing human interference (Grieco et al. 2021). Automated metrics are the specific quantitative measures of behavior that HCM devices collect (e.g., movement distance or feeding duration), whereas key performance indicators (KPIs) are higher-level measures of experimental success or efficiency that these metrics inform (e.g., time savings, data quality, or predictive power of a model). In other words, metrics are the raw objective readouts, while KPIs reflect how those data improve experimental outcomes. Establishing this distinction is important to evaluate how HCM technology benefits translational research.

Common behavioral metrics captured by HCM include:

- *Locomotor Activity*: Continuous tracking of movement levels (distance traveled, speed, bouts of activity vs. rest). This can be measured via video tracking, RFID-based tracking or sensors and provides a baseline of overall activity (Kahnau et al. 2023). Locomotor activity is probably the best analytically validated parameter in HMC. High-resolution activity metrics allow detection of changes in mobility or lethargy that might indicate health deterioration, disease progression in animal models or drug effects.
- *Circadian Rhythm and Rest Patterns*: Because HCM is continuous, it captures diurnal variations in behavior. Metrics like daytime vs. nighttime activity, sleep duration or fragmentation, and phase shifts in routine are commonly derived. These reveal an animal's circadian rhythm stability and any disturbances. For instance, HCM identified that ALS model mice showed abnormal daytime activity (when they should be resting) well before overt symptoms, reflecting sleep disturbances like those seen in patients (Golini et al. 2020). Such metrics directly relate to KPIs like data richness and biological relevance, since capturing full circadian cycles improves the translational validity of the model, while rodents are assessed on their normal nocturnal schedule rather than only during human working hours (Mingrone et al. 2020).
- *Social Interactions*: In group-housed settings, HCM can quantify social behavior metrics such as proximity between animals, frequency of interactions, or dominance behaviors. Traditional tests assess social novelty or aggression in short sessions, but HCM allows observation of natural social dynamics over days. While tracking individuals in groups is technically challenging, advances (e.g., RFID tags or multi-animal video tracking) enable measuring time spent together vs. alone, social grooming, or aggression bouts (Hohlbaum et al. 2024). These metrics inform welfare-related KPIs—for example, ensuring animals can be group-housed while still collecting individual data (Terry et al. 2023). Enhanced social behavior data can reduce the need for separate social interaction tests, thus saving experiment time.

- *Feeding and Drinking Behavior*: Many HCM systems log food and water intake using hopper sensors or weight transducers. Metrics include the number of feeding bouts, total food consumed, drinking frequency, etc. (Hohlbaum et al. 2024). Changes in feeding patterns can be early signs of illness or drug side effects. Automating their measurement yields KPIs of improved data quality (objective consumption data versus sporadic weighing of food) and animal welfare (animals are not singly caged for metabolic tests but can be monitored in a home cage). For instance, continuous monitoring of food/water intake in home cages has revealed subtle changes in appetite that correlate with drug tolerability (Terry et al. 2023), alerting investigators to potential toxicity sooner than weekly body weight checks.
- *Subtle or Complex Behaviors*: HCM can detect micro-behaviors or composite metrics that are hard to measure by human observation. Examples include grooming duration, rearing events, nesting quality, or spatial patterns of cage use (such as preference for corners indicating thigmotaxis). Sophisticated analyses can yield metrics like an animal's use of cage zones (e.g., percentage of time along walls vs. center) or a "rest disturbance index" quantifying abnormal activity during the usual rest phase (Golini et al. 2020). These nuanced metrics greatly increase sensitivity to changes reflected in KPIs like earlier detection of on-set disease and more predictive modeling. Indeed, automated home-cage solutions has been shown to identify subtle changes (e.g., slight increases in restlessness or repetitive motions) that precede overt clinical signs, thereby improving the predictive power of preclinical models (Bains et al. 2018; Mingrone et al. 2020).

Each of the above metrics drives improvements in experimental KPIs. Continuous locomotor and circadian data translate to time saved and reduced labor, because experiments run 24/7 without an experimenter present, and large behavioral datasets are gathered without manual scoring. This automation also reduces handling of animals, an important refinement that lowers stress and variability in results. Continuous longitudinal metrics leverage more predictive models, as they capture treatment effects and disease progression in greater detail over time. Social and subtle behavior metrics contribute to data richness, giving a multidimensional view of an animal's state (motor, social, cognitive) in an integrated manner. In sum, by exploring these metrics, HCM technology feeds into KPIs such as enhanced efficiency (continuous data collection, fewer personnel hours), improved animal welfare (minimal disturbance, group housing), and increased translational relevance of the data (behavior measured in an undisturbed, naturalistic context).

3.2 HCM-Derived KPIs for Compound Efficacy Profiling and Early Adverse Effect Detection

Unlike traditional end-point assays, HCM captures changes continuously, often revealing drug effects that would be missed with infrequent observations. Below, we illustrate these advantages with examples across neurological, psychiatric, inflammatory, and aging-related disease models:

Neurodegenerative Disease (ALS) In amyotrophic lateral sclerosis (ALS) models, home-cage behavioral readouts have proven valuable for early disease onset signals. A landmark study demonstrated that using running wheels in the home cage allowed daily monitoring of motor function in SOD1-G93A ALS mice, detecting onset of decline as early as around 40 days of age, the same time as the gold-standard rotarod test, but with far less variability. The reduced variability meant researchers could use smaller group sizes to achieve statistical power, thereby reducing the number of animals required (Bennett et al. 2014). This exemplifies an HCM-driven KPI: improved sensitivity leading to both refinement (less manual testing) and reduction in animal usage, without compromising detection of drug effects.

Psychiatric and Behavioral Models Automated HCM has been championed as a way to improve the translational validity of psychiatric drug studies. Traditional tests for anxiety or depression-like behavior are short and environment-dependent, often failing to predict clinical results (Mingrone et al. 2020). In contrast, HCM allows longitudinal efficacy profiling of psychoactive compounds in a stable environment. For example, in chronic anxiety models, an anxiolytic drug's effect might manifest as a gradual increase in nocturnal exploratory activity or more regular sleep patterns over weeks. These are subtle changes that HCM can quantify, but standard tests might miss. One study showed that home-cage monitoring after chronic antidepressant treatment revealed increased regularity in daily activity cycles and reduced restlessness, changes that aligned with therapeutic effects and occurred well before improvements would be evident in a forced swim test (Kaffman et al. 2019). Thus, behavioral signatures over time serve as KPIs for a compound's efficacy profile: drugs can be differentiated by whether they restore normal circadian rhythmicity, social interaction frequency, or other sustained behaviors, rather than just acute test performance.

Inflammation and Disease Severity Monitoring In models of inflammatory disease or chronic illness, HCM-derived metrics often track the course of disease and treatment response more continuously than clinical scoring. For instance, in a colitis inflammatory bowel disease model (Zentrich et al. 2021), automated activity monitoring detected decreases in movement corresponding with disease onset and identified stress-related behavioral changes due to handling of the animals. Researchers showed that an algorithm combining HCM activity data with body weight could classify mice into "burdened" (disease-active) vs. "not burdened" groups, matching the clinical colitis scoring. This suggests HCM can potentially serve as an automated severity assessment tool, a KPI relevant to both scientific rigor and animal welfare. HCM thus helps distinguish effective vs. ineffective treatments in inflammation models by providing objective, high-frequency readouts of disease severity and recovery. Similarly, HCM can catch early signs of systemic adverse effects: for example, if an anti-inflammatory drug causes malaise or pain, mice might show decreased nocturnal activity or abnormal restlessness even before any weight loss occurs, alerting researchers to the problem. The ability to quantify welfare conditions continuously is a transformative KPI and studies can be adjusted in real-time (e.g., providing supportive care or euthanizing to prevent suffering) and drug effects (beneficial or harmful) are not missed between scheduled checks.

Aging Models and Frailty Index Long-term HCM in aging studies has revealed subtle changes in behavior that signify health span or emerging frailty, offering a window to evaluate interventions (Moore et al. 2024). For example, Moore et al. (2024) tracked mice from middle age to old age in digital home-cages and found that overall activity levels declined steadily up to ~14 months old, then unexpectedly rose again in very old mice. This observation suggests compensatory hyperactivity or stereotypies in aged animals. HCM thus enabled early detection of these maladaptive behaviors, highlighting a welfare concern (animals in prolonged housing developing repetitive behaviors) that could be mitigated. In terms of efficacy profiling, if testing an anti-aging or neuroprotective therapy, scientists could monitor whether treated mice maintain a younger activity pattern (e.g., sustained high dark-phase activity and solid rest during light phase) compared to controls that might show fragmented rest or declining activity. These metrics improve the predictivity of how an intervention affects quality of life, not just lifespan, bridging clinical geriatric outcomes like sleep quality and daily activity levels.

4 Return on Investment (ROI) and Business Considerations

4.1 Detection of Rare Events

Animal models that exhibit pathological behavioral readouts occurring infrequently over time present challenges for use in drug discovery. For instance, in Scn1a+/A1783V (PFC) mice, approximately one-third of the animals experienced spontaneous seizures, with a frequency of 1.33 seizures per day (Riga et al. 2024). Manual observation, whether live or via video recordings, is often impractical or prohibitively labor-intensive.

HCM, combined with appropriate data analysis algorithms, enables continuous tracking of pathological behaviors over extended periods, as well as assessment of pharmacological treatment effects. As such, HCM facilitates the use of animal models in drug discovery even when behavioral abnormalities occur infrequently.

4.2 Refined KPIs: Impact on Predictivity, Animal Welfare, and Project Outcomes (ALS Case Study)

Shifting to an HCM fundamentally changes key performance indicators for preclinical studies. Instead of relying on sparse end-point measures, researchers obtain a continuous stream of high-quality data, which can streamline workflows and improve decision-making. Important KPIs that are refined by HCM include: personnel effort (full-time equivalent, FTE) reduction, data richness and quality, facility utilization efficiency, speed of decision-making, predictive validity, and animal welfare improvements. We illustrate these with a head-to-head case study of an ALS drug efficacy experiment run with and without HCM, as shown in Figs. 2 and 3.

This experiment in Fig. 2 outlines a 40-week ALS mouse study design using traditional assessments only. Timepoints for periodic functional tests (FT1, FT2), such as grip strength and gait analysis, imaging sessions, and biological sample collections (blood, CSF, histology), are indicated. The table below shows the approximate hands-on time required for each task type per week and per month, summing to ~192 hours/month of labor (~1.2 FTE). Over a 6-month span, the study demands ~1150 hours (~7.2 FTE) of the researcher's time. Because data are only collected during weekly tests or periodic imaging, the overall dataset is relatively sparse ("single snapshots" of behavior) and important changes between timepoints may be missed. In this scenario, several KPIs are suboptimal: *Resources*: The study is time-consuming, with significant personnel hours dedicated to handling mice for tests and measurements. *Data Quantity*: Each mouse yields limited data (e.g., one score per week for a grip strength test), leaving gaps in the disease timeline. *Data Quality and Variability*: Results can vary depending on technician skill and the animals' stress during handling, potentially reducing reproducibility. *Clinical Translatability*: Intermittent tests provide a narrow view of the disease, which may not capture symptoms like disrupted sleep that are relevant to patients. *Animal Wellbeing*: Mice must be repeatedly removed from their cage and trained for tasks, which elevates stress. The process thus imposes a burden on the animals, and signs of disease onset might only be recognized after they become pronounced, potentially delaying interventions to reduce suffering.

In the HCM-enhanced design of Fig. 3, animals are continuously monitored in their home cages throughout the 40-week study, in addition to the same periodic tests and endpoints as the control scenario. The DVC® home-cage activity monitoring system, for example, logs movement 24/7 without human intervention. The table of task times shows a stark reduction in effort for certain endpoints: because behavior is tracked automatically, the reliance on some manual tests or long imaging sessions is reduced (here, the frequency or duration of tasks like FT1, FT2, Image 1/2 can be cut in half). Total labor drops to ~101 hours/month (~0.6 FTE), amounting to ~607 hours over 6 months (~3.7 FTE), roughly a 50% reduction in personnel time compared to Fig. 2. Several refined KPIs emerge in this scenario: *Resource Optimization*: Only half the staff time is needed, freeing researchers to conduct other tasks and/or allowing more studies to run in parallel. This improved efficiency directly lowers costs and speeds up research timelines. *Data Quality and Quantity*: Instead of single data points per week, the experiment yields a rich behavioral dataset comprising continuous activity measures, circadian rhythm profiles, etc., for each cage. This leads to an increased statistical power and potentially reduces the number of animals needed to detect effects, because each cage serves as its own control over time

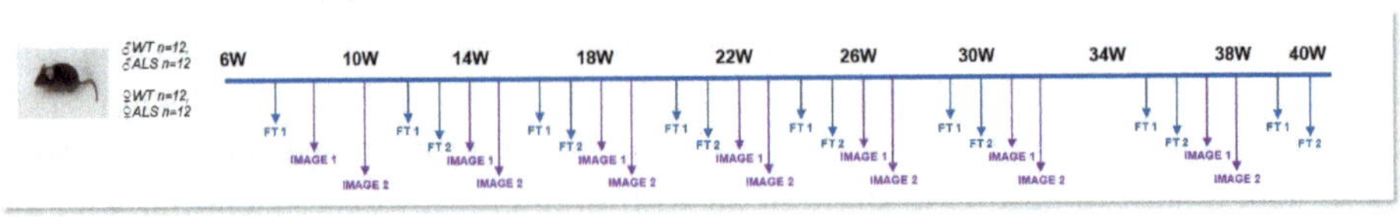

Fig. 2 Conventional ALS Study without HCM

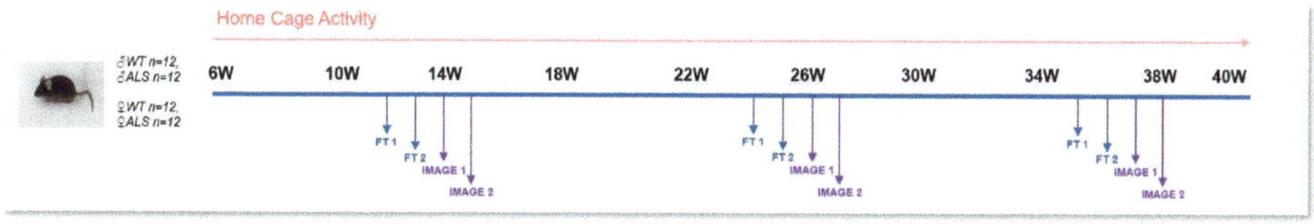

Fig. 3 ALS study with HCM

with many repeated measures. *Enhanced Sensitivity and Predictivity*: Continuous monitoring means early subtle changes (like an emerging limb weakness at 18 weeks, or an unusual activity drop at night) are recorded immediately. This improves predictive modeling: researchers can foresee which animals are starting to decline or respond to treatment before conventional measures signal it. In our ALS example, HCM activity data could show the therapeutic benefit of a drug (e.g., treated mice maintain normal nightly activity levels) weeks before a conventional clinical score difference is apparent. Such sensitivity facilitates early decision-making, allowing investigators to adjust dosing or cull ineffective compounds sooner in the pipeline. *Higher Translatability*: The mobility metrics captured continuously have higher analogs in human clinical observation (such as actigraphy for patient activity). This alignment offers better clinical relevance. As noted in the HCM figure, continuous activity monitoring improved detection of disease onset and provided a more continuous disease readout, which correlates better with how human neurodegenerative diseases progress, and can be considered as a translational digital biomarker. *Animal Welfare Gains*: Perhaps most importantly, the HCM approach keeps mice in their home environment for assessments, drastically reducing handling stress. Mice are monitored in-cage, which minimizes distress and avoids the confounding effects of handling on behavior. Additionally, welfare alerts mean that if an animal's condition worsens, researchers can identify this and implement humane endpoints or treatments promptly, rather than waiting for the next scheduled check. In summary, the HCM-integrated study achieves scientific and operational excellence: more data of better quality, gathered with less effort and animal strain.

To achieve meaningful reductions in animal numbers and cage usage when using HCM technology, it is essential to apply an appropriate study design tailored to its capabilities. This includes considerations such as randomization, blocking, and leveraging continuous behavioral data, which together allow for more efficient group sizes and reduced experimental burden without compromising scientific quality.

The upper panel of Fig. 4 illustrates a conventional four-week study involving 84 mice housed in 21 cages, with three animals per cage. Experimental groups are defined by sex (female and male) and genotype (wild-type and knockout), with seven cages per group. Behavioral testing is conducted manually once per week over four sessions, with imaging in weeks 1 and 4 and histological analysis at study end. The design lacks randomization and blocking, and behavioral data are limited to discrete timepoints. Manual testing requires repeated animal handling and transfers to specialized equipment, increasing labor

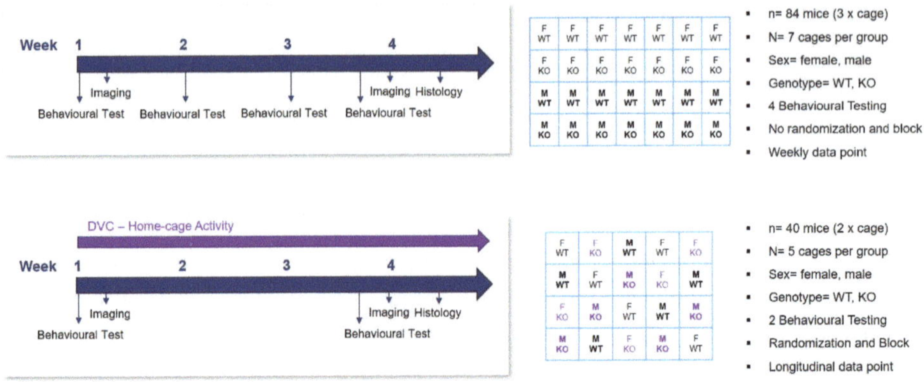

Fig. 4 Traditional vs. HCM integrated study designs in a neurodegenerative mouse model. Comparison of two experimental study designs evaluating behavioral and physiological outcomes in a neurodegenerative mouse model, one using a traditional approach and the other integrating HCM technology

needs and potentially introducing stress-induced variability, which is particularly problematic in neurodegenerative disease models.

The lower panel of Fig. 4 presents a refined study design that incorporates HCM to continuously monitor spontaneous activity in the home cage. In this setup, the number of animals is reduced from 84 to 40, a 52% reduction, and the number of cages from 21 to 10, also a 52% reduction. Each group contains five cages with two animals per cage. The design includes proper randomization and blocking. Behavioral testing is reduced to two sessions, while longitudinal behavioral data are captured automatically without disturbing the animals. Imaging and histology follow the same schedule as in the traditional design.

The difference in cage usage and consumable demand between the two designs has notable implications for operational efficiency and return on investment. Over the four-week period, the traditional setup shown in the upper panel requires 84 cage-weeks, calculated as 21 cages over 4 weeks. Assuming each cage consumes 150 g of food pellets and 100 g of bedding per week, the total material use reaches approximately 12.6 kg of food and 8.4 kg of bedding. With cage changes performed every 2 weeks, the 21 cages require 42 cage change events over the study duration.

In contrast, the HCM-integrated design shown in the lower panel uses only 10 cages across 4 weeks, resulting in 40 cage-weeks. Material consumption is therefore reduced to 6.0 kg of food and 4.0 kg of bedding, representing a 52% reduction in both categories. The number of cage changes also drops to 20 events, reflecting a 52% reduction compared to the traditional setup.

This reduction in cage numbers and associated consumables translates into fewer cages requiring cleaning, sterilization, and handling, significantly lowering water and energy consumption, technician labor hours, and wear on facility infrastructure such as washers, autoclaves, and IVC systems.

From a facility management and return on investment perspective, this shift toward HCM enables substantial cost savings in operational resources and maintenance cycles. These benefits are realized without compromising scientific integrity. On the contrary, HCM enhances data quality by delivering continuous, high-resolution behavioral insights with minimal animal handling. Thus, the integration of HCM supports both ethical research principles and strategic facility optimization.

4.3 Application to the Clinic

When an HCM-derived parameter is applicable in both preclinical and clinical settings, it is referred to as a translational digital biomarker. As discussed earlier in this chapter, biomarkers generally enhance the success rate of clinical trials, and translational digital biomarkers are no exception. These biomarkers can support internal decision-making regarding the progression of clinical trials. When such a biomarker is accepted by the FDA or other regulatory agencies for use in drug approval processes, it is designated a surrogate endpoint, a substitute for a direct clinical endpoint such as survival or symptom improvement.

An example of preclinical HCM in a Parkinson's Disease rat model has been provided by Requejo et al. (2020), who used a dopamine-depletion rat model that mimics the early prodromal stage of the disease. HCM revealed behavioral changes in response to dopamine depletion, including hyperactivity during the light phase and hypoactivity during the dark phase. Such a disruption of the circadian rhythm has also been described in PD patients. The effects of experimental drugs in preclinical R&D can be translated to clinical development. An example of pharmaceutical companies exploring this is illustrated by the ongoing clinical study conducted by Koneska Health, Merck Sharp and Dohme, and Regeneron Pharmaceuticals. Here, digital biomarkers in patients (www.clincialtrials.gov: NCT06219629) are being explored. This longitudinal, observational study aims to assess the usability, analytical and clinical validity, and biomarker discovery for wearable and mobile device measurements of disturbed sleep and neurological disorders.

5 Applications in Safety and Toxicology

5.1 How HCM Can Align with Safety Pharmacology Studies, Complementing Telemetry and Other In-Life Measures

The guidelines ICH M3(R2) on non-clinical safety studies state that studies for clinical development trials and marketing authorization should be performed in two species (one rodent and one non-rodent) (ICH 2025). According to Europe's statistics on the use of animals for scientific purposes in 2022, 499,931 animals were used for "Toxicity and other safety testing including pharmacology" in the "regulatory use purposes" category. The main species used in this category were mice (33.6%) and rats (26.9%) (European Commission 2024).

The use of HCM has been mentioned in the literature since the 1980s (Stoff et al. 1983; Tamborini et al. 1989; Evans 1989). But even if the conclusion was that HCM should be included in toxicity screening, its application in routine safety and toxicology studies did not spread. With the emergence of the automation of HCM data analysis and live data visualization, the integration of HCM is worth considering. The validation of HCM data has been reported in the literature over the past years. They are not considered standard yet, and HCM still needs to be integrated in CROs study catalogue.

As mentioned in the part on pharmacological validation of HCM systems, HCM can at least complement, if not replace, other measures.

Telemetry Telemetry implants allow animal monitoring in their home-cage environment but require surgical intervention. Non-invasive jacketed telemetry tools do not require surgery but add some restraint to the animals. Mösch et al. (2023) published the evaluation of an HCM system for mice and rats, allowing the monitoring of parameters usually assessed via telemetry, such as heart rate, respiratory rate, and body temperature, besides tracking of movement and circadian rhythm (Mösch et al. 2023). If used in preclinical safety pharmacology studies, this kind of system would provide data on unanesthetized and unrestrained animals and help in refining the experimental procedure by reducing the need to perform surgery for telemetry implant or the restraint on animals for jacketed telemetry tools.

Food and Water Intake These measures are not systematically included in the in-life observations of safety and toxicology study designs if no impact is expected or are performed at a predefined frequency, which may be associated with a delayed detection of an impact on the animals. However, changes in these behaviors can be drug-related, either due to a drug effect on the appetite or thirst, or to a more global health deterioration. The automated monitoring of food and water intake represents valuable additional data, without being time-consuming during the experimental procedure.

Locomotor Activity HCM data on locomotor activity can be used as an early sensor of health deterioration and give insights on potential toxic effects and reversibility (Baran et al. 2020; Berridge et al. 2024; Vagima et al. 2020).

5.2 Detection of Subtle Behavior Changes—Signal of Emerging Toxicity or Off-Target Effects

As HCM allows continuous monitoring, it is more susceptible to detecting subtle changes. The following Table 1 gathers some examples of HCM contributions on this topic.

Table 1 Examples of subtle behavior changes detected by HCM systems in pharmacology or toxicology studies

Species	Drug/therapeutic area	Study design	HCM data	Non-HCM data	HCM system	Subtle changes—HCM data input	Reference
Mouse	Valproic acid (VPA, antiepileptic) in drinking water	VPA exposure in adult VPA fetal exposure Group control vs VPA	Water consumption Food consumption Running wheel	Clinical observation Open field (pups)	Phenotyper (Noldus Information Technology)	Diminution of total active state time without alteration of the mean duration of active states or voluntary wheel-running behavior No evidence of social withdrawal with continuous monitoring, which differs from results with short-scored assays of social exploration	Bass et al. (2020)
Rat	Sodium valproate (antiepileptic), intraperitoneally	Fetal exposure Group control vs treated group	Water consumption Locomotor activity	Blood samples Gene expression assay Juvenile social play Maternal Deprivation-Induced Ultrasonic Vocalization	IntelliCage system (manufactured by TSE Systems, Bad Homburg, Germany)	Psychogenic polydipsia, decreased exploration, altered circadian rhythm	Pelsőczi et al. (2020)

(continued)

Table 1 (continued)

Species	Drug/therapeutic area	Study design	HCM data	Non-HCM data	HCM system	Subtle changes—HCM data input	Reference
Mouse	Voluntary ethanol consumption in drinking water	Water group vs low-level prenatal alcohol exposure group	Water consumption Food consumption Locomotor activity	Body weight Blood samples (ethanol) Forelimb grip strength test Beam walk Open-field testing Acoustic startle responses and Prepulse inhibition Motor skill training	Do it yourself system	No alteration of locomotor activity in a familiar environment in chronic low-level prenatal alcohol exposure	Chaudoin et al. (2023)
Mouse	Paroxetine, sub-cutaneous	Saline group vs paroxetine group	Activity Sleep	NA	Continuous Open Mouse Phenotyping of Activity and Sleep Status (COMPASS)	Subtle changes in sleep structure persist for up to a week after discontinuation, which could serve as a biomarker for selective serotonin reuptake inhibitor discontinuation syndrome	Collins et al. (2023)
Mouse	LPS (model of sickness behavior, including pain-like behavior) Indomethacin (anti-inflammatory drug)	Control group vs LPS-treated group	Locomotor activity Behaviors (climbing, rearing, immobility) Water intake Food consumption	Open-field test	LABORAS (Laboratory Animal Behavior Observation, Registration and Analysis System)	More pronounced behavioral changes during the dark phase	Hasriadi et al. (2021a)

Mouse	Carrageenan (inflammatory pain) Indomethacin (anti-inflammatory drug)	Control group vs Carrageenan-treated group	Locomotor activity Behaviors (climbing, rearing, immobility) Water intake Food consumption	Open-field test Rotarod test von Frey filaments and plantar test	LABORAS (Laboratory Animal Behavior Observation, Registration and Analysis System)	Strong correlation between traditional reflexive pain measures and non-reflexive locomotor behaviors which includes long-term locomotor activity data	Hasriadi et al. (2021b)
Mouse	Lycorine (alkaloid analgesic), intraperitoneally	Vehicle group vs chlorpromazine-treated or lycorine-treated groups	Locomotor activity Water intake Food consumption	Rotarod test Body weight Formalin test	LABORAS (Laboratory Animal Behavior Observation, Registration and Analysis System)	CNS safety profile of lycorine	Hasriadi et al. (2024)

Table 2 Examples of HCM data that can be integrated into the clinical or behavioral endpoints

Endpoints	HCM data
General behavior	Food intake Water intake Grooming Aggression Communication/Vocalization
In-cage activity level	Locomotor activity Circadian rhythm Resting Wheel running
Heart activity	Heart rate
Breathing pattern	Respiratory rate
Body condition	Temperature

5.3 Integrating HCM with Physiological Endpoints for a More Holistic Understanding of Compound Safety Profile

For HCM systems in standard housing, with no required additional experimental space, HCM can be implemented by default in toxicology and safety studies if enough equipped cages are available (Table 2).

HCM data can be integrated into the clinical or behavioral endpoints and contribute to the improvement of health monitoring and the refinement of experimental procedures, even more with live data visualization. Implementing HCM in early toxicology studies can generate valuable data for future safety studies. For instance, the detection of health impairments, whether occurring without visible clinical signs or preceding their manifestation, might give critical insights for designing subsequent study protocols. HCM technology-based decisions are already implemented in some laboratories.

6 Implementation of HCM in the Daily Routine

6.1 Overcoming Initial Skepticism

In the process of evaluating and validating HCM systems, it is easier to obtain the support of study directors and technicians if the new systems do not add constraints on the already established study designs. HCM systems that do not need extra experimental space around the home cage and are compatible with the regular housing rooms have better chances to be included in future studies.

When performing pilot studies, a limited number of trained people is required. When deploying HCM systems, the population undergoing training for these systems must be clearly identified.

6.2 Lessons Learned and Best Practices

The sources of interference and/or data variability must be identified and considered in the study design if need be. The home cage environment must be standardized, which can include the type and amount of bedding, the enrichment used and its location in the cage. It is well known that the cage change has an impact on the locomotor activity (Pernold et al. 2019), so the day of the cage change should not be the same as the day of the study start or during the time window of expected drug effect. For video-tracking systems, the camera's field of view must be clear, not be hindered by nesting material, and have a fixed position.

If the HCM system does not provide automated reports or alerts, setting up quality control by checking the hardware and the data collection, before and after the dark phase or the time window of interest, is a good practice that ensures that there is no loss of data during the study. For HCM systems enabling live visualization of data, checking every morning what happened during the last 24 hours is also a good practice, which can uncover early health deterioration or anomaly.

7 Future Outlook and Conclusions

Despite significant technological advancements in recent years, both in hardware and software, HCM remains in its early stages. A number of systems are currently available, developed either by commercial technology providers or as custom-built solutions utilizing open-source software. Most of these technologies have been developed using mice as the primary model organism. It is anticipated that some of these systems will eventually be adapted for use in larger species, including dogs and non-human primates. However, as previously noted, mice remain the predominant species used in experimental research, making them a more economically viable focus for development. Moreover, non-rodent species (i.e., dogs, non-human primates and mini-pigs) are primarily employed in safety studies where GLP regulation represents a higher barrier for implementation.

The miniaturization of sensors and the integration of recorded data with AI/ML are expected to lead to HCM systems that incorporate multiple sensor technologies. At present, systems are typically based on video, Radio-Frequency Identification (RFID), or embedded electronics, such as those used in Tecniplast's DVC® system. These approaches can be complemented by established technologies like telemetry, including ElectroEncephaloGram (EEG), ElectroCardioGram (ECG), blood pressure, and body temperature monitoring.

Ultrasound recording represents another valuable technique. Initially, it was employed to assess anxiety-related behavior in mouse pups using bat detectors. However, advances in high-end microphones and frequency analysis have demonstrated that ultrasonic vocalizations can also be used in adolescent and adult rodents to investigate the neurobiology of socio-affective communication (Wöhr and Schwarting 2013). Although the analysis of these vocalizations has traditionally been time-consuming, AI/ML tools have significantly improved efficiency (e.g., Pessoa et al. 2020). The use of sound cameras or the integration of vocalization data with RFID or video-based identification of individual animals could yield highly informative compound fingerprints or facilitate disease model characterization. Nevertheless, it remains uncertain whether these technologies can be effectively combined into a unified HCM approach and whether such integration would be financially scalable.

The cost of implementing HCM technologies will remain a key factor influencing their adoption in standard animal facilities, even when based on single-sensor systems. Not only is the expense of the hardware significant, but the demand for computing power and data storage should also not be underestimated.

We anticipate that, in the near future, animal facilities in industrial settings will expand their HCM capabilities, likely incorporating a variety of different systems. Depending on the specific requirements of each animal experiment, the most suitable HCM approach can be selected to ensure an optimal balance between cost and benefit. A key consideration is whether data should be collected at the level of individual animals or as cage-level averages. While cage-level data acquisition is generally more cost-effective, both in terms of hardware requirements and computational resources such as processing time and data storage, individual-level data offers greater statistical power per cage, which may, in turn, allow for a reduction in the overall number of animals required per experimental group.

Ongoing reductions in hardware size and cost, along with the increasing availability of (open-source) AI/ML-based algorithms, are expected to accelerate the integration of HCM in both industrial and academic environments. Ultimately, the value proposition of HCM will increase substantially once clear examples emerge demonstrating its utility as a translational digital biomarker in clinical settings. The integration HCM has received positive feedback from regulatory authorities. While its implementation is acknowledged as an advancement in animal health assessment, incorporating HCM technology into drug development submissions necessitates an additional validation process. This process must ensure compliance with Good Laboratory Practice (GLP) computerized systems requirements (OECD 1995). Consequently, HCM technologies are more likely to find widespread adoption in non-GLP preclinical studies, where they can accelerate drug candidate selection, rather than being incorporated into market authorization submissions.

References

Bains RS, Wells S, Sillito RR, Armstrong JD, Cater HL, Banks G, Nolan PM (2018) Assessing mouse behaviour throughout the light/dark cycle using automated in-cage analysis tools. J Neurosci Methods 300:37–47. https://doi.org/10.1016/j.jneumeth.2017.04.014

Baran SW, Gupta AD, Lim MA, Mathur A, Rowlands DJ, Schaevitz LR, Shanmukhappa SK, Walker DB (2020) Continuous, automated breathing rate and body motion monitoring of rats with paraquat-induced progressive lung injury. Front Physiol 11:569001. https://doi.org/10.3389/fphys.2020.569001

Baran SW, Bolin SE, Gaburro S, van Gaalen MM, LaFollette MR, Liu C-N, Maguire S, Noldus LPJJ, Bratcher-Petersen N, Berridge BR (2025) Validation framework for in vivo digital measures. Front Toxicol 6:1484895. https://doi.org/10.3389/ftox.2024.1484895

Bass JS, Tuo AH, Ton LT, Jankovic MJ, Kapadia PK, Schirmer C, Krishnan V (2020) On the digital psychopharmacology of valproic acid in mice. Front Neurosci 14:594612. https://doi.org/10.3389/fnins.2020.594612

Bennett EJ, Mead RJ, Azzouz M, Shaw PJ, Grierson AJ (2014) Early detection of motor dysfunction in the SOD1G93A mouse model of Amyotrophic Lateral Sclerosis (ALS) using home cage running wheels. PLoS One 9(9):e107918. https://doi.org/10.1371/journal.pone.0107918

Berridge BR, Baran SW, Kumar V, Bratcher-Petersen N, Ellis M, Liu C-N, Robertson TL (2024) Digitalization of toxicology: improving preclinical to clinical translation. Front Toxicol 6:1377542. https://doi.org/10.3389/ftox.2024.1377542

Califf RM (2018) Biomarker definitions and their applications. Exp Biol Med (Maywood) 243(3):213–221. https://doi.org/10.1177/1535370217750088

Chaudoin TR, Bonasera SJ, Dunaevsky A, Padmashri R (2023) Exploring behavioral phenotypes in a mouse model of fetal alcohol spectrum disorders. Dev Neurobiol 83(5–6):184–204. https://doi.org/10.1002/dneu.22922

Collins HM, Pinacho R, Tam SKE, Sharp T, Bannerman DM, Peirson SN (2023) Continuous home cage monitoring of activity and sleep in mice during repeated paroxetine treatment and discontinuation. Psychopharmacology (Berl) 240(11):2403–2418. https://doi.org/10.1007/s00213-023-06442-3

Coravos A, Goldsack JC, Karlin DR, Nebeker C, Perakslis E, Zimmerman N, Erb MK (2019) Digital medicine: a primer on measurement. Digit Biomark 3(2):31–71. https://doi.org/10.1159/000500413

Crabbe JC, Wahlsten D, Dudek BC (1999) Genetics of mouse behavior: interactions with laboratory environment. Science 284(5420):1670–1672. https://doi.org/10.1126/science.284.5420.1670

European Commission (2024) Summary report on the statistics on the use of animals for scientific purposes in the Member States of the European Union and Norway in 2022. https://data.consilium.europa.eu/doc/document/ST-12496-2024-INIT/en/pdf

European Medicines Agency (2017) Guideline on strategies to identify and mitigate risks for first-in-human and early clinical trials with investigational medicinal products. https://www.ema.europa.eu/en/documents/scientific-guideline/guideline-strategies-identify-and-mitigate-risks-first-human-and-early-clinical-trials-investigational-medicinal-products-revision-1_en.pdf

Evans HL (1989) Behaviors in the home cage reveal toxicity: recent findings and proposals for the future. J Am Coll Toxicol 8(1):35–52. https://doi.org/10.3109/10915818909009092

Golini E, Rigamonti M, Iannello F, De Rosa C, Scavizzi F, Raspa M, Mandillo S (2020) A non-invasive digital biomarker for the detection of rest disturbances in the sod1g93a mouse model of als. Front Neurosci 14:896. https://doi.org/10.3389/fnins.2020.00896

Grieco F, Bernstein BJ, Biemans B, Bikovski L, Burnett CJ, Cushman JD, van Dam EA, Fry SA, Richmond-Hacham B, Homberg JR, Kas MJH, Kessels HW, Koopmans B, Krashes MJ, Krishnan V, Logan S, Loos M, McCann KE, Parduzi Q, Pick CG, Prevot TD, Riedel G, Robinson L, Sadighi M, Smit AB, Sonntag W, Roelofs RF, Tegelenbosch RAJ, Noldus LPJJ (2021) Measuring behavior in the home cage: study design, applications, challenges, and perspectives. Front Behav Neurosci 15:735387. https://doi.org/10.3389/fnbeh.2021.735387

Hasriadi H, Wasana PWD, Vajragupta O, Rojsitthisak P, Towiwat P (2021a) Automated home-cage monitoring as a potential measure of sickness behaviors and pain-like behaviors in LPS-treated mice. PLoS One 16(8):e0256706. https://doi.org/10.1371/journal.pone.0256706

Hasriadi H, Wasana PWD, Vajragupta O, Rojsitthisak P, Towiwat P (2021b) Automated home-cage for the evaluation of innate non-reflexive pain behaviors in a mouse model of inflammatory pain. Sci Rep 11(1):12240. https://doi.org/10.1038/s41598-021-91444-4

Hasriadi H, Wasana PWD, Thongphichai W, Sukrong S, Towiwat P (2024) Exploring the safety of lycorine in the central nervous system and its impact on pain-like behaviors in mice. Sci Rep 14(1):16856. https://doi.org/10.1038/s41598-024-64410-z

Hohlbaum K, Andresen N, Mieske P, Kahnau P, Lang B, Diederich K, Palme R, Mundhenk L, Sprekeler H, Hellwich O, Thöne-Reineke C, Lewejohann L (2024) Lockbox enrichment facilitates manipulative and cognitive activities for mice. Open Res Eur 4:108. https://doi.org/10.12688/openreseurope.17624.2

ICH (2025) In: International Council for Harmonisation Official web site. https://www.ich.org/

Kaffman A, White JD, Wei L, Johnson FK, Krystal JH (2019) Enhancing the utility of preclinical research in neuropsychiatry drug development. Methods Mol Biol 2011:3–22. https://doi.org/10.1007/978-1-4939-9554-7_1

Kahnau P, Mieske P, Wilzopolski J, Kalliokoski O, Mandillo S, Hölter SM, Voikar V, Amfim A, Badurek S, Bartelik A, Caruso A, Čater M, Ey E, Golini E, Jaap A, Hrncic D, Kiryk A, Lang B, Loncarevic-Vasiljkovic N, Meziane H, Radzevičienė A, Rivalan M, Scattoni ML, Torquet N, Trifkovic J, Ulfhake B, Thöne-Reineke C, Diederich K, Lewejohann L, Hohlbaum K (2023) A systematic review of the development and application of home cage monitoring in laboratory mice and rats. BMC Biol 21(1):256. https://doi.org/10.1186/s12915-023-01751-7

Louis-Maerten E, Rodriguez Perez C, Cajiga RM, Persson K, Elger BS (2024) Conceptual foundations for a clarified meaning of the 3Rs principles in animal experimentation. Anim Welf 33:e37. https://doi.org/10.1017/awf.2024.39

Mingrone A, Kaffman A, Kaffman A (2020) The promise of automated home-cage monitoring in improving translational utility of psychiatric research in rodents. Front Neurosci 14:618593. https://doi.org/10.3389/fnins.2020.618593

Moore JL, Kennedy J, Hassan A-A (2024) Automated home cage monitoring of an aging colony of mice—implications for welfare monitoring and experimentation. Front Neurosci 18:1489308. https://doi.org/10.3389/fnins.2024.1489308

Mösch L, Kunczik J, Breuer L, Merhof D, Gass P, Potschka H, Zechner D, Vollmar B, Tolba R, Häger C, Bleich A, Czaplik M, Pereira CB (2023) Towards substitution of invasive telemetry: an integrated home cage concept for unobtrusive monitoring of objective physiological parameters in rodents. PLoS One 18(9):e0286230. https://doi.org/10.1371/journal.pone.0286230

Motahari-Nezhad H, Péntek M, Gulácsi L, Zrubka Z (2021) Outcomes of digital biomarker-based interventions: protocol for a systematic review of systematic reviews. JMIR Res Protoc 10(11):e28204. https://doi.org/10.2196/28204

OECD (1995) The application of the principles of GLP to computerised systems. OECD

Pelsőczi P, Kelemen K, Csölle C, Nagy G, Lendvai B, Román V, Lévay G (2020) Disrupted social hierarchy in prenatally valproate-exposed autistic-like rats. Front Behav Neurosci 13:295. https://doi.org/10.3389/fnbeh.2019.00295

Pernold K, Iannello F, Low BE, Rigamonti M, Rosati G, Scavizzi F, Wang J, Raspa M, Wiles MV, Ulfhake B (2019) Towards large scale automated cage monitoring – Diurnal rhythm and impact of interventions on in-cage activity of C57BL/6J mice recorded 24/7 with a non-disrupting capacitive-based technique. PLoS One 14(2):e0211063. https://doi.org/10.1371/journal.pone.0211063

Pessoa D, Petrella L, Castelo-Branco M, Teixeira C (2020) Automatic segmentation of ultrasonic vocalizations in rodents. In: Henriques J, Neves N, de Carvalho P (eds) XV Mediterranean conference on medical and biological engineering and computing – MEDICON 2019. Springer International Publishing, Cham, pp 37–46

Petersen N, Adank DN, Raghavan R, Winder DG, Doyle MA (2023) LIQ HD (lick instance quantifier home cage device): an open-source tool for recording undisturbed two-bottle drinking behavior in a home cage environment. eNeuro 10(4):ENEURO.0506-22.2023. https://doi.org/10.1523/ENEURO.0506-22.2023

Piilgaard L, Rose L, Justinussen JL, Hviid CG, Lemcke R, Wellendorph P, Kornum BR (2023) Non-invasive detection of narcolepsy type I phenotypical features and disease progression by continuous home-cage monitoring of activity in two mouse models: the HCRT-KO and DTA model. Sleep 46(9):zsad144. https://doi.org/10.1093/sleep/zsad144

Requejo C, López-de-Ipiña K, Ruiz-Ortega JÁ, Fernández E, Calvo PM, Morera-Herreras T, Miguelez C, Cardona-Grifoll L, Cepeda H, Ugedo L, Lafuente JV (2020) Changes in day/night activity in the 6-OHDA-induced experimental model of Parkinson's disease: exploring prodromal biomarkers. Front Neurosci 14. https://doi.org/10.3389/fnins.2020.590029

Riga MS, Pérez-Fernández M, Miquel-Rio L, Paz V, Campa L, Martínez-Losa M, Esteban FJ, Callado LF, Meana J, Artigas F, Bortolozzi A, Álvarez-Dolado M (2024) Scn1a haploinsufficiency in the prefrontal cortex leads to cognitive impairment and depressive phenotype. Brain 147(12):4169–4184. https://doi.org/10.1093/brain/awae167

Robinson L, Riedel G (2014) Comparison of automated home-cage monitoring systems: emphasis on feeding behaviour, activity and spatial learning following pharmacological interventions. J Neurosci Methods 234:13–25. https://doi.org/10.1016/j.jneumeth.2014.06.013

Sertkaya A, Beleche T, Jessup A, Sommers BD (2024) Costs of drug development and research and development intensity in the US, 2000–2018. JAMA Netw Open 7(6):e2415445. https://doi.org/10.1001/jamanetworkopen.2024.15445

Stoff DM, Stauderman K, Wyatt RJ (1983) The time and space machine: continuous measurement of drug-induced behavior patterns in the rat. Psychopharmacology (Berl) 80(4):319–324. https://doi.org/10.1007/BF00432113

Tamborini P, Sigg H, Zbinden G (1989) Quantitative analysis of rat activity in the home cage by infrared monitoring. Application to the acute toxicity testing of acetanilide and phenylmercuric acetate. Arch Toxicol 63(2):85–96. https://doi.org/10.1007/BF00316429

TEATIME Action (2025) Home cage monitoring technologies. https://www.cost-teatime.org/about/technologies/

Terry S, Gommet C, Kerangueven A-C, Leguet M, Thévenin V, Berthelot M, Begoud L, Windenberger F, Lainee P (2023) Activity in group-housed home cages of mice as a novel preclinical biomarker in oncology studies. Cancers (Basel) 15(19):4798. https://doi.org/10.3390/cancers15194798

Tse K, Sillito R, Keerie A, Collier R, Grant C, Karp NA, Vickers C, Chapman K, Armstrong JD, Redfern WS (2018) Pharmacological validation of individual animal locomotion, temperature and behavioural analysis in group-housed rats using a novel automated home cage analysis system: a comparison with the modified Irwin test. J Pharmacol Toxicol Methods 94(Pt 1):1–13. https://doi.org/10.1016/j.vascn.2018.03.008

Vagima Y, Grauer E, Politi B, Maimon S, Yitzhak E, Melamed S, Achdout H, Gur D, Aftalion M, Shemesh A, Hasson A, Yitzhaki S, Shapira SC, Mamroud E (2020) Group activity of mice in communal home cage used as an indicator of disease progression and rate of recovery: effects of LPS and influenza virus. Life Sci 258:118214. https://doi.org/10.1016/j.lfs.2020.118214

Voehringer P, Nicholson JR (2020) Minimum information in in vivo research. In: Bespalov A, Michel MC, Steckler T (eds) Good research practice in non-clinical pharmacology and biomedicine. Springer International Publishing, Cham, pp 197–222

Wöhr M, Schwarting RKW (2013) Affective communication in rodents: ultrasonic vocalizations as a tool for research on emotion and motivation. Cell Tissue Res 354(1):81–97. https://doi.org/10.1007/s00441-013-1607-9

Wong CH, Siah KW, Lo AW (2019) Estimation of clinical trial success rates and related parameters. Biostatistics 20(2):273–286. https://doi.org/10.1093/biostatistics/kxx069

Wouters OJ, McKee M, Luyten J (2020) Estimated research and development investment needed to bring a new medicine to market, 2009–2018. JAMA 323(9):844. https://doi.org/10.1001/jama.2020.1166

Zentrich E, Talbot SR, Bleich A, Häger C (2021) Automated home-cage monitoring during acute experimental colitis in mice. Front Neurosci 15:760606. https://doi.org/10.3389/fnins.2021.760606

Commercializing Home Cage Monitoring: From Prototype to Global Access

Michael Florea, Noah Weber, Christopher K. Adams, John Lighton, Robbin Turner, Matt Ruiter, and Stefano Gaburro

Abstract

Even the greatest invention is useless if it does not become widely accessible. This chapter presents a practical framework for commercializing and scaling automated home cage monitoring (HCM) systems used in laboratory animal research. It traces the path from prototype to industrial-grade, globally deployable product, integrating principles of engineering, manufacturing, software development and compliance.

The chapter outlines how product-market fit is achieved through user need identification, pilot validation, and economic feasibility. It details the process of productization and manufacturability, covering lean prototyping, material selection and transition to scalable industrial methods. Key manufacturing topics include process standardization, automation and quality systems aligned with ISO 9001, GLP, and CE/FCC requirements.

The chapter also covers the software and data infrastructure that underpin HCM technologies, including embedded firmware, secured cloud architectures and Software

M. Florea (✉) · N. Weber
Olden Labs, South San Francisco, CA, USA
e-mail: michael@oldenlabs.com

C. K. Adams
Columbus Instruments, Columbus, OH, USA

J. Lighton · R. Turner
Sable Systems International, North Las Vegas, NV, USA

M. Ruiter
Unified Information Devices, Kenosha, WI, USA

S. Gaburro
Tecniplast S.p.A, Buguggiate, VA, Italy

S. Gaburro, S. Mandillo (eds.), *Home Cage Monitoring in Rodents: A Global Effort*,
https://doi.org/10.1007/978-3-032-19781-8_6

as a Service (SaaS) models for scalable analytics. Sustainability, ethical sourcing, and lifecycle design are integrated throughout.

Finally, the chapter examines global deployment strategies: resilient supply chains, interoperable data systems and open science principles, which together ensure reproducibility, reliability, and long-term access.

Keywords
Manufacturing · 3D printing · Entrepreneurship · Customer service · AI · Automation · Physiological Monitoring

1 Introduction

Home Cage Monitoring (HCM) systems represent a significant advancement in preclinical research, mechanistic studies, and animal husbandry. However, moving from functional prototypes to globally deployed, dependable, and affordable systems presents a distinct challenge.

The translation of an academic prototype into a commercial product requires an understanding of user needs, manufacturability, compliance, and long-term support. Academic designs often function as bespoke instruments built for a single study, optimized for flexibility, and maintained by expert users. Commercial systems must, first and foremost, fulfill the need of a wide variety of users. They must operate continuously across many installations and conditions and be durable, serviceable, and supported by a supply chain that ensures uptime and consistency of performance.

This chapter describes the complete lifecycle required to bring automated monitoring systems from concept to scalable access. It begins with an examination of market needs and the process of establishing product-market fit. It then outlines the transition from prototype development to productization, focusing on manufacturability, materials, and design principles. The discussion moves through scaling production, standardizing processes, and maintaining quality assurance in complex supply chains. Later sections address the software and data infrastructure that enable large-scale operation, along with regulatory, ethical, and sustainability considerations. The final sections focus on customer support, multigenerational product planning, and strategies for long-term access and adoption.

2 Product-Market Fit

2.1 Identifying Needs

Often, first prototypes are developed to fulfill the immediate need of the author. Building a product, however, requires establishing whether this need matches that of many other people. If it does, the product has the potential to achieve Product-Market Fit (PMF) and become widely used. Most products fail at this stage, even though engineering, marketing, and sales may continue for years after launch. Therefore, understanding the user's need *precisely and deeply* is critical, before any engineering is done.

The core users for HCM are neuroscientists, pharmacologists, toxicologists, behavioral scientists, sleep researchers, longevity researchers, animal facility managers, and anyone who requires reproducible animal health or cage condition data.

2.2 Validating Customer Pain Points

Understanding user requirements requires structured engagement with stakeholders across the research pipeline. A great way to do this is by following the structure outlined in the book The Mom Test (Fitzpatrick 2013)—structured but informal asking about a prospective user's pain points without any mention of the possible product in mind. This reduces bias and enables identification of whether the supposed problem is even a real problem worth solving. In animal research, facility managers emphasize robustness, ease of cleaning, and compatibility with standard cage formats. Scientists focus on data quality, analysis workflows, and integration with laboratory information systems. Technicians value reliability, serviceability, and intuitive operation. Feedback on hindrances to adoption of existing HCM systems frequently highlights high costs, excessive data volume, nonintuitive software interfaces, or hardware designs that complicate cage handling and washing.

2.3 Pilot Deployments

Mapping customer profiles and their pain points and engineering of prototype devices should be followed by rapid pilot installations in selected beta users' facilities. Entrepreneurs sometimes delay this step, fearing reputational damage or simply sobering feedback; however, these deployments provide empirical evidence of value in authentic laboratory conditions. A successful pilot validates that the proposed solution truly addresses the user need, despite the likely existence of many technical limitations. Getting *real, external* user feedback as fast and with as few resources as possible is the key driver of learning and the key concept behind the Lean Startup paradigm (Ries 2011). Therefore, prototyping and pilot deployments should be viewed as essential experiments that give feedback on where development is most needed and whether the design concept is ready for the next stage—a fully functional prototype ready for paying users.

2.4 Iterating on Design

Until user's need is solved, based on evidence, pilots should continue to iterate as rapidly as possible, removing key technical deficiencies. Sustained iteration transforms a technical success into a dependable laboratory instrument. Until the entrepreneur is confident that their system solves the key need, a minimum viable product (MVP) has not been created—even if the system is complex and advanced.

In the case of HCM systems, key requirements are simplified cage integration, sealed electronics for washing, ease of use and cleaning, and improved lighting geometry for imaging and automated data processing pipelines.

2.5 Solving for Economics

A key part of the design is understanding economics and user purchasing capabilities and behaviors. A solution is only a solution if users can actually buy it. In general, for a system to spread widely, it must either (a) reduce costs, (b) give new capabilities, or (c) improve the quality and rigor of existing methods. Often, for adoption to occur, it must offer all three to overcome adoption barriers. The pricing and sales model must reflect these realities. The price that users can afford (while net saving money compared to alternatives) dictates the upper bound of the cost of manufacturing a system. This price ceiling dictates design in all aspects. Therefore, understanding economics of the industry directly influences the design of the system.

For the case of HCM systems, the commercial model must reflect how institutions can acquire and maintain scientific equipment. Generally, larger laboratories prefer direct purchase of hardware upfront or sometimes combined with annual software or service agreements. Smaller research groups often benefit from leasing programs that distribute costs over time while including maintenance and software updates. Academic labs and pharma often prefer upfront payments (due to grant funding and institutional bureaucracy), while biotech companies and Contract Research Organizations (CROs) prefer lower upfront costs and spread of the costs across time or their internal users.

Early experimentation with these models clarifies both financial viability and adoption barriers, allowing commercialization strategies to evolve in parallel with product refinement.

3 Productization and Design for Manufacturability

Productization is the process of turning a functioning prototype into a reliable, manufacturable instrument that can be deployed across research facilities. The goal is to move from a one-off laboratory built to a system that can be produced consistently, cleaned and serviced easily, and used for years without degradation. This consists of prototyping, translation, design refinement, material selection, and industrialization. Each stage adds structure and repeatability to what began as an experimental tool.

3.1 Prototyping: Speed

Early development should prioritize speed and learning. The objective is to build devices that answer specific questions with the least time and cost. Using 3D printing, laser cutting, and outsourced metal work to fabricate mechanical parts and relying on off-the-shelf sensors, microcontrollers, and cameras to avoid unnecessary engineering are generally the fastest ways to achieve this. Prototype assemblies should be simple, modular, and repairable by hand. Components should be screwed together rather than be glued or permanently fixed, allowing reconfiguration in hours rather than weeks.

Low-volume, lean methods make it possible to build, test, and iterate quickly. A prototype that records stable animal activity for 1 week provides more useful data than a perfect design that never reaches a cage. Each prototype cycle should test core functions: sensor reliability, cage compatibility, durability under cage changes, and ease of cleaning. By tracking material costs and assembly time, these early builds also reveal the practical limits of future production cost. Understanding these constraints early shapes every later design decision.

3.2 Translating Prototypes into Products

Once a prototype reliably solves a scientific problem, it must be transformed into a repeatable product. The focus shifts from experimentation to scalability, manufacturability, and stability. A deployable system must withstand bedding dust, humidity, vibration, chewing by animals, and exposure to disinfectants. Ideally, it should integrate seamlessly with existing cage bottoms for improved cleaning workflows. Design elements should support quick installation, minimal maintenance, and operation by animal care staff with standard training.

Design for Manufacturing and Assembly (DFMA) often requires substantial redesign of the original system to reduce complexity and costs and increase robustness and redundancy of supply chain (Juniani et al. 2022). This process, however, must retain the key features that enable solution of the user need, including the price point that can effectively be adopted. Steps in this process can involve redesigning parts for volume manufacturing (below), reducing the number of components, simplifying each subsystem so that it can be built, tested, and cleaned easily, integrating related parts into single assemblies, reducing the number of fasteners and tools needed for assembly, and other steps. Ideally, the user should be able to service the unit with minimal tools provided by you. If this is not the case, the future support and maintenance load will be high.

For HCM systems, it is a good practice to design with testing and cleaning in mind, including access points for calibration and inspection, avoiding deep recesses where bedding or liquids can collect. As possible, smooth curves and seal joints to extend lifetime and simplify sanitation. Each unit should be testable before shipment using a short, repeatable validation routine that confirms sensor response, image quality, or connectivity. Good

DFMA practice lowers cost, improves yield, and increases confidence that all units will perform identically.

3.3 Materials and Durability

A key consideration in the choice of materials is whether a component will come into contact with animals or not, whether it must be washable/disinfectable, and whether it must be autoclavable. For many components of HCM systems, they must survive daily use in humid, abrasive, and chemically active environments. Materials should be chosen to resist mechanical wear, heat, and cleaning agents. Early-stage plastics such as PLA are acceptable for prototypes or single-use designs but not suited for scalable manufacturing. When using 3D printing, be mindful to avoid toxic filaments or resins, such as ABS (Wojtyła et al. 2017). Long-term systems should use polycarbonate, Ultem, anodized aluminum, or stainless steel. Nontoxic 3D printed filaments can be used for single-use products, but this should be limited to low-medium volume (up to 1000/year) products due to the scalability limitations of 3D printing.

Durability testing should simulate real facility conditions: cage wash cycles, exposure to ammonia, and repeated handling by staff. Connectors and seals must tolerate moisture, and optics should resist fogging. Every component should maintain calibration and structural integrity through months of operation. Selecting the correct materials at this stage prevents downstream failures and reduces maintenance costs across installations.

3.4 Transition to Industrial Methods

When prototypes mature and demand increases, production must move to industrial fabrication. Injection molding is the standard for large-volume plastic parts, producing consistent, cleanable components such as cage adapters, housings, and mounting brackets. Machining is ideal for medium-volume parts that require precision, stiffness, or heat resistance, including enclosures and load-bearing frames. Laser cutting and bending are efficient for structural sheet components and mounting plates.

Industrialization requires detailed specifications—tolerances, surface finishes, and assembly procedures—to ensure repeatability across suppliers. Finishes such as electropolishing, anodizing, and powder coating improve chemical resistance and cleanability (Groover 2020). The goal is not only to scale production, but to maintain scientific reliability across every deployed unit. A well-documented, industrially manufactured system becomes a true research instrument: reproducible, serviceable, and trusted in long-term studies.

4 Manufacturing and Quality Systems

The journey from "new product" to becoming a household name is epic. Fundamentally, a product cannot grow from prototype to being market leader without scalability. Generally speaking, sales grow manufacturing, manufacturing grows service, and service grows sales. Some of these are more scalable than the others, and manufacturing is the most challenging of them all. As demand increases, so does the speed at which parts must be made, assembled, and tested for quality and function.

4.1 Manufacturing of Parts

Once the design is perfected, it must be scaled for everyday use. For HCM equipment, it must survive being scratched, chewed, dropped, cage-washed, autoclaved, and vaped. Many of the plastics used for 3D printing lack the robustness to survive all these conditions. As a general rule, the more robust the plastic, the more difficult it is to 3D print (Groover 2020). As a product transitions from prototype to production, alternative materials and methods must be adopted. The CAD drawings used for 3D printing can be mostly applied to injection molding, machining, laser cutting, and metal bending; however, sometimes, modifications to the designs are required to be compatible with these higher-volume processes. The step of going from a 3D printed or low-volume design to a mass-manufacturable design often requires specialized expertise and in-depth knowledge of specific machines used for production.

Various manufacturing technologies can be used to produce consistent "rubber stamp" parts with the exceptional strength and longevity. Many different production methods exist and covering them is beyond the scope of this chapter. However, the main ones are:

Injection Molding To withstand the rigors of routine use and washing, injection molding of thermoplastic is used to produce all cage bottoms used in laboratories around the world. Injection molding has notoriously high startup costs because the molds are very expensive to make, normally in the order of $10,000–$100,000 per part. But beyond the initial cost, injection molding is ideally suited for high volume production of precision pieces that need high durability with a low per-unit price point. "High volume" may be an understatement, as tens or hundreds of thousands of units must be sold to recoup the initial startup investment and offer a worthwhile return.

Laser-Cutting Stainless steel and aluminum offer the highest durability but at an increased direct and *indirect* cost. The precision and consistency of parts produced by laser-cutting are unmatched, but unlike injection molding, it's a multistep process to the finished product. Sharp edges are typically smoothed by a tumbler machine. This vibrates the parts in an abrasive compound and is ideal for deburring a large quantity of parts all at once. Once freed of sharp edges, the metal surface must be finished to protect against corrosion. There are many options for this, but quality products typically use one of these three:

Electropolishing Stainless steel parts are placed in an electrolyte bath and then a DC current is applied to dissolve a thin layer of the metal at the surface. The finished product is highly corrosion-resistant. The process removes free iron particles from the surface, increasing the concentration of chromium, leaving it corrosion-resistant. Electropolishing also micro-deburrs the surface, leaving it perfectly smooth and safe for animal use. It also has undeniable esthetic appeal with its shiny, chrome-like appearance.

Anodizing Aluminum parts are a different electrolytic process that produces an oxide-protective coating, typically 5 to 25 μm in thickness, and is used to give improved surface resistance to wear and corrosion. An esthetic advance to anodizing is the vast array of colors and finishes available for the final piece.

Powder Coating Stainless steel can be protected more economically with powder coating. This is an electrostatically applied dry powder that is then heated and bonded to the material. It offers more robust protection than paint. Powder coat can be applied to aluminum, but it does not offer the same level of protection as anodizing. The anodizing is part of the metal and cannot peel or chip, whereby powder coating is adhered to it. The costs are similar, with anodizing being more cost-effective for small runs and powder coating being more efficient for large batches.

CNC Machining Specialty parts made at a more moderate volume are more effectively produced in a machine shop. Specialty tools like robotic routers, CNC mills, lathes, and waterjets can make complex parts with great precision in a relatively short time. Their programming is an extension of the CAD drawings used for the prototype to ensure consistency. There is also a wide variety of materials that can be machined, like stainless steel, aluminum, polycarbonate, PVC, and acrylic. The tools are a substantial investment, take up a lot of space, and are often cost-prohibitive but offer the widest flexibility in material choice, complexity of design, and speed in which the piece can be produced.

4.2 Assembly

A product requires assembly and quality control in addition to parts. At volume, assembly inefficiencies compound quickly. Assembly must therefore be organized as a repeatable, standardized process. Each step should be clear, measurable, and optimized for time, motion, and quality. The objective is to achieve consistent output with minimal variation, regardless of who performs the task.

For HCM systems, assembly involves integrating optical modules or other sensor modules, food hoppers, water bottle holders, test objects, and enclosures into units that function identically across hundreds of cages.

Well-designed assembly requires purposeful design of the assembly process, accurate documentation, and standard operating procedures that are robust to variations in components and variations in workforce availability and workforce level of training. Every unit should be traceable through its serial number, with records showing which components were installed, by whom, and when. This ensures accountability and supports long-term reliability. Efficiency in assembly also depends on the flow of materials. Delays from missing components or disorganized inventory can halt production entirely. The Bill of Materials (BOM) must list every component, from screws to sensors, with clear specifications and suppliers. Each part should have two independent vendors to prevent supply chain bottlenecks. Regular audits of parts, tools, and consumables prevent production stalls and maintain delivery timelines.

A scalable assembly line for automated animal monitoring technology focuses on precision and cleanliness as much as throughput. Every subassembly—camera module, lighting unit, or sensor base—should be individually tested before final integration. End-of-line testing must confirm full system function, connectivity, and calibration. These checks ensure that units are ready for immediate use upon delivery to research facilities. Finally, the assembled product must be sterilized and packaged in a sterile setting.

A new assembly line for a new product should always start with human workers. Once an assembly process has been developed and time-tested, automation can be considered to reduce the highest labor bottlenecks or most dangerous tasks. Only then and if supported by sufficient volume should end-to-end automation be considered.

The assembly line must be quantified and embedded into automatic recordkeeping systems that join inventory management, ordering, and product fulfillment information into a single system. This enables identification of failure trends (whether a fault arises from a specific supplier batch, assembly procedure, or testing step), informs accounting by capturing true costs associated with scrap, rework, and warranty replacements, and ensures timely orders for parts. Digital tracking tools, such as manufacturing execution systems (MES) or integrated spreadsheets for smaller operations, can provide part-level accountability and improve accuracy in both technical and financial reporting.

4.3 Process Standardization: SOPs and Reproducibility for High-Quality Production

Establishing uniform assembly protocols is crucial for maintaining consistency, quality, and efficiency in manufacturing processes. Standard Operating Procedures (SOPs) serve as comprehensive guidelines that delineate each step of the manufacturing process, ensuring that all personnel adhere to the same methods and quality standards. The reality of the assembly floor is that the worker turnover can be high. Therefore, individual steps of the assembly must be clearly documented and be effective even in the hands of minimally trained workers. Comprehensive quality checks at the end of line are required to identify any assembly errors. This standardization minimizes variability, reduces the likelihood of errors, and ensures that each HCM system produced meets predetermined quality benchmarks.

4.4 Automation: Robotics and AI

As production matures, automation can become an important factor in ensuring consistent output, long-term efficiency, and lower costs. Once human-driven assembly lines are fully defined and stable, selective automation can replace repetitive, labor-intensive, or precision-critical tasks. Robotics can be introduced to handle standardized steps such as component placement, fastening, and inspection, sensor calibrations, and part placement, improving accuracy while reducing fatigue-related errors.

Additionally, use of computer vision and AI can speed up quality control through inspection of parts. However, it is prudent to perform a cost-benefit analysis at each automated step, since automation can introduce complexity and require its own maintenance.

4.5 Quality Assurance and Compliance

Robust Quality Management Systems (QMS) are essential to ensure that HCM (HCM) systems meet international standards, maintain reliability, and support scientific integrity. Frameworks such as ISO 9001, Good Laboratory Practice (GLP), and regional certifications like CE and FCC establish the foundation for consistent quality and compliance across all stages of product development and manufacturing.

A well-structured QMS integrates quality into every process—from design and supplier management to assembly, calibration, and service. ISO 9001 emphasizes documentation, internal audits, and continuous improvement, ensuring that nonconformances are identified and corrected systematically. For HCM systems, this means controlled workflows, qualified suppliers, and standardized testing procedures that guarantee reproducibility and reduce variability across installations.

Alignment with GLP principles ensures that devices meet the same standards of data integrity required in regulated research. Each system must have validated performance records, calibration logs, and verifiable audit trails linking hardware, software, and analytical outputs. Compliance with CE and FCC requirements further certifies that all electrical and wireless components are safe, low-emission, and suitable for continuous operation in laboratory environments.

Traceability forms the backbone of both quality and compliance. Serial numbers, batch tracking, and digital build histories link each product to its materials, assembly, and test data. Modern systems connect these records to inventory and quality databases, enabling real-time tracking of defects, warranty claims, and supplier performance. Regular audits, risk assessments, and corrective action programs close the loop, ensuring that every issue leads to measurable improvement.

4.6 Balancing Standardization and Flexibility

Standardization is critical for ensuring reproducibility, particularly in scientific research and manufacturing. Implementing standardized processes ensures that each HCM system is produced consistently, facilitating reliable performance across different units and studies.

While standardization offers numerous benefits, over-standardization can pose risks by limiting flexibility and hindering the ability to customize manufacturing processes to meet specific requirements. An overly rigid adherence to standardized procedures may stifle innovation and prevent the adaptation of processes to accommodate unique project needs or emerging technologies. In practice, this can be achieved by not designing an assembly system overly reliant on narrow automation.

In summary, the industrialization and scaling of HCM systems involve a multifaceted approach that integrates advanced manufacturing technologies, standardized processes, automation, and robust quality management. By thoughtfully balancing these elements, manufacturers can produce high-quality, reliable HCM systems that meet the evolving needs of scientific research and animal welfare.

5 Software, Data Infrastructure, and Cybersecurity

Hardware makes up only one part of a HCM system. The product of the system is data. Specifically, scientifically valuable and sometimes sensitive data. Therefore, the robustness of software, encryption, data privacy, and ease of use are as important as the correct hardware in providing a fully functional solution.

5.1 Embedded Software Development

Software starts at the device level. Embedded firmware coordinates sensors, cameras, and environmental controls to ensure stable and synchronized operation. It manages timing, data integrity, and power consumption. Firmware must be version-controlled, validated, and field-updatable to ensure consistent function across long-term studies and multiple installations. Data should ideally be recorded on the HCM itself in addition to the final database in case connectivity issues occur.

5.2 Data Management and Analytics Pipelines

HCM systems generate continuous data streams that require structured handling for storage, transfer, and analysis. Some HCM systems can generate very large files, more than hundreds of gigabytes per day for high resolution video data. Data pipelines must be robust to such volumes. Firmware should also include monitoring and alerts of device health and connectivity to enable automatic detection of anomalies and post-failure troubleshooting.

5.3 Local vs Cloud Storage

Choosing between local and cloud storage affects scalability, accessibility, and compliance. Local storage provides full control, fast access within secure networks, and easier compliance with institutional data policies. It is preferred when data privacy or bandwidth limitations restrict cloud transfer. However, local systems demand ongoing maintenance, backup management, and physical redundancy.

Cloud storage supports scalability and centralized analysis across facilities. It enables remote monitoring, collaborative research, and integration with cloud-based analytics or SaaS platforms. Proper encryption, anonymization, and controlled access are essential to maintain data security. Hybrid models, where raw data are cached locally and synchronized with the cloud for processing, combine the control of local infrastructure with the flexibility of cloud computing and can offer an optimal balance for research-scale deployments.

5.4 Data Governance and Security

Data governance ensures privacy, traceability, and ethical compliance. All datasets should carry metadata linking them to device IDs, firmware versions, and calibration logs to preserve reproducibility. Encryption, access control, and authentication protocols protect sensitive research data from unauthorized use. Regular cybersecurity audits, vulnerability testing, and incident response planning further reinforce system integrity. Governance policies should be aligned with institutional and regional standards, ensuring compliance with data protection regulations such as GDPR or equivalent frameworks.

5.5 Software as a Service (SaaS) Models

Cloud-based Software as a Service (SaaS) models are increasingly used for HCM analytics. These systems deliver automated software updates, centralized support, and access to advanced analytics without requiring local infrastructure. Subscription-based models reduce maintenance costs and ensure all users operate on standardized, validated software versions. SaaS also provides integrated data governance, compliance tracking, and multi-institutional collaboration through unified access control and audit logging.

Together, these components form a secure, scalable software and data ecosystem. By combining robust local control, efficient cloud integration, and disciplined governance, modern HCM systems achieve reproducible, automated, and compliant research at scale.

6 Regulatory and Sustainability Considerations

Modern manufacturing of HCM systems must balance performance, compliance, and environmental impact. Sustainable practices begin with material selection, favoring recyclable plastics, low-toxicity coatings, and metals with established recycling streams. Energy efficiency in fabrication, machining, and assembly reduces both cost and carbon footprint. Supply chain responsibility is equally critical; sourcing components from ethical suppliers with transparent labor and environmental practices ensures long-term sustainability. Manufacturers increasingly adopt environmental management standards such as ISO 14001 to quantify energy use, waste generation, and emissions. Packaging and logistics should be designed for minimal material waste and optimized shipping volume, reducing total embodied energy across the product lifecycle.

Sustainability extends beyond production into the full product lifecycle. Lifecycle assessment (LCA) evaluates environmental impact from raw material extraction through disposal, guiding design decisions that reduce waste and resource consumption. HCM systems should be modular and serviceable, allowing components—such as sensors, power modules, or enclosures, to be replaced or upgraded without discarding the entire unit. Designing for disassembly simplifies recycling and repair, while standardized components reduce spare-part waste. Long product lifetimes, combined with refurbishing and component reuse programs, further minimize environmental footprint.

Implementing these principles aligns environmental responsibility with operational efficiency. A sustainable HCM platform not only meets research demands, but also supports institutional goals for responsible innovation, regulatory compliance, and reduced laboratory waste.

7 Serviceability, Customer Support, and Multigenerational Product Planning

HCM systems incorporate electronic and mechanical components that are subject to eventual failure. These failures typically occur during active use, leading to experimental interruptions and initiating a cascade of frustrations for both customers and suppliers. Since hardware failure is inevitable, the manufacturer's service response becomes the critical determinant of a product's long-term success and sustainability in the market.

As product adoption increases, so too does the demand for technical support. This support cost must factor into the cost of the device. However, while manufacturing capacity can scale predictably, service capacity often cannot. Service operations are inherently difficult to scale. Effective service requires personnel with extensive experience, and companies recognized for high-quality support often rely on their most seasoned staff. Yet, it is not possible to acquire service experience at the same pace as sales growth. Consequently, service delays may increase, potentially damaging the product's reputation unless measures are taken to alleviate the support burden. Recruiting individuals with expertise in such specialized equipment is exceptionally difficult. Therefore, transitioning to a *Multigenerational Product Planning (MGPP)* strategy can be a highly effective approach for reducing service demands.

MGPP is a product development framework focused on the continuous evolution and improvement of a technology. It adopts a long-term perspective, with each new generation building upon the successes and shortcomings of previous iterations to better meet customer needs and adapt to evolving market conditions. In the context of service and product growth, well-executed MGPP can significantly reduce the time and effort required to resolve service issues, thereby helping support operations keep pace with increasing sales. Improvements may include mechanical redesigns that minimize time spent at client sites or reduce the number of service visits required.

Other effective strategies include implementing service plans for components with predictable lifespans and offering training programs to address knowledge gaps and reduce user anxiety associated with maintaining and servicing equipment. Each HCM system has its unique strengths and limitations, so optimal strategies may differ across manufacturers. As the user base grows, particularly locally at customer sites, service demands can also decrease due to accumulated institutional knowledge at the site. For these reasons, making the device simple to operate and use is a critical factor in long-term effectiveness of a system as well as its cost.

8 Scaling Access and Global Deployment

8.1 Supply Chain Strategy

Expanding access to HCM systems requires a supply chain that is both dependable and adaptable. Centralized manufacturing offers the advantage of consistent quality and cost efficiency, but regional assembly brings flexibility, allowing faster delivery, lower taxes, local customization, and reduced shipping emissions. If the user base is sufficiently large, a balanced model works best, where key components are produced centrally and final assembly and quality control occurs closer to the end user. Building relationships with multiple trusted suppliers is key to prevent shortages and keep production resilient to global disruptions.

8.2 Data Infrastructure Scaling

As installations spread across research institutions and continents, the data infrastructure must grow alongside them. Scalable cloud systems such as AWS, Google Cloud, or Microsoft Azure, paired with regional data centers, ensure that researchers everywhere have fast, reliable access to their data while meeting local data protection laws. Some facilities prefer hybrid solutions, where data are processed locally but synchronized with the cloud for analytics and backup. These setups maintain high uptime and data integrity, even when internet access is limited. Additionally, centralized monitoring tools such as MQTT allow administrators to track the status of every device, push software updates, and manage performance remotely, ensuring consistent user experience across thousands of systems.

8.3 Open Science and Data Interoperability

Scientific progress depends on collaboration and data sharing. To achieve this, HCM systems must produce data that can easily integrate with laboratory information management systems (LIMS) and major research databases. Adopting open standards and shared metadata formats enables researchers to compare results across studies, species, and institutions. Interoperable data pipelines also support the FAIR principles—making data findable, accessible, interoperable, and reusable. When HCM data flow freely between platforms, it becomes easier to validate findings, combine datasets for meta-analyses, and accelerate discovery. Open, connected systems turn individual experiments into part of a broader scientific network, strengthening both reproducibility and collaboration on a global scale.

9 Conclusion

In conclusion, commercializing and scaling HCM systems is a long-term journey that requires a staged, disciplined approach.

Product-Market Fit Successful systems begin with precise definition of user needs. This is achieved by interviewing stakeholders, testing early prototypes in pilot deployments, and iterating until the core scientific problem is solved in practice. Economic viability is established in parallel, ensuring the solution can be purchased, supported, and justified by research groups.

Productization and Manufacturability A functioning prototype is converted into a reliable instrument through lean modular prototyping, design for manufacturing and assembly, durable material selection, and attention to cleaning and serviceability. The design is then adapted for industrial processes such as injection molding, machining, and laser cutting so that it can be produced consistently at scale.

Manufacturing and Quality Systems Scaled production depends on controlled part fabrication, standardized and testable assembly workflows, and progressive use of automation once processes are stable. Quality systems based on ISO 9001, GLP, and CE or FCC requirements, together with full traceability, ensure reproducibility and regulatory compliance while avoiding overrigid processes that block adaptation.

Software and Data Infrastructure Embedded firmware, secure data pipelines, governed local or cloud storage, and in many cases SaaS delivery models support continuous monitoring, automated analysis, and repeatable study workflows across institutions.

Sustainability and Lifecycle Design Environmental responsibility is addressed through responsible sourcing, energy conscious production, modular design for service and upgrade, and planning for repair, reuse, and end of life recovery.

Serviceability and Long-Term Support Field reliability is driven by ease of service, training of users, and multigenerational product planning. Designing for rapid maintenance and predictable replacement of high wear components reduces downtime and support burden as deployments grow.

Global Deployment Reaching scale requires resilient supply chains that balance centralized manufacturing with regional assembly, scalable data infrastructure that operates across sites and jurisdictions, and interoperable data standards that support open, comparable, and auditable science.

Together, these methods define a full commercialization pathway that turns a single lab prototype into a validated, reproducible, serviceable, and globally available research platform.

Contributions Michael Florea contributed to most subchapters.
Noah Weber contributed to subchapters 2–3.
Matt Ruiter contributed to Automation subchapter.
John Lighton and Robbin Turner contributed to Regulatory Compliance and Quality assurance subchapters.
Christopher Adams contributed to Product growth and Legacy subchapters.
Stefano Gaburro supervised the redaction.

- Competing Interests While the following did not fund or contribute directly to the research presented here, the work aligns with their scope of activity and may indirectly increase their visibility. Michael Florea and Noah Weber are employees and shareholders of Olden Labs
- Christopher K. Adams is an employee of Columbus Instruments

- Matt Ruiter is an employee of Unified Information Devices
- John Lighton and Robbin Turner are employees of Sable Systems
- Stefano Gaburro is an employee of Tecniplast S.p.A

References

Fitzpatrick R (2013) The mom test: how to talk to customers & learn if your business is a good idea when everyone is lying to you

Groover MP (2020) Fundamentals of modern manufacturing: materials, processes, and systems, 7th edn. Wiley

Juniani AI, Singgih ML, Karningsih PD (2022) Design for manufacturing, assembly, and reliability: an integrated framework for product redesign and innovation. Designs 6(5):88. https://doi.org/10.3390/designs6050088

Ries E (2011) The lean startup: how today's entrepreneurs use continuous innovation to create radically successful businesses. Currency, New York

Wojtyła S, Klama P, Baran T (2017) Is 3D printing safe? Analysis of the thermal treatment of thermoplastics: ABS, PLA, PET, and nylon. J Occup Environ Hyg 14:D80–D85. https://doi.org/10.1080/15459624.2017.1285489

Technologies for Home Cage Monitoring in Preclinical Research

Damien Huzard, Christopher K. Adams, Julio Alvarez, Michael Florea, Stefano Gaburro, Thomas Lorimer, Paul Mieske, Matt Ruiter, Oliver Sturman, Noah Weber, and Davor Virag

Abstract

This chapter provides a comprehensive overview of technological solutions for home cage monitoring (HCM) in biomedical research. It outlines various monitoring needs and the corresponding technologies, including video-based systems, RFID, electromagnetic field technology, motion sensors, load cells, telemetry, metabolic monitoring, environmental sensors, and acoustic monitoring. The chapter discusses the

Christopher K. Adams, Julio Alvarez, Michael Florea, Stefano Gaburro, Thomas Lorimer, Paul Mieske, Matt Ruiter, Oliver Sturman and Noah Weber contributed equally with all other contributors.

D. Huzard (✉)
Neuronautix, Montpellier, France

Metadatapp (MAPP), Montpellier, France

C. K. Adams
Columbus Instruments, Columbus, OH, USA

J. Alvarez
Data Sciences International (DSI), Harvard Bioscience, Inc., Saint Paul, MN, USA

M. Florea · N. Weber
Olden Labs, South San Francisco, CA, USA

S. Gaburro
Tecniplast S.p.A., Buguggiate, VA, Italy

T. Lorimer · O. Sturman
ETH Zurich 3R Hub, ETH Zurich, Zürich, Switzerland

S. Gaburro, S. Mandillo (eds.), *Home Cage Monitoring in Rodents: A Global Effort*,
https://doi.org/10.1007/978-3-032-19781-8_7

technological overview, use and measurements, pros/cons, and specific considerations of each system. It also addresses future trends, combinations of systems, emerging technologies (such as AI-based computer vision), and aspects to consider when driving innovation in HCM technologies. The aim is to guide scientists in selecting appropriate tools and understanding the complexities of data collection and analysis in the HCM world.

Keywords

Technological solutions · Monitoring systems · Sensor integration · Behavioral analysis · Physiological monitoring

1 Introduction

Home-cage monitoring (HCM) systems are an integrated set of technologies that continuously and automatically observe and record animal behavior, physiology, and environmental features within an animal's home cage. Combining hardware (sensors and actuators) and software, HCM systems collect data with minimal human intervention. These systems ensure basic animal needs are met while enabling long-term monitoring, providing reliable, reproducible data for improved biomedical research.

In behavioral and physiological research, selecting the right toolset begins with a clear definition of the scientific question. Instead of focusing on the technologies themselves, researchers should first identify the type of monitoring required—e.g., locomotor activity, individual differentiation, physiological readouts, and environmental parameters—and then choose the appropriate methods to address their goals. Table 1 exemplifies this approach, categorizing available technologies based on the specific monitoring tasks they enable. By aligning experimental needs with the appropriate tools, this framework ensures that the data collected are both relevant and robust, streamlining the path from question to discovery.

HCM technologies offer a diverse array of tools tailored to specific experimental objectives, enabling detailed behavioral and physiological studies in laboratory animals. These tools range from video-based systems, capable of tracking individual or group behaviors with high accuracy and performing 3D pose reconstruction using multicamera setups, to RFID systems, which provide robust individual identification in group-housed conditions

P. Mieske
Bundesinstitut für Risikobewertung (BfR), Berlin, Germany

M. Ruiter
Unified Information Devices, Inc. (UID), Lake Villa, IL, USA

D. Virag
Department of Pharmacology and Croatian Institute for Brain Research, University of Zagreb School of Medicine, Zagreb, Croatia

Table 1 Overview of HCM technologies categorized by monitoring needs, measured parameters, and compatible technologies

Type of monitoring need	Measurements needed (parameters)	Available technologies
Continuous cage tracking	Locomotion (circadian activity)	Video, RFID, beam-break, passive infrared sensors, capacitive electrostatic sensing, load cell, running wheel, telemetry implants, EMF
	Positional preference, social grouping	Video, RFID, capacitive electrostatic sensing
	Bouts of specific behaviors (sleeping, rearing, grooming, social interaction)	Video, 2 layers of IR sensors for rearing, load cells for scratching, EMF (for single-housed animals), acoustic monitoring (USV)
	Differentiation of individuals	Video, RFID
Recording events in the cage	Eating	Video, RFID, beam-break, passive infrared sensors, (to some extent) load cells
	Drinking	Video, capacitive electrostatic sensing
	Location in cage	Video, RFID, beam-break, passive infrared sensors, EMF
	Interactions with devices	Video, capacitive electrostatic sensing, beam-break, lever, touchscreen
Wearable / implantable devices	Bioelectric signals (e.g., ECG or EEG) *High sampling rates required*	Telemetry implants
	Biochemical signals (blood glucose), body temperature	Various: telemetry implants Temperature: IR camera, RFID implants
	Movement data	Accelerometers, gyroscopes
Environmental data	Temperature, humidity, light intensity, noise levels	Various sensors
Welfare	Biomarkers	EMF (urination), video (for posture analysis)

The table highlights available tools for continuous cage tracking, event-based recording, wearable sensing, environmental monitoring, and welfare assessment in laboratory animals. This list is not exhaustive

by detecting animals as they move through specific areas or interact with objects. Beam-break sensors and passive infrared sensors offer simple, event-based monitoring for activities like nose pokes or general locomotion, although they lack individual identification. Advanced methods like capacitive electrostatic sensing and load cells enable precise spatial tracking or unique measurements such as body weight, albeit with complex calibration and data processing requirements. Wearable/implantable devices like accelerometers and gyroscopes further extend monitoring capabilities, offering potential insights into fine-grained movement and equipment interactions. Table 1 organizes these technologies by their type of monitoring, guiding researchers to match their experimental needs (measurements needed), ensuring the available technologies match their scientific goals.

HCM technologies integrate various components to capture and analyze animal behavior in their natural environment. As summarized and simplified in Fig. 1, hardware

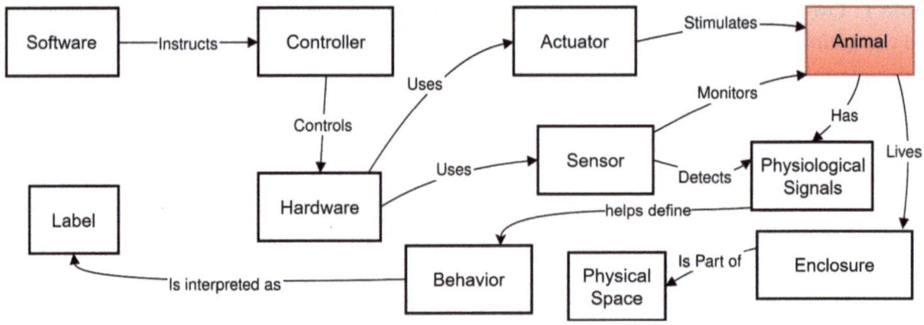

Fig. 1 HCM definition, adapted and simplified from TEATIME's Olog definition (Bains et al. 2025)https://www.cost-teatime.org/about/hcm-definition/. Specialized software controls hardware systems with sensors that monitor animal physiology and behavior. Actuators complement sensors to stimulate responses for dynamic experiments. Interpreted sensor data define labeled behaviors for analysis, yielding research insights. The system operates within an enclosure mimicking natural conditions, ensuring accurate tracking, stimulation, and interpretation for preclinical and behavioral studies

systems, controlled by specialized software, deploy sensors to monitor animals' physiological signals (e.g., ECG and EEG) and movements (e.g., locomotion and rearing). These sensors are often complemented by actuators, which interact with the animals to stimulate or influence specific responses, enabling more dynamic and precise experiments. The collected data are interpreted to define behaviors based on signals or movement patterns, which researchers label and analyze to derive experimental insights. The entire system operates within an enclosure (e.g., cage) designed to mimic the animal's natural living conditions, forming part of the broader physical space. This seamless interaction between sensors, actuators, and software ensures accurate tracking, stimulation, and behavioral interpretation, providing valuable data for preclinical and behavioral studies.

2 HCM Technologies

In this section, an overview of the technological landscape currently shaping the HCM field is provided. Rather than offering a comprehensive catalog, as was already organized by the COST ACTION TEATIME (CA20135) consortium (thebehaviourdatabase.org), we aim to highlight a representative selection of technologies—ranging from commercially available platforms to emerging open-source or experimental setups—that illustrate the diversity and evolution of approaches. Our analysis focuses on key dimensions relevant to both researchers and developers, including data output and scalability, accuracy and resolution, energy and computational efficiency, ease of use, cost, ethical considerations, modularity, and throughput capacity. While not exhaustive, this review strives to be both accurate and up to date, offering a structured framework to assess HCM technologies.

2.1 Video-Based Monitoring Systems

Among the various HCM technologies, video-based monitoring systems stand out for their ability to noninvasively capture a rich array of behavioral data. Furthermore, video systems can also directly monitor environmental variables, such as water or food availability and intake, flooding events, cage presence or absence in the rack, cage ID, and metadata (e.g., precise timestamps of light cycling or personnel entrances). This can greatly reduce the complexity of the sensor suites required for HCM solutions at scale.

2.1.1 Technology Overview

Video-based monitoring systems leverage standard video recording techniques alongside specialized methods such as infrared (IR, e.g., Kinect cameras) and thermal imaging (e.g., FLIR cameras) to monitor animals around the clock. Standard cameras capture high--resolution, color images during the day, while infrared cameras facilitate nocturnal monitoring (while still being fully functional in daylight), ensuring that observations continue seamlessly throughout the light–dark cycles. The typical configuration involves one (or more) cameras strategically mounted above (and/or around) the home cage. This setup is often enhanced by automated tracking and analysis software that employs computer vision and machine learning (ML) algorithms to quantify behaviors. Such algorithms are designed to identify and track individual animals, analyze their movements, and classify behavioral patterns. This technology not only enables the precise quantification of basic activities, such as locomotion and grooming but can also can be adapted to capture more complex social interactions and subtle postural changes, key aspects in preclinical research.

The main considerations when designing video monitoring systems relate to visibility. It is important to have high image clarity, no blind spots, and appropriate illumination (visible or IR) with as few reflections and shadows as possible. As home cages are typically required to be autoclavable, video monitoring systems are best placed outside the cage. In single-camera recording systems, this raises important geometric considerations to avoid blind spots, such as the viewing angle of the lens, relative position and size of the window, and location of occluding objects, like water bottles or food grids. Blind spots can be particularly challenging in cages with climbing enrichments, where ceiling surfaces and floor surfaces may need to be monitored simultaneously.

Because video systems produce very large amounts of data, the downstream processing and connectivity need to be designed into the setup. Where will storage and/or processing take place? Locally in the cage? On a rack-based server? In the cloud? What limits on the near-real-time availability of insights does this imply? How will video acquisition schedules be controlled? It is always tempting to aim for increasingly more data, but a video monitoring system that performs 24/7, high-resolution, 30 frame/s, full behavioral analysis can face very different computational hardware design bottlenecks from a system that performs scheduled analyses and occasional health and environment checks.

Real-time analysis also presents data bottleneck issues: video data compression is far more efficient when performed on sections of video rather than individual frames. Several models of camera popular in mouse behavioral analysis transmit video in an uncompressed format, which dramatically changes downstream hardware requirements when scaling to a whole-rack HCM system. In most HCM applications, this kind of ultralow video latency is not needed, and compression can be designed into the system.

2.1.2 Use and Measurements of Video Technologies

Video technology in HCM offers a noninvasive approach to measure a diverse range of behavioral and physiological parameters. Researchers utilize video recordings to assess the following:

- Locomotion and Activity Patterns: Detailed tracking of movement patterns provides insights into general activity levels, circadian rhythms, changes in locomotor behavior over time, and information on body postures (such as *rearing* or *climbing* behaviors).
- Social Interactions: Group-housed animals can be observed to study social hierarchies, mating behaviors, and aggression, all of which are crucial in behavioral studies.
- Grooming and Self-Care Behaviors: Video technology can quantify grooming frequency and duration, which are often indicators of stress or neurological conditions.
- Sleep and Resting States: Video monitoring, particularly with infrared technology, allows for accurate detection of sleep and resting without disturbing the animals.
- Eating and Drinking Behaviors.
- Physiological Parameters via Thermal Imaging: Thermal cameras can detect variations in body temperature, which may reflect underlying physiological changes such as fever, stress, or metabolic shifts.

In addition, advanced systems are exploring the integration of video data with other sensor modalities, potentially enabling the derivation of parameters such as respiratory rates or even subtle heart rate fluctuations when combined with high-resolution imaging and advanced analytical algorithms.

2.1.3 Keypoint Tracking Methods

Due to the difficulty of directly extracting measures from image data, the video analysis approach usually includes tracking the movement of keypoints of interest across the timespan of the video. This is done using background subtraction, or neural networks. Background subtraction methods for video analysis in HCM operate by comparing each video frame to a static reference frame, or background model, and identifying changes in pixel values. These changes are assumed to represent moving objects, ideally the animal. First applied to behavioral analysis in the late 1990s, this computationally efficient algorithm requires minimal setup, with static parameters like thresholds set once and applied across the entire dataset. Its predictability in terms of time investment is a key advantage. However, background subtraction alone is limited to single-animal tracking, typically tracking the center of mass of the animal's silhouette. It necessitates a significant visual distinction between the animal and the background and is highly susceptible to background changes, such as shifts in bedding. These limitations make it practically unsuitable for most complex home cage monitoring scenarios (Pennington et al. 2021).

Neural networks (NNs) offer a more advanced approach to video analysis, employing "black-box" models trained on researcher-labeled data. This iterative process involves labeling representative images from videos (typically 100–1000), training the NN, evaluating its performance, and then labeling additional images, often focusing on edge cases, before retraining. This continues until satisfactory performance is achieved. While this workflow has an unknown time investment and requires significant computational resources, including graphical processors (often found in gaming computers or institutional high-performance computing centers), a well-trained NN can achieve high accuracy in labeling diverse features, including specific body parts. The errors produced by NNs are usually pronounced and easily identifiable, and the variability in labeling between researchers can be quantified to ensure robust training data as well as a scale on which the model's accuracy can be gauged. Furthermore, NNs can be used for sophisticated tasks such as skeleton reconstruction, 3D pose estimation, and multianimal tracking (Pereira et al. 2022; Mathis et al. 2018; Lauer et al. 2022). See additional info in Sect. 3.5.

2.1.4 Pros of Video-Based Monitoring

One of the primary advantages of video technology in HCM is its ability to capture extensive and nuanced behavioral data without physical interference. Key benefits include

- Rich Behavioral Data: Video recordings provide a comprehensive visual record, allowing for detailed post hoc analysis of behavior. This is particularly useful for studying complex behaviors that are difficult to quantify with other sensors.
- Non-Invasive Monitoring: By relying on cameras instead of implanted devices or direct contact sensors, video systems minimize stress and discomfort, ensuring that the animals' natural behaviors are not altered by the monitoring process.
- Adaptability and Flexibility: Video systems can be easily integrated into various experimental setups. Whether it is a single camera for a small-scale study or a multicamera array for large group-housed studies, the technology scales according to experimental needs.
- Automated Analysis: Advances in machine learning and computer vision have led to robust software capable of automatically detecting and quantifying behaviors. This reduces manual labor and potential human error in data interpretation.

2.1.5 Cons and Challenges of Video-Based Monitoring

Despite the numerous advantages, video-based monitoring comes with its own set of challenges:

- Large Data Storage Requirements: Continuous video recording generates vast amounts of data, necessitating substantial storage capacity and efficient data management solutions.

- High Computational Demands: The processing and analysis of high-resolution video, particularly when using advanced ML algorithms, require significant computational power. This can be a bottleneck in studies involving long-term monitoring.
- Potential for Tracking Errors: Automated tracking systems may occasionally lose individual identities, especially in group-housed or environmentally enriched scenarios.
- Video Encoding Issues: High-quality video encoding is essential to preserve data fidelity, but it also increases computational overhead.

2.1.6 Future Developments

Looking ahead, the integration of video with other emerging technologies presents exciting possibilities. For instance, ongoing developments aim to incorporate physiological measurements such as respiratory patterns and body weight assessments from video data using computer vision (Guzman et al. 2024). Experimental setups are being designed to monitor not only adult rodents but also pups, thereby expanding the utility of video systems across different developmental stages (Lapp et al. 2023).

2.2 Systems Using RFID Technology

Radio frequency identification (RFID) uses radio waves for contactless data transmission, evolving from radar in the 1940s to wireless data exchange by the 1970s. It transmits information from a reader-powered transponder ("microchip") to a reader via radio waves, enabling the transmission of small amounts of data. Unlike other methods, RFID does not require a clear line of sight, allowing transponders to be embedded.

2.2.1 Technology Overview

There are three main types of RFID technology used today: low frequency (124–135 kHz), used for implantable devices like animal microchips due to its ability to penetrate tissue and water, which offers a read range of up to several meters. High frequency (13.56 MHz), suitable for vial labels in freezing conditions, enabling anti-collision reading in the short range (1–2 cm); however, it is unsuitable for implants. Ultrah-high-frequency (433–960 MHz) RFID, used in toll systems and retail security for its long range (up to 30 m) and active RFID systems with the highest range (up to 100 m) and fast data transmission, yet again not suitable for implantation or close contact.

For over three decades, LF RFID microchips have been utilized for animal identification, offering a permanent, reliable identification method. By implanting a transponder under the skin of laboratory animals and using compatible readers, researchers can achieve precise identification and tracking across various species. With microchips ranging from 1.2 mm to 2.1 mm in diameter and 6 mm to 13 mm in length, they are ideal for use in small animals such as mice and rats.

LF RFID systems typically consist of a reader equipped with wire coils that generate an electromagnetic signal. When a transponder comes into the range of the reader's signal, it absorbs energy from the electromagnetic field and modulates the signal to transmit stored data. The range and effectiveness of the system depend on factors such as the properties of the coil (diameter and number of windings), reader power, and the frequency of the signal. LF RFID microchips use either full duplex (FDX) or half duplex (HDX) communication methods. ISO 11784/85, more specifically FDX-B (134.2 kHz), is the most common communication standard in animal identification, offering an optimal read range and data transmission capabilities, making it ideal for laboratory animal tracking.

2.2.2 Use and Measurements of RFID Systems

Over the past decade, advancements in RFID technology have enabled the tracking of mice and rats in their home cage environments, opening new avenues for scientific exploration. One example is the study by researchers at Pfizer Worldwide Research, which combined RFID with home cage monitoring technology to track respiratory rates in laboratory animals (Winn et al. 2021). A reader plate was placed under the animal's home cage to track individual animals' data throughout the experiment. Another example is the Live Mouse Tracker (LMT, more details at https://micecraft.org/lmt/), which can automatically extract the (social) behavior of group-living mice by combining RFID and video data from an IR camera (de Chaumont et al. 2019; Huzard et al. 2022). Utilizing an implantable microchip and a specialized reader system allows for undisturbed monitoring of animals in their home cage. Previously, such evaluations relied solely on visual observation or required removing the animals from their cages, which introduced external stress and potential experimental variability.

The ISO 11784/85 standard provides a universal pet identification system for global compatibility, primarily for border crossing and lost pet recovery. Modern RFID technology extends this standard with increased memory to store additional data like temperature alongside identification (https://www.uidevices.com/laboratory-animal-temperature/). RFID technology's ability to monitor and track animals in real time has revolutionized behavioral studies and home cage monitoring. For instance, Sass et al. (2024) used RFID to track the thermogenic responses and metabolic rates of group-housed mice in response to neurokinin 2 receptor activation. RFID systems allowed researchers to monitor individual animals' activity levels and body temperature without the confounding effects of restraint or stress (Sass et al. 2024).

Another example of tracking animal movement and activity from cage to cage can be achieved using a tunnel reader. In the research study by Habedank et al., an RFID-based tracking system was used to determine the position of laboratory mice in a preference test (Habedank et al. 2022). The researchers described the process of using commercially available RFID components and an Arduino microcontroller to identify the mice as they pass through a tunnel in a housing system combined with two standard cages.

RFID has been used in seminaturalistic housing environments to collect detailed information on animal behavior while generating only small and manageable amounts of data. For example, a study using 29 RFID antennas tracked 20 mice, generating over 186,000 data points in 7 days while maintaining a compact total data volume of only 10.1 MB

(Mieske et al. 2021). These data can be analyzed using AI or specific scripts to monitor activity, temperature fluctuations, and behavioral patterns in real time, providing valuable insights into animal welfare and overall health.

2.2.3 Considerations with RFID Implants

RFID microchips should be implanted subcutaneously in the mid-scapular region (between the shoulder blades) using a caudal-to-cranial needle insertion to minimize infection and dislodging, typically resulting in a 1–2% fall-out rate for experienced researchers. Needle size guidelines vary based on microchip dimensions (e.g., ~12.5G for 2.1 mm × 12 mm). In postweaned animals, anesthesia is often unnecessary (acceptable in the US for >15 g mice with ≤15G needles and > 30 g rats with ≤12G needles), although European Directive 2010/63/EU classifies unanesthetized implantation as mild stress. Optimal RFID performance also depends on antenna size and positioning; tube antennas should match tube dimensions, while 3″ circular cage-side antennas offer a 3–4″ read range. Do-It-Yourself (DIY) antenna winding is technical and requires precise tuning to the reader, making consultation with RFID specialists advisable for proper functioning through inductance and capacitance adjustments.

For HCM, RFID can be used as a complementary tool alongside other technologies. The main benefit of RFID is its ability to track individual animals within a group-housed setting. While video systems can track a large number of animals using ear tags or other markers, they have limitations when animals are huddled together or out of the camera's view. RFID overcomes these challenges by detecting animals through bedding, nonmetallic enrichment devices, and water, making it a reliable identification method. When combined with temperature-sensing microchips, RFID also enables continuous animal welfare monitoring, as temperature is a key indicator of health and stress. Recent advances are pushing the development of newer implants combining various sensors (thermometer, accelerometer, and photoplethysmograph) within the RFID chip and allowing the recording of a wider range of behavioral, as well as health parameters (https://micetracking.com/). New data open new fields of research in medicine, pharmacology, and animal well-being.

2.2.4 Challenges, Limitations, and Future of RFID Technology

While RFID technology offers significant benefits, it also presents certain challenges, such as imaging interference and anti-collision signal interference. First, although most RFID microchips are compatible with MRI, X-ray, NMR, or body composition analysis, they can produce imaging artifacts. Researchers should assess the impact on their specific area of interest to ensure that image quality remains uncompromised. Second, when two or more microchips are present within the same antenna field, the reader may scan microchips A, B, or neither during a given scan. This occurs due to the nature of the LF RFID signals and how the reader interprets individual readings. When mice are huddled together, the reader may register one animal or none. To enhance data reliability, combining RFID monitoring for identification and temperature tracking with complementary methods such as video analysis can provide a powerful research solution.

RFID technology has proven to be an invaluable tool for tracking and identifying laboratory animals, providing precise and reliable data without the need for visual contact. Advances in RFID capabilities and applications in animal research continue to grow, enabling innovative methodologies for studying behavior, health, and welfare. By selecting appropriate equipment, optimizing implantation techniques, and adhering to ethical standards, researchers can fully leverage RFID technology while prioritizing animal welfare.

Combining RFID technology with additional sensors represents a significant advancement, enabling the simultaneous and continuous collection of diverse data. This integration in a single RFID implant ensures multiple measurements, highly repeatable experiments, and strong correlation with external factors (e.g., day/night cycle and temperature) and activities (e.g., sleeping and eating). For instance, continuous photoplethysmography (PPG) measurements allow the calculation of physiological parameters like heart rate, blood pressure, respiratory rate, and blood oxygen saturation using digital signal processing (DSP) and machine learning (ML) techniques. Furthermore, the integration of chemistry-free sensors into a surgery-free RFID implant provides an ethical and cost-effective approach compared to traditional methods (https://micetracking.com/).

2.3 Electromagnetic Field Technology

Electromagnetic field (EMF) technology has emerged as a compelling solution for HCM, offering a noninvasive, continuous, and scalable method to capture various animal behavioral and physiological parameters. By integrating EMF sensors within the cage setup, systems such as Tecniplast's DVC® enable researchers to monitor group-housed animals in real time, collecting group data on activity levels and indicators like rest/wake bouts and polyuria patterns (Voikar and Gaburro 2020; Brachs et al. 2025).

2.3.1 Technology Overview

EMF-based HCM systems utilize an array of magnetic or capacitive sensors placed underneath or along the walls of standard animal cages. These sensors detect subtle perturbations in the local electromagnetic field caused by an animal's movement or presence. When an animal moves across the cage floor, its body—characterized by high water content—alters the local dielectric properties, modifying the field strength and distribution. The sensor outputs, typically voltage fluctuations, are recorded and processed to infer movement and position. For instance, the DVC® system from Tecniplast employs multiple electrodes to monitor changes in conductance as animals traverse the cage, providing quantitative measurements of activity and spatial positioning (Iannello 2019).

2.3.2 Applications and Measured Parameters

The EMF technology in HCM is designed to capture a range of measurements with minimal human intervention. Key parameters include

- Activity Levels: Continuous tracking of general locomotion allows researchers to assess patterns such as distance traveled and average speed.
- Social Interactions: Group-housed settings benefit from the ability to record interactions such as fights or aggressive encounters with minimal precision since the system cannot know which animals are implicated in this magnetic field fluctuation.
- Sleep Patterns: Changes in activity can serve as a proxy for sleep, as periods of inactivity during the dark phase of the circadian cycle often indicate rest.
- Wetness and Urination Events: Variations in the electromagnetic signal can also reveal the presence of fluids such as urine, which may indicate both normal physiology and recovery postsurgery, or indicate flooding of the cage.
- Environmental Room Conditions: Real-time conditions (humidity, temperature, human presence, noise, and vibration) can be monitored with a rack-based tool (see Sect. 2.8).

By providing data on these aspects, the DVC system supports refined phenotyping and welfare assessments without the need for continuous human observation.

2.3.3 Noninvasive and Continuous Monitoring

EMF technology offers noninvasive, 24/7 monitoring, minimizing stress and complications. Its low data storage needs (4 MB/cage/day with 4 Hz sampling) enable long-term studies and automated, continuous data collection, crucial for observing natural behaviors in group-housed animals while minimizing human interaction.

2.3.4 Group Housed Data Collection and Social Interactions

EMF-based monitoring tracks group-housed animals in ventilated rack cages, monitoring over 10,000 cages simultaneously without disturbance. It provides a comprehensive activity profile for each cage, revealing social dynamics like aggressive encounters and detecting subtle behavioral shifts (e.g., stress indicators from increased daytime movement in nocturnal species). This group-level data, when correlated with other parameters, offers insights into animal welfare. However, it lacks individual animal data or precise social dynamic details.

2.3.5 Pros of EMF

- Continuous, Real-Time Monitoring: EMF sensors provide ongoing surveillance, capturing rapid behavioral changes without gaps in data collection.
- Low Data Storage Requirements: The simplicity of the data (voltage fluctuations) means that even long-term recordings produce manageable data volumes.
- Suitability for Group Housing: EMF systems can monitor multiple animals simultaneously, preserving the social environment and reducing handling stress.

- Non-Invasive Measurement: avoiding surgical interventions improves welfare outcomes.
- Versatility in Measurement: EMF systems can capture data on rest/wake bouts and even detect wetness, which can be critical for monitoring the onset of hyperglycemia (Brachs et al. 2025).
- Ideal for combination with other technologies.

2.3.6 Cons and Limitations of EMF

- Limited Behavioral Resolution: While EMF sensors accurately record gross activity, they typically lack the detailed resolution required to distinguish fine-grained behaviors (e.g., grooming or subtle postural changes).
- Potential for Signal Interference: External electromagnetic noise or overlapping signals from closely interacting animals might lead to data artifacts. This can be particularly challenging in settings with high ambient interference or when cages are not properly shielded.
- Need for Specialized Cage Setups: Cages must be compatible with the sensor arrays to maximize the effectiveness of EMF sensors. Retrofitting existing cages might require modifications to ensure proper sensor placement and signal capture.
- Group Data Aggregation: Although group monitoring is an advantage, it also means that individual behavior is sometimes obscured, limiting the capacity for individual-level analysis in social housing scenarios.

2.3.7 Comparison with Other Technologies

Compared to video-based monitoring, which can offer detailed behavioral insights through advanced computer vision techniques, EMF-based systems prioritize high scalability and low invasiveness. Video systems tend to generate large amounts of data and require significant computational resources to process high-resolution images continuously. In contrast, EMF systems produce simpler data that are easier to store and analyze, making them more practical for large-scale, high-throughput studies. Similarly, while RFID systems excel at individual identification and tracking, they typically require the implantation of chips, which is invasive and may affect animal welfare. By operating externally, EMF technology avoids these drawbacks while still delivering valuable group-level data.

2.3.8 Perspectives and Conclusion

Looking ahead, improvements in sensor design, data processing algorithms, and refined analysis could help overcome some current limitations of EMF-based HCM systems. For instance, integrating machine learning approaches to deconvolve overlapping signals better could enhance behavioral resolution, enabling the system to differentiate between complex activities. Advances in sensor miniaturization and shielding could reduce the impact of external electromagnetic interference, improving data accuracy even in challenging environments. Additionally, combining EMF data with other noninvasive monitoring technologies—such as videos or microphones—could provide a more comprehensive understanding of animal behavior. Such systems might leverage the strengths of each method: EMF for continuous, low-data monitoring and video for detailed behavioral classification. This integrative approach holds promise for future research to refine phenotyping methods and enhance experimental reproducibility. Finally, improving scientists' ability to discover insights from existing datasets could be achieved by validating and refining EMF algorithms using AI models trained on data from systems that integrate multiple technologies.

EMF technology enables continuous, noninvasive home cage monitoring of activity, some social interactions, sleep, and urination. While less detailed than video tracking, its low data storage requirements and suitability for group housing make it valuable in HCM. Its scalability and easy integration benefit researchers designing large-scale, high-throughput studies. Ongoing development aims for improved animal welfare and research reliability. Despite limitations in detailed behavioral analysis and potential interference, EMF's noninvasiveness and scalability make it a preferred preclinical method.

2.4 (Other) Motion-Sensing Technologies

Alongside EMF (and, in some uses, RFID technology), implantable accelerometers, passive infrared (PIR) sensors, and infrared beam break systems represent fundamental technologies used in HCM systems to quantify locomotor activity, assess circadian rhythms, and broadly capture movement-related behaviors in laboratory animals. These tools are especially valued in research settings where minimizing human interaction is essential for reducing stress and experimental artifacts while ensuring that animals' daily activities and behaviors are continuously monitored (Goulding et al. 2008). Similarly to EMFs, implantable accelerometers' complex raw output is attractive as it could be used to infer occurrences of various specific behaviors. On the other hand, PIR and beam break sensors have simple data outputs, but their simplicity and cost make them attractive options. Motion, proximity, or presence sensing using radar-like time-of-flight measurements (ultrasound or microwaves) are not present in HCM systems. Ultrasonic sensors are unsuitable due to rodent sensitivity. Microwave sensors, while having similar drawbacks to infrared sensors, also have higher complexity and cost, explaining their absence. Motion sensing can also monitor voluntary activity like running wheel usage in home cages.

2.4.1 Implantable Accelerometers in HCM

Accelerometers have been designed to detect and record subtle movements of the animal (S. Venkatraman et al. 2010). These sensors are embedded within implantable telemetry devices and provide high temporal resolution, making them ideal for studies where precise quantification of movement patterns is necessary (Ouyang et al. 2024). These devices capture detailed acceleration and orientation data across multiple axes, providing researchers with comprehensive activity profiles. High sampling rates (up to 1 kHz) record even minor movements, enabling accurate activity assessments over various timescales.

Accelerometer data are used to evaluate circadian rhythms by tracking patterns of activity and rest across the day–night cycle. In addition, they provide information about gross locomotor activity—essential for studies in behavioral neuroscience and physiology where changes in movement can be indicative of underlying conditions or responses to interventions (Seibenhener and Wooten 2015; Crawley 2007, 2023). Because the data generated by these sensors are relatively compact, storage and data processing demands are significantly reduced compared to more data-intensive methods like continuous video monitoring. This makes accelerometer-based HCM systems efficient and cost-effective for long-term studies.

Implantable accelerometers minimally impact animal behavior, allowing for natural movement recording after surgical placement. Although invasive, the procedure yields reliable, long-term movement data. Calibration is necessary for accurate acceleration reflection, and long-term studies must consider battery type (batteryless or rechargeable).

2.4.2 Infrared Beam Break Systems in HCM

Infrared (IR) beam break systems monitor animal movement via IR beam interruptions in a cage, offering basic 3D data on locomotion and rearing. Their advantage lies in continuous, high-sensitivity monitoring with minimal data storage, suitable for long-term studies where video is impractical. These systems integrate well with other technologies, enhancing HCM implementations.

IR beam break systems have limitations, notably their inability to provide detailed behavioral information. They detect movement but struggle to differentiate specific behaviors beyond beam interruptions. Early systems struggled with this, but Columbus Instruments later developed a system using microprocessors to classify beam breaks as ambulatory or stereotypic based on interruption sequences (Czekajewski et al. 1982). Initially, data collection was limited, but systems with integrated computers enhanced data output and enabled automated scoring (Sulaiman et al. 1986). Using a grid arrangement, animal position can be mapped using Cartesian coordinates, and based on beam break patterns, states like resting, sleeping (Pack et al. 2007), genotypic, and ambulatory (Kelley 1993) can be classified.

Locomotor movement is the movement from one position to another (Kelley 1993). Sometimes, stereotypic movement is scored incorrectly as locomotor movement, and with sophisticated software, "stereotypic filtering" can be employed. Software-based stereotypic filtering uses an imaginary fence to classify movements. Movements within the fence are stereotypic. If the subject's centroid exits, the state becomes ambulatory, and the fence is erased and redrawn upon stopping. Abrupt ambulation from rest might initially classify steps within the fence as stereotypic, even if the path becomes ambulatory. Short periods of stereotypic movement immediately preceding ambulation can be reclassified as ambulatory if shorter than a set threshold.

Today, more data tools are becoming available for actigrams, heatmaps, and automated sleep scoring (Keenan et al. 2020). While IR beams have become excellent at recording locomotion, they still remain limited in two ways: animals must be singly housed, and the sensors lack sensitivity to further classify stereotypic movements into specific behaviors (grooming, feeding, or seizures).

2.4.3 Passive Infrared Sensors in HCM

Unlike beam break sensors, passive infrared (PIR) sensors do not emit infrared light—they are sensitive to the rodent's own infrared emissions. Usually, such a sensing element is part of a module with a specialized integrated circuit, which detects, amplifies, and thresholds the signal, finally outputting a logical 1 when the threshold is crossed, i.e., movement is detected. Such data require little storage space and compresses well.

Owing to the PIR sensor modules' simplicity, low cost (less than 20€ for a calibrated, industrial variant, 1€ for a hobbyist variant), and simple data output, this approach is especially attractive for DIY HCM, and Chap. 9 contains full instructions for building a simple prototype.

While PIR and beam break sensors have similar pros and cons, PIR sensors are better for larger areas and easier to install, often requiring just one sensor per cage for general activity. Beam break sensors need a horizontal beam, which can be obstructed by bedding or enrichment items. However, beam breaks excel at detecting presence at specific points, especially in small spaces like shelter or nosepoke openings.

2.4.4 Future Directions

Core sensing technologies like PIR, beam break sensors, and accelerometers have reached a maturity level limiting further innovation in the sensors themselves. Future advancements will likely stem from applying computational methods, such as machine learning for behavioral biomarker extraction from raw sensor data (as Tecniplast does with DVC system) and multimodal data integration. Innovation is shifting toward data fusion, advanced modeling, and behavioral inference algorithms.

2.5 Load Cells and Pressure Sensors

HCM systems offer a nonintrusive, continuous way to observe and record animal behavior without disturbing the animals. In this context, load cells and pressure sensors play a crucial role by capturing subtle weight shifts and changes in weight distribution that may reflect various behaviors. These sensors, typically placed under the cage or integrated into its floor, provide real-time data on locomotion and activity-related behaviors, such as scratching bouts (LABORAS system from Metris) — behaviors that are often challenging to capture with video-based systems alone.

2.5.1 Technical Overview and Operating Principles

Load cells and pressure sensors, integrated into cage floors, use strain gauge technology to detect minute weight or force changes as electrical signals. This noncontact method allows for the unobtrusive, continuous monitoring of animal behavior in a natural setting, detecting subtle weight distribution shifts for detailed analysis, although the exact cause of these variations may not always be identifiable.

2.5.2 Applications in Monitoring Behavioral and Physiological Parameters

Load cells and pressure sensors have a broad range of applications in HCM systems:

- Activity Levels: These sensors continuously track weight shifts, providing precise data on animal locomotion, including movement patterns, rest, and activity bursts, offering insights into circadian rhythms and behavioral changes.
- Body Weight Estimation: Integrated systems can estimate overall body weight from continuous data, reducing stressful handling and weighing (e.g., TSE AnimalGate).
- Detection of Fine Motor Behaviors: Advanced calibration and AI algorithms enable sensors to detect behaviors like scratching, often difficult to validate via video. This is valuable in studies where grooming or scratching indicates stress or neurological conditions (Huzard et al. 2024).

These sensors monitor group-housed animals, providing a reliable overview of group dynamics and activity trends through aggregated data, although individual identification may require additional technology.

2.5.3 Pros

Several key benefits make load cells and pressure sensors attractive for HCMs:

- Non-Intrusive and Continuous Monitoring: These contactless sensors allow for noninterfering behavioral recording, reducing stress variability and improving data reliability.
- Simplicity and Ease of Setup: Load cells easily integrate into existing cage systems, requiring minimal structural changes, making them a cost-effective and scalable solution for large studies.
- Versatility in Data Collection: Load cells offer valuable insights into behaviors like feeding, drinking, and scratching, making them versatile for diverse research, from metabolic studies to behavioral neuroscience.

2.5.4 Cons

Despite their many advantages, the use of load cells and pressure sensors comes with several caveats:

- Sensitivity to Environmental Vibrations: These systems are highly sensitive to vibrations, with environmental movements or cage disturbances causing data noise. Researchers must isolate the setup and use signal-processing algorithms to filter vibrations.

- Potential for Inaccurate Measurements: Inconsistent bedding or cage movement can skew weight measurements by altering sensor pressure. Regular calibration and correction factors are crucial to address this.
- Calibration and Data Processing: Accurate initial calibration and robust data systems are essential for reliable weight change monitoring from continuous sensor data, avoiding external interference and data loss.
- Integration with Other Modalities: Load cells are best combined with other sensors (e.g., video tracking, RFID, and telemetry) for comprehensive analysis, increasing complexity but improving behavioral interpretations.
- Group Data Aggregation: While these sensors can effectively estimate bulk activity and behavioral patterns in group-housed environments, it is difficult to discern readings of individual animals in these conditions.

2.5.5 Better Load Cell Data and Practical Examples

Recent advancements in sensor technology have led to improved load cell designs with enhanced sensitivity and better vibration isolation. A system like LABORAS has demonstrated the capability to not only monitor general activity levels but also detect specific behaviors that were previously challenging to measure, such as scratching (LABORAS system from Metris). Additionally, PASTA (Platform for Acoustic STArtle)—despite not being a full HCM system—is an open source example that demonstrates the ease of interfacing with load cells in a DIY setup (D. Virag et al. 2021). In the PASTA proof-of-concept experiment, periodic breathing as a result of the startle response was detected in video-validated PASTA output.

Integrating load cell data with telemetry or video tracking enhances understanding of animal behavior by correlating physiological and behavioral observations. This multimodal approach offers a holistic view, reducing reliance on single measurements and improving data accuracy. For example, combining telemetry's cardiovascular data with load cells' physical activity insights creates a more complete picture of an animal's well-being.

2.6 Telemetry Systems

2.6.1 Advantages of Telemetry in Research

Implantable telemetry is the most humane technique for collecting physiological signals from undisturbed, fully conscious, and freely moving laboratory animals (Kramer 2001) in different behavioral settings (Huzard et al. 2019). This wireless technology refines physiological monitoring in biomedical research since animal experiments are performed under stress-free conditions (B. P. Brockway et al. 1992), including home cage environments. As a result, experimental artifacts and stress-induced and intersubject variability are minimized, leading to increased accuracy, reliability, and predictive value of the data relative to studies using anesthetized or restrained animals (Kramer and Kinter 2003). Through refinement, telemetry helps to reduce the number of animals needed per study (Kinter 1996). Furthermore, telemetry assists researchers in identifying essential operational and experimental aspects to improve animal welfare (Toth et al. 2015; Meijer 2006). Telemetry implantation requires invasive surgery by skilled professionals following strict aseptic and ethical guidelines to minimize complications and distress. Training, standardized protocols, and refined techniques are crucial for scientific integrity and animal welfare.

2.6.2 Components and Functionality of Telemetry Systems

Telemetry uses implantable sensors to collect and transmit animal physiological signals to a remote transceiver. This transceiver then relays the data to software that saves raw data and generates derived parameters based on user instructions (Kramer 2001). Telemetry systems monitor multiple rodents simultaneously. A typical rodent study may utilize six to ten animals, but telemetry platforms are scalable and can accommodate more test subjects for larger-scale studies (Pedraza et al. 2025). The implantable sensors (or transmitters) are the key to conferring a high degree of modularity and versatility to the technique. Telemetry transmitters offer varying battery lives (1–12 months) and can measure signals like biopotentials, pressure, and blood glucose (Kramer et al. 2021). Transmitter type and surgical methods determine study length and which physiological signals (e.g., ECG, BP, EEG, EMG, glucose, temperature, and activity) can be recorded.

Cardiovascular evaluations via telemetry are accomplished by placing the body of the transmitter intraperitoneally or subcutaneously. For ECG measurements in rodents, the positive and negative electrodes are placed subcutaneously (Gkrouzoudi et al. 2023; Sgoifo et al. 1996). In this setting, proper electrode positioning is critical to acquiring quality ECG data from mice or rats. For BP recordings in mice, the less invasive method is placing the BP catheter into the carotid artery (Mills 2000). In contrast, surgical approaches using the abdominal aorta or femoral artery are more suitable for rats (Mattes and Lemmer 1991). The pressure-sensing technology also permits the assessment of left ventricular pressure, an indicator of cardiac contractility. Common cardiovascular investigations utilizing telemetry in rodents include heart rate variability analysis, physiological and mechanistic examinations, disease modeling, pharmacological testing, and circadian rhythms.

On the other hand, the typical use of rodent telemetry in neuroscience research includes seizure and sleep studies, neuropharmacology, phenotyping, and chronobiology (Kramer et al. 2021). In this regard, the most assessed physiological signals in rodents are EEG and EMG. Electrodes are attached to the skull for EEG measurements, with the leads placed epidurally or connected to deep electrodes (Lundt 2016). For combined EEG and EMG recordings, another set of electrodes is sutured to the neck muscles to obtain EMG signals. The body of the transmitter is generally placed subcutaneously.

2.6.3 Other Physiological Parameters Measured Via Telemetry

Another widespread practice of rodents instrumented with telemetry transmitters is to monitor body temperature and activity, crucial for pharmacology, infectious disease, and behavior studies. Continuous glucose telemetry improves welfare (Brockway 2015) via glucose oxidase enzyme catheters, aiding in understanding homeostasis and biomarker evaluation. Innovative telemetry applications include deriving respiratory rates from EMG or pressure signals and measuring pressures like intracranial, arterial, or ventricular. Telemetry integrates with phenotyping (Sommer 2005), fear conditioning (Gaburro 2011), and metabolic cages (Gaigé 2014). However, excessive multiparameter data collection may negate home cage advantages.

2.6.4 Challenges, Considerations, and Future Developments of Telemetry Implementation

Telemetry, an invasive method requiring surgical transmitter implantation, offers benefits but presents implementation challenges. Minimizing discomfort and complications hinges on appropriate animal body weight and transmitter type, alongside skilled surgical staff for successful implantation and reduced postoperative issues. Following proper care and recovery, rodents tolerate transmitters well, enabling longitudinal studies (Baumans 2001). Second, telemetry enables scheduled or continuous data acquisition, usually at sampling rates between 600 and 1000 Hz. Raw data from telemetry signals can generate large files. For example, a rodent experiment that collects data continuously for 7 days is estimated to render approximately 1.5 gigabytes of information per subject. Reasonable computing capacity (8 Gb RAM minimum, Intel® Core™ i7) and sufficient disk drive storage space (250 Gb) are needed, and competent software modules that automate data analysis and event detection are beneficial, especially for long-term studies. Last, the acquisition of a telemetry system involves strategic budgeting, capital allocation, and planning and running costs for transmitters. Nevertheless, the cost is generally wholly recovered through reduced animal use (Kramer et al. 2021). Additionally, users often leverage the versatility of telemetry to provide research services to maximize returns on the investment.

Telemetry technology continues to progress. Modern telemetry platforms count on group housing capabilities to monitor groups of rodents in their home cages (Martin 2024) and extended transmission ranges to accommodate high-density caging environments with minimal signal interference. Further advancements could witness the development of new sensors to measure additional parameters, cloud-based data collection, smaller transmitters, and longer battery life.

2.7 Metabolic Monitoring Systems

Metabolic technology, particularly indirect calorimetry, is a crucial part of home cage monitoring for studying energy balance, obesity, and metabolic health. It measures oxygen consumption and carbon dioxide production to determine metabolic rate, energy expenditure, and homeostasis. Additional sensors track activity and food intake, providing context without stressing the animals. These measurements also reveal diurnal changes in RER, indicating whether carbohydrates (RER closer to 1.0) or fats (RER nearer 0.7) are being metabolized (Deuster and Heled 2008). This level of detail is crucial for studies examining metabolic flexibility, the impact of dietary interventions, and the progression of metabolic disorders. However, indirect calorimetry requires the isolation of animals, and it would be challenging to adapt it to the group-housed context, as all subjects in the cage would be judged as one biomass.

2.7.1 Integration with Activity Data for Comprehensive Metabolic Profiling

Physical activity significantly contributes to energy expenditure. HCM technology offers many options for tracking home-cage locomotor activity, with IR beam activity meters being the gold standard for accuracy, scalability, and compact size. Analyzing metabolism correlated to activity is nuanced due to the causal relationship between activity, behavior, and metabolism. Modern metabolic phenotyping systems can align activity events with increased energy expenditure, and specialized software can analyze TEE differences based on activity levels, enhancing data robustness and experimental repeatability (Škop et al. 2023).

2.7.2 Integration with Feeding Data for Comprehensive Metabolic Profiling

Modern metabolic HCM systems integrate calorimetric data with feeding and water intake records for comprehensive analyses, correlating energy expenditure with nutritional intake. This integration is vital for understanding metabolism, behavior, and environmental factors, enabling energy balance calculations crucial for obesity research and metabolic syndrome studies (Rubio et al. 2023).

HCM systems use specialized software to analyze real-time metabolic data, providing immediate insights and enhancing the predictive value of experimental data by identifying patterns like circadian rhythms or dietary responses.

2.7.3 Pros of Metabolic Monitoring in HCM

- Rich Data Collection: The ability to monitor oxygen consumption, carbon dioxide production, and feeding behavior simultaneously provides a multidimensional view of an animal's metabolic state. This is crucial for studies focused on energy balance and the pathophysiology of obesity.
- Reduced Stress Artifacts: While isolation for indirect calorimetry can cause stress, home-cage metabolic sensors reduce this by shortening separation times. Future methods may enable group measurements using stable isotopes but currently face technical and cost challenges.

- Enhanced Experimental Relevance: Continuous and long-term monitoring allows for the detection of subtle physiological changes over time, making it possible to assess the effects of chronic interventions or the progression of metabolic disorders.

2.7.4 Cons of Metabolic Monitoring in HCM

- Complex Setup and Maintenance: Implementing indirect calorimetry in a home-cage setting involves sophisticated hardware and software integration. The system must be meticulously calibrated to account for environmental factors, such as bedding materials, cage design, and ambient temperature.
- Potential Housing Limitations: While the integration of metabolic monitoring into HCM systems is advancing, many setups still require individual housing to ensure precise measurements. This can limit the study of social behaviors and may necessitate modifications to standard HCM configurations.
- Data Management Challenges: Continuous data acquisition results in large datasets that require robust computational resources and specialized analysis modules to process and interpret effectively.

2.7.5 Commercial Examples and Innovations

Several commercial systems have been developed to meet the demands of metabolic monitoring in home-cage environments. Examples include the Sable Promotion, TSE PhenoMaster, and Oxymax-CLAMS (Comprehensive Lab Animal Monitoring system). These platforms are designed to integrate indirect calorimetry with additional behavioral and environmental monitoring tools. The CLAMS system, for instance, has been successfully used in collaborative research to evaluate the interplay between bedding, metabolic rates, and feeding behavior, providing a model for comprehensive metabolic profiling in a naturalistic setting (Speakman 2013; Eynaud et al. 2024; Hu et al. 2023; Škop et al. 2020).

Additionally, plethysmography—while conceptually attractive for respiratory monitoring—faces significant practical limitations in a full-volume home-cage setting. Accurately recording tidal volume becomes infeasible once the cage airspace exceeds a few liters, and although the breathing rate can still be tracked, the signal-to-noise ratio is poor. In fact, Columbus Instrument is currently the only commercial provider to offer respiratory frequency in a home-cage context, but it is planned to phase it out due to these technical challenges. Previously, smaller CLAMS "center-feeder" cages (with roughly half the internal volume) yielded more reliable plethysmographic signals, but those formats are no longer in widespread use.

2.7.6 Enriching HCM with Advanced Metabolic Insights

Recent advances have greatly improved HCM metabolic monitoring. Sensor technology offers enhanced sensitivity and accuracy, with cloud-based data and real-time analytics enabling remote monitoring. Algorithms and machine learning now automatically classify metabolic events, linking them to behavior or environment for deeper physiological insights. Miniaturized sensors reduce invasiveness and allow for group housing integration, with ongoing research addressing accuracy challenges to create more versatile and scalable HCM systems.

2.7.7 Future Perspectives

The future of metabolic technology in home-cage monitoring promises less invasive, more precise, and broader data collection. Wireless, battery-free sensors could enable continuous monitoring, akin to advancements in physiological telemetry. Integrating metabolic data with video-based behavioral analysis and environmental sensing will create multiparametric platforms, streamlining experiments, and reducing animal numbers per study by providing comprehensive datasets.

2.7.8 Conclusion

Integrating metabolic technology, particularly indirect calorimetry (VO_2, VCO_2, and RER) and feeding data, into home-cage monitoring advances biomedical research. Despite setup and data management challenges, the benefits of enhanced experimental relevance and reduced stress make it invaluable for studying metabolism, obesity, and animal welfare. Technological innovations and multimodal integration will ensure that metabolic HCM systems play a key role in future preclinical research.

2.8 Environmental Monitoring

Environmental factors like illumination, humidity, and temperature significantly impact rodent behavior and physiology yet are often overlooked in studies. Broadly, there are three options for environmental monitoring systems. First, there is a commercial, lab-oriented system, e.g., Pallidus.io. This system is composed of battery-powered, cage top-mounted units that send activity, humidity, and temperature data to a real-time cloud dashboard. Second, there is a segment of the home automation market for wireless, networked sensors for home air quality data, such as Aqara, AirGradient, Apollo AIR-1, or Sonoff, which could ostensibly be repurposed for laboratory use. Finally, there are lab-developed open-source solutions, such as the MIROSLAV device with the EnviroSLAV addition to the main unit, which also provides real-time wireless data transmission to one or multiple logging devices (Virag et al. 2025). While the EnviroSLAV addition was originally developed to monitor habitat conditions, attaching the main MIROSLAV unit to cage tops is feasible. For example, recently, a group developed a real-time ambient sensing tool, MyVivarium, based on IoT and the Raspberry Pi system, allowing the recording and logging of environmental measures in a cloud-based application (Vidva et al. 2025). DIY systems offer significant appeal due to their lower cost and broader customization options compared to limited commercial solutions (see Chap. 9). However, open-source projects may face abandonment or lack of ongoing support due to the unpredictable nature of academic research trajectories.

Generally, any study, especially those utilizing HCM technologies, can benefit greatly by also implementing sensors for illumination, temperature, humidity, noise, pressure, and a passive infrared sensor to acquire precise timestamps of personnel entrances. These sensors have good durability, do not require frequent calibration, and can produce time-series data that can be correlated with other in-cage events, such as home cage activity (Virag et al. 2024; Hu et al. 2023).

Affordable, high-quality sensors like the Sensirion SHT45 (temperature/humidity) and ams OSRAM TSL25721 (light) are readily available, enabling accurate and low-maintenance environmental monitoring at the cage level, which can control for a major source of variability. Sensors for gases like carbon dioxide, ammonia, and volatile organic compounds (VOCs) are available (€60–€300) but often need maintenance. Some, like the Telaire T6713 for CO2, offer long, calibration-free lifespans using infrared dispersion. While useful for ventilated cages, their effectiveness in open-top cages is questionable due to airflow variations.

2.9 Acoustic Monitoring (USV)

Integrating ultrasonic vocalization (USV) recording into HCM systems would significantly enhance our understanding of rodent communication, social behavior, and emotional states. Rodents communicate via USVs (18–110 kHz), which are inaudible to humans. These vocalizations are context dependent, with variations in frequency, duration, and modulation reflecting different emotional states like anxiety, pain, or positive social interactions. While visual monitoring has advanced, USV interpretation has lagged. Incorporating audio monitoring would provide researchers with a more comprehensive behavioral repertoire for assessing animal welfare and stress responses (Portfors 2007; Lefebvre et al. 2020). Consequently, the detection and analysis of USVs have become a marker of animal welfare and an indirect indicator of the internal state of the subject.

USV detection in HCM requires specialized microphones with a broad, ultrasonic frequency response. Captured audio is analyzed using advanced software to identify and categorize call types based on spectral and temporal features. Commercial systems like Avisoft, Dodotronic, and Sonotrack provide dedicated solutions that can be integrated with HCM setups. Similarly, platforms such as those offered by METRIS, Noldus (e.g., UltraVox XT), and BatSound extend these capabilities by combining audio data with other behavioral measures. Additionally, using a 'bat microphone' (Petterson M500-USB, https://batsound.com/product-category/usbmicrophones/) and open source recording software (e.g., Audacity®) is also a viable and significantly cheaper solution to record USVs in laboratory settings.

Integrating ultrasonic audio recording into HCM requires sensitive microphones (18–110 kHz) to convert acoustic waves into electronic signals. Software must synchronize audio capture with other sensor data. Advanced algorithms and machine learning filter noise, segment recordings, and classify call types, automating analysis for affective states and social interactions (Coffey et al. 2019; de Chaumont et al. 2021). Data, audio, video, telemetry, and sensor inputs are integrated to create a comprehensive view of animal behavior, enhancing assessment reliability.

2.9.1 Applications in Behavioral and Welfare Studies

The integration of ultrasonic vocalization detection within HCM systems has several valuable applications. (i) USVs are integral to understanding the dynamics of rodent communication during group housing. Analysis of these vocalizations can elucidate the nuances of social hierarchy, mating behavior, and affiliative interactions (D'amato 1991; Egnor and Seagraves 2016). (ii) Changes in vocalization patterns often indicate stress responses. For instance, alterations in call frequency or intensity may signal discomfort or distress, enabling researchers to assess the impact of experimental conditions on animal welfare (A. Venkatraman et al. 2024). (iii) In drug discovery and testing, monitoring USVs provides an additional behavioral endpoint to evaluate the efficacy and side effects of novel therapeutics. Indeed, subtle shifts in vocalization profiles may reveal the impact of pharmacological agents on central nervous system function (Brudzynski 2015; Simola 2015; Premoli et al. 2023). (iv) Tracking the evolution of USVs over time can offer insights into the developmental trajectory of communication skills in rodents, contributing to studies on neurodevelopmental disorders (Castellucci et al. 2018; Granata et al. 2022).

2.9.2 Pros of USV Systems

- *Non-Invasive Monitoring*: Audio recording is entirely noninvasive, ensuring that animals are not disturbed by the monitoring process.
- *Additional Behavioral Context*: USV data complement other monitoring modalities, such as video or telemetry, by providing an auditory dimension to behavioral analysis.
- *Real-Time Data Collection*: Continuous audio recording enables the capture of spontaneous and transient vocalizations, which might otherwise be missed in periodic assessments.
- *Enhanced Welfare Assessment*: Monitoring USV patterns can provide an early warning system for stress and discomfort, enabling timely interventions to improve animal welfare.

2.9.3 Cons

- *Background Noise Interference*: A major challenge is the potential for background noise, both environmental and equipment-generated, to interfere with the detection of ultrasonic signals.
- *Varying recording quality*: Microphone orientation and distance relative to the animal are crucial. Minor obstructions, like plastic houses, can significantly attenuate USV intensity.
- *Automated Analysis Challenges*: Despite software advances, parsing complex vocalizations and distinguishing individual animals in groups remains challenging.

- *Amount of Data*: Recording ultrasound vocalizations at high sampling rates generates vast datasets, even over short periods, creating real-time analysis and storage challenges. This necessitates limiting continuous observation or incurring higher costs for storage and high-performance technology.
- *Cost Considerations*: High-quality ultrasonic microphones and associated data acquisition systems can be expensive, particularly when multiple recording channels are needed.
- *Individual Identification Limitations*: Single-microphone audio recording alone cannot reliably identify vocalizing animals, unlike RFID or video. This remains a significant limitation, as multimicrophone systems and complex computational methods still struggle with USV emitter identification and incur high costs (de Chaumont et al. 2021; Waidmann et al. 2024). To clearly link vocalizations to individuals, recordings are usually made individually or in specific arenas. However, this often removes the social group and home cage context.

2.9.4 Integration and Future Directions

Integrating ultrasonic vocalization detection into HCM systems is a significant advance in behavioral phenotyping. Future efforts will likely focus on improving audio resolution and developing more sophisticated, real-time analytical algorithms. Emerging technologies may include

- Enhanced Signal Processing: Algorithms that better differentiate between overlapping calls and effectively filter out background noise, possibly using deep learning methods.
- Multimodal Data Fusion: Closer integration of audio data with video and telemetry outputs, allowing for a synchronized analysis of vocalizations alongside movement, physiological parameters, and environmental factors.
- Wireless and Miniaturized systems: As with telemetry, there is ongoing development of smaller, wireless audio recording systems that can be easily incorporated into home cages without interfering with animal behavior.
- Wearable devices with custom circuit boards that can be fitted to individual mice and connected to a variety of existing USV recording systems are currently under development and reached an accuracy of 90% when attributing vocalizations to a specific animal, based on the relative amplitude differences (Waidmann et al. 2024).
- Cloud-Based Data Analysis: Leveraging cloud computing to process and store large volumes of audio data, facilitating large-scale studies and collaborative research efforts.

Audio technology in HCM offers insight into rodent communication, enhancing our understanding of social behavior, stress, and animal welfare. By capturing USVs, researchers gain a rich dataset that complements traditional measures, advancing behavioral neuroscience.

Integrating ultrasonic vocalization detection enriches HCM experimental tools, providing an additional data layer that, combined with other monitoring, offers nuanced interpretations of animal behavior. As technology evolves, improvements in sensitivity, data integration, and analysis will solidify audio monitoring as a fundamental component of home-cage behavioral studies.

2.10 Operant Technology in the Home Cage

Operant systems not only observe *but also directly impact animal* behavior, coupling sensors that detect an animal's voluntary action with actuators that deliver cues, rewards, or punishments to elicit a response. The interaction can be described by three consecutive one-way interactions: (i) the device presents *a cue* to the animal, (ii) the animal exhibits *a response* detected by the device, and (iii) the device provides *a consequence* (reward or punishment) to the animal. The specific behaviors a device can elicit and measure in user-defined operational protocols depend on the electronic components the system is equipped with. Integrating this closed-loop system into the social cage transforms it into an interactive environment for continuous learning and decision-making with minimal human intervention.

2.10.1 The Cue

Cues activate animal senses via electronic components. Components offering wider range and finer control enhance protocol design flexibility. For example, addressable RGB LEDs offer precise light control for varied cues, unlike incandescent bulbs. Protocols must account for animal sensory limits (e.g., mice hear 2–70 kHz, humans 20 Hz-20 kHz).

2.10.2 The Response

A sensor, the main electronic component, translates physical phenomena into electronic impulses, recorded as data. Thus, nearly any sensing technology in this chapter could apply, depending on the behavior scientists aim to recognize as a response to a presented cue.

- Video detection (see Sect. 2.1) uses simple algorithms for presence/movement. Neural networks can also recognize behaviors or body parts; the latter, combined with algorithms (e.g., distance-based interaction), classifies behavior. Real-time neural network inference makes this technically complex.
- RFID tagging (see Sect. 2.2) can be used to detect the presence of one specific animal in a defined area, which can, for example, trigger the start of a test.
- Capacitive sensors can be used to detect touch or licking and function on the same principle as electromagnetic field systems (see Sect. 2.3).
- Infrared motion sensors can be used to detect an animal's presence in an area, while beam-break sensors are commonly used to detect nosepokes in a designated opening (see Sect. 2.4).

- Similar to electromechanical microswitches, load cells and pressure sensors (see Sect. 2.5) can be used to detect an animal pressing on a lever or for area presence detection.
- Ultrasonic vocalization (see Sect. 2.9) can be detected to elicit a consequence. A specific type of vocalization could be filtered using digital signal processing (DSP) algorithms, with or without a machine learning classifier.

Skinner boxes, originally using electromechanical levers, now primarily employ nosepoke openings with beam-break sensors. Levers for rats need to be low and wide for activation, as thin, high levers only elicit sniffing. Nosepokes are better for isolating individual responses in multianimal settings. Ideally, the initial action (e.g., sniffing a nosepoke, standing on a platform) should be neutral before reinforcement or punishment.

2.10.3 The Consequences (Reward Versus Punishment)

Operant conditioning *rewards* often use automated food/water dispensers, with liquid rewards requiring more maintenance. Servo-controlled gates allow diverse reward types. Animal preferences vary, and sugars can complicate experiments. *Punishment*, using air puffs or mild electric shocks, yields consistent reactions and avoids food or water deprivation issues but raises ethical concerns due to stress.

2.11 Benefits of the Home Cage-Based Approach

Conventional operant conditioning is time-consuming (1 month for 1-h daily sessions), limiting its use in adolescence or disease models. For example, assessing ADHD-related impulsivity in rodents is restricted to adulthood due to long training. Home cage setups drastically reduce training time (e.g., <7 days for 5-CSRTT), enable 24/7 testing with many trials (Bruinsma et al. 2019), and may improve learning in a familiar, human-free environment. Shorter training and automation make water gating a more viable reward. Scheduled unattended testing, e.g., 3-h sessions, is possible. Ongoing work hints that food/water deprivation may not be necessary to induce operant learning, at least in rats (Augier et al. 2017). Home cage operant conditioning offers increased statistical power, reduced experimenter workload, and allows testing younger animals and across circadian cycles.

2.11.1 Cognitive Domains Assessed

Operant conditioning protocols assess attention and impulse control (5-CSRTT training in <7 days), cognitive flexibility (IntelliCage reversal/rule-switch protocols), and motivation/effort cost (progressive-ratio hoppers/nose-poke panels). Sensory discrimination and sequence learning are evaluated using PsiBox (tone/frequency discrimination within 2 weeks).

2.11.2 Home Cage Implementation

Configurable home cage operant systems allow for various testing protocols, but translating standard operant tasks to the home cage is not a 1:1 process. For example, a rat home cage 5-CSRTT task showed different impulsivity results and more performed trials when testing was restricted to 2.5 h versus 24/7. These findings highlight new aspects of executive function and the need to reoptimize protocols for the home cage.

2.11.3 Data Acquisition Architecture in Operant Systems

Operant conditioning devices, particularly home cage systems, require precise synchronization and prolonged unattended operation, necessitating robust measures against data loss. While common in embedded systems and automation through redundancy and failure detection, commercial HCM operant systems often rely on a single PC, creating a point of failure. Open-source systems like FED3 (Matikainen-Ankney et al. 2021) offer more resilience by logging to SD cards, but simultaneous, redundant logging and networked architectures with remote alerts would be ideal for preventing data loss and enabling real-time monitoring and control, as demonstrated by nonoperant HCM systems like Tecniplast DVC and MIROSLAV (Virag et al. 2024). Integrating local storage with network logging would further enhance reliability. Given the severe consequences of data loss in animal research, increased adoption of such preventative measures is ethically crucial as HCM systems become more complex.

2.11.4 Pros

- 24/7 Sampling: hundreds of trials across the circadian cycle boost statistical power.
- Voluntary, self-paced interaction keeps stress hormones low and eliminates the experimenter effect.
- Faster acquisition: learning complete in days rather than weeks.
- Group scalability: high-throughput pipelines exist (www.micecraft.com).
- Systems integration: operant event clocks aligned with telemetry, video pose, or environmental sensors enable comprehensive phenotyping.

2.11.5 Cons

- Equipment in contact with animals more prone to malfunction:
  - Dust or bedding on lick spouts: false lick detections and corrupted data.
  - Cable chewing: data loss or hardware failure.
- More severe consequences of equipment malfunction:
  - Servo miscalibration on pellet hoppers: unintended food restriction.
  - Power outages: unsignaled deprivation of food or water and loss of data.

Open-source dashboards bundled with devices like *LIQ-HD* display live lick counts, so anomalies are detected without disturbing the cage (Petersen et al. 2023). Weekly calibration scripts, version-controlled task code, and hardware health checks are recommended best practices.

2.11.6 Implementation Notes for Researchers

When designing an operant HCM cage, link the cue (LEDs/speakers), action (nose-poke/lickometer), and reinforcer (pellets/water) to specific hardware. For cues, use spectrally distinct LEDs or calibrated speakers. For actions, nose pokes localize responses, while lickometers measure precise contact but need water scheduling; combining both distinguishes trial initiation from choice. For reinforcers, use optical gates for pellet verification and daily purging for water lines. Scheduling tasks during the initial dark phase maintain motivation without deprivation, as seen in the 5-CSRTT "time-restricted" protocol.

2.11.7 Data Handling and Analysis

Operant events (subject ID, timestamp, and code) are appended to the HCM log and can be aligned with video pose or telemetry to relate internal state to behavior. A single mouse generates ≈1 MB day^{-1} of event data; automated scripts that bin trials by light phase or stimulus difficulty reduce file sizes and feed dashboards for rapid QC.

3 Combinations of Systems, Emerging Technologies, and Future Considerations

Modern HCM research is moving from single-modality "black boxes" toward interoperable ecosystems in which multiple sensors, actuators, and analytical pipelines talk to each other in real time. This section surveys the technical and conceptual shifts that enable that transition, from hardware miniaturization to metadata standards, and it discusses how ethical and logistical constraints shape the next generation of platforms.

3.1 Aspects to Consider When Driving Innovation in HCM Technologies

- *Miniaturization and Efficiency*: Advancements in nanotechnology and materials science are leading to smaller, more efficient sensors that can be easily integrated into the homecage environment. These sensors can measure a wider range of parameters with greater accuracy and lower power consumption.
- *Integration with Big Data and AI*: Combining sensor data with advanced analytics and machine learning algorithms allows for deeper insights into animal behavior and physiology. Cloud computing and data storage solutions facilitate the management and analysis of large datasets generated by HCM systems.
- *Wearable Technologies*: Flexible electronics and wearable sensors offer the potential for noninvasive, continuous monitoring of physiological parameters in freely moving animals. These technologies can be integrated into lightweight, comfortable devices that minimize stress and behavioral disruption.

- *Personalized and customized monitoring systems*: The development of modular, open-source HCM platforms allows researchers to tailor monitoring systems to their specific research questions and experimental needs. This flexibility enables greater innovation and collaboration within research.

3.2 Key Drivers of Innovation

Advancements in nanofabrication and low-power ASIC design enable sugar-cube-sized multisensor nodes to record locomotion, temperature, and ECG for weeks using harvested energy. These devices, paired with cloud-based GPU clusters, transform home cages into “data lakes” for machine learning to uncover subtle phenotypes. Additionally, open-source modular chassis allow labs to build custom rigs, speeding up iteration and reducing costs (see Chap. 9).

3.3 Retrofitting Versus Green-Field Set-Ups

Where budgets or animal-facility regulations limit new infrastructure, solutions such as Olden Labs’ cage-lid modules (https://oldenlabs.com/) or the iMouse retrofit camera system (https://imouse.info/) allow researchers layer monitoring onto standard shoebox cages and commercial racks (Tecniplast, Allentown, …). Conversely, fully integrated arenas like MouseVUER (Salem et al. 2024), LMT (de Chaumont et al. 2019), TSE’s Phenomaster (Gallage et al. 2024), or Noldus Phenotyper 2 (Grieco et al. 2021) trade initial capital expenses for richer 3D viewpoints, environmental control, and simplified cabling—at the cost of lower throughput per square meter. Choosing between these extremes depends on the study’s spatial footprint, biosafety class, and anticipated life-span of the experiment.

3.4 Embedding Neuroscience Toolchains

Optogenetic stimulators, wireless headstages for calcium imaging, and miniaturized photometry fibers can now be docked inside the home cage so that brain activity, behavior, and environmental cues are recorded synchronously. Proof-of-concept work with 2D-Neuro’s wireless optogenetic implants allows freely moving mice to receive pattern-locked stimulation within their home cage settings (https://2dneuro.com/).

3.5 Computer Vision and AI-Based Systems

In recent years, artificial intelligence (AI) has become a cornerstone of next-generation HCM systems, enabling fully automated, high-throughput analysis of complex behavioral and physiological data. By integrating AI with the tools, data, and sensors used in HCM, researchers can extract richer insights, reduce human bias, and accelerate discovery. In the following sections, we describe how AI advances across two primary tasks (identification and interpretation), the evolving role of transformer-based architectures, multicamera 3D solutions, and the trade-offs inherent in edge versus cloud computing deployments.

3.5.1 Identification Task: From Frames to Quantitative Data

The identification task converts raw video frames into numerical representations—animal centroids, body-part keypoints, or object masks—that feed downstream analyses. Early breakthroughs came from repurposing human-pose architectures: DeepLabCut repackaged DeeperCut into an end-to-end toolkit for animal researchers, democratizing markerless pose estimation with just dozens of labeled frames (Insafutdinov et al. 2016; Mathis et al. 2018). Building on this, (Lauer et al. 2022) introduced multianimal pipeline enhancements for faster training and real-time inference, and SLEAP demonstrated robust multianimal tracking in complex arenas (Pereira et al. 2022).

Complementary to pose estimation, object detection networks such as YOLO have been adopted for rapid cage-wide animal localization (Redmon et al. 2015). YOLO's single-pass architecture allows real-time processing on consumer-grade GPUs, making it ideal for large cage racks where dozens of video streams must be monitored simultaneously. Together, these CNN-based tools provide a modular "plug-and-play" identification layer that can be tailored to specific HCM tasks—locomotion quantification, enrichment interaction, or social proximity mapping—while maintaining minimal hardware requirements.

3.5.2 Semantic Segmentation and the Transformer Revolution

While pixelwise semantic segmentation has historically lagged in HCM—due to the laborious annotation of object polygons—recent transformer-based models are poised to change this landscape. The Segment Anything Model (SAM) delivers zero-shot segmentation of previously unseen objects, allowing rapid adaptation to new cage configurations or lighting conditions without manual mask labeling (Kirillov et al. 2023). By prompting SAM with minimal cues, researchers can obtain precise object boundaries—critical for measuring fine-scale interactions with manipulanda or nest materials—without incurring prohibitive annotation costs. This shift from convolutional to transformer architectures (Vaswani et al. 2017) also underpins novel self-supervised methods that learn from vast amounts of unlabeled video. In the near future, HCM platforms may employ such models to discover latent environmental or postural features—beyond predefined keypoints—that correlate with physiological events, further enriching the scope of home-cage analytics.

3.5.3 Three-Dimensional Tracking: Multicamera Integration

Extending AI-driven identification into three dimensions enhances the fidelity of behavioral measures—especially for activities like vertical rearing or climbing. Libraries such as OpenCV have long offered undistortion and stereo-triangulation tools (Bradski 2000), but specialized pipelines streamline 3D pose estimation in rodents. DeepLabCut 3D integrates per-camera keypoints and performs triangulation to reconstruct 3D trajectories (Nath et al. 2019). Building on this, Anipose unifies multicamera calibration and triangulation workflows, simplifying setup across three or more viewpoints (Karashchuk et al. 2021).

Advanced approaches like DANNCE leverage geometric reasoning to resolve occlusions and improve volumetric reconstructions (Dunn et al. 2021), while s-DANNCE introduces scalability optimizations for denser camera arrays (Klibaite et al. 2025) and allows for better social behavior discrimination. Despite the clear benefits of 3D data—precise kinematics and enriched behavioral grammar—the increased hardware complexity and per-cage cost mean that most commercial HCM systems still favor single-camera setups, reserving 3D rigs for specialized studies.

3.5.4 Interpretation Task: From Keypoints to Behavior

Once quantitative features are extracted, the interpretation task employs AI to translate these time series into meaningful behavioral or physiological categories. Supervised classifiers—including support vector machines and deep sequence models—map pose trajectories or raw video clips to ethologically defined behaviors (e.g., grooming, digging, and rearing). While powerful, these methods demand extensive labeled datasets and are limited to prespecified behaviors visible to human observers.

To address annotation bottlenecks and observer bias, unsupervised segmentation algorithms have gained traction. B-SOiD clusters high-dimensional pose dynamics to segment behavior sequences without labels and then derives compact classifiers for real-time use (Hsu and Yttri 2021). Similarly, VAME leverages variational autoencoders to learn latent representations of movement motifs (Luxem et al. 2022), and BehaviorFlow statistically compares behavioral state transition matrices that can be based on any discrete segmentation of behavior, although typically are based on clustering of time-series-embedded gait features (von Ziegler et al. 2024). More recently, Keypoint MoSeq integrated motion sequencing with hidden Markov models to automatically discover hierarchical behavioral modules (Weinreb et al. 2024). These unsupervised methods not only reveal novel patterns—such as subtle gait alterations preceding motor deficits—but also reduce reliance on human-defined ethograms, improving reproducibility.

3.6 Ethical Considerations

- Minimizing Stress and Discomfort: Homecage monitoring systems should be designed and implemented in a way that minimizes stress and discomfort for the animals. Noninvasive or minimally invasive technologies are preferred whenever possible.
- Impact of Monitoring Devices: Researchers should carefully assess the potential impact of monitoring devices on animal behavior and welfare. This includes considering the size and weight of devices, their placement on the animal, and any potential for interference with normal activities.

- Regulatory Compliance: All homecage monitoring studies must adhere to relevant ethical guidelines and regulations for the care and use of laboratory animals.
- Balancing Data Needs with Animal Welfare: Researchers must carefully balance the need for scientific data with the welfare of the animals. Open and transparent communication with ethical review boards and the public is essential for maintaining public trust and support for animal research.
- Be careful to not reduce welfare and limit the translational and physiological relevance of the extended amount of data recorded by trying to integrate too much at a time. Welfare should be a priority, not just a set of rules constraining the development of the technologies.

3.7 Interoperable Metadata Across HCM Systems

As described in Chap. 11, it is more than critical that systems and different technologies are able to communicate efficiently with each other. In addition, they should provide standardized and fully interoperable set of metadata schemas. It is therefore highly recommended that both academics developing DIY solutions (Chap. 9) and manufacturers work together toward a consensus for (meta)data management as recently proposed and described (Bains et al. 2025). For example, when companies develop new technologies, they should now prioritize the interconnectivity of their solutions with already existing systems. This could be simplified by developing and offering open APIs that could allow scientists to integrate and combine their variations in system databases. Offering TTL communications is also a great way to facilitate the use and communication between systems, but integrating interoperability at the software level should become a reflex as well. For example, individual solutions are currently being developed with the goal of offering a unified metadata management system, integrating, standardizing, and unifying metadata at the level of project elaboration, mouse management, and data publication (Metadatapp (MAPP), www.metadatapp.net).

Acknowledgments The authors wish to thank Michael Girand for his valuable contribution to the text of the Telemetry section of this chapter and Yves Eray for his contribution to the RFID implants section.

Author Contributions DH supervised the redaction and participated in the entire chapter redaction. DV contributed to most of the sections (Intro, Video, Other Motion Sensors, Load Cells, Environment Monitoring, Operant Systems) and writing of the entire manuscript. CA contributed to the motion sensors section, the Environmental Monitoring section, the Load Cells and Pressure Sensors section, and the Metabolic monitoring section. OS, TL, and NW contributed to the Video section and Computer Vision and AI section. PM and MR contributed to the RFID section. SG contributed to the EMF section. JA contributor to the Telemetry section. Competing Interests While the following did not fund or contribute directly to the research presented here, the work aligns with their scope of activity and may indirectly increase their visibility. Damien Huzard is the owner of NeuroNautix (registered as sole proprietorship in France) and the creator of Metadatapp, a metadata management solution. Julio Alvarez is working for DSI, a company manufacturing telemetric implants. Christopher K. Adams is working for Columbus Instruments. Matt Ruiter is working for UIDevices. Michael Florea is the CEO of Olden Labs. Stefano Gaburro is working for Tecniplast S.p.A. Davor Virag, Oliver Sturman, Paul Mieske, and Thomas Lorimer work with HCM technologies but do not have industrial conflicts of interest.

References

Augier E, Dulman RS, Singley E, Heilig M (2017) A method for evaluating the reinforcing properties of ethanol in rats without water deprivation, saccharin fading or extended access training. J Vis Exp 119(January):e53305

Bains RS, Huzard D, McCutcheon JE, Boguszewski P, Virag D, Restivo L, Lewejohann L et al (2025) Too big to lose—a FAIR repository for biomedical data derived from home-cage monitoring. Open Sci Framework. https://doi.org/10.31219/osf.io/fsg83_v1

Baumans V (2001) Intra-abdominal transmitter implantation in mice: effects on behaviour and body weight. Anim Welf 10:291–302

Brachs S, Dall M, Zimbalski L-K, Santin Y, Oeing C, Mai K, Parini A, Gaburro S, Nielsen TS (2025) Robust non-invasive detection of hyperglycemia in mouse models of metabolic dysregulation: the novel urination index biomarker. bioRxiv. https://doi.org/10.1101/2025.04.02.646666

Bradski G (2000) The OpenCV library. Dr Dobb's J Softw Tools 25(11):120–123

Brockway R (2015) Fully implantable arterial blood glucose device for metabolic research applications in rats for two months. J Diabetes Sci Technol 9(4):771–781. https://doi.org/10.1177/1932296815586424

Brockway BP, Hassler CR, Hicks N (1992) Minimizing stress during physiological monitoring. Refin Reduct Anim Test 17:18

Brudzynski SM (2015) Pharmacology of ultrasonic vocalizations in adult rats: significance, call classification and neural substrate. Curr Neuropharmacol 13(2):180–192

Bruinsma B, Terra H, de Kloet SF, Luchicchi A, Timmerman AJ, Remmelink E, Loos M, Pattij T, Mansvelder HD (2019) An automated home-cage-based 5-choice serial reaction time task for rapid assessment of attention and impulsivity in rats. Psychopharmacology 236(7):2015–2026

Castellucci GA, Calbick D, McCormick D (2018) The temporal organization of mouse ultrasonic vocalizations. PLoS One 13(10):e0199929

Coffey KR, Marx RE, Neumaier JF (2019) DeepSqueak: a deep learning-based system for detection and analysis of ultrasonic vocalizations. Neuropsychopharmacology 44(5):859–868

Crawley JN (2007) What's wrong my mouse? behavioral phenotyping transgenic knockout mice. Wiley

Crawley JN (2023) Twenty years of discoveries emerging from mouse models of autism. Neurosci Biobehav Rev 146(March):105053

Czekajewski JA, HL Hill, KJ Kober (1982) Animal activity monitor and behavior processor. USPTO 4337726. US Patent, filed July 7, 1980, and issued July 6, 1982. https://patentimages.storage.googleapis.com/ff/51/8a/d6bd5935b9fa28/US4337726.pdf

D'amato FR (1991) Courtship ultrasonic vocalizations and social status in mice. Anim Behav 41(5):875–885

de Chaumont F, Ey E, Torquet N, Lagache T, Dallongeville S, Imbert A, Legou T et al (2019) Real-time analysis of the behaviour of groups of mice via a depth-sensing camera and machine learning. Nat Biomed Eng 3(11):930–942 de Chaumont F, Lemière N, Coqueran S, Bourgeron T, Ey E (2021) LMT USV toolbox, a novel methodological approach to place mouse ultrasonic vocalizations in their Behavioral contexts—a study in female and male C57BL/6J mice and in Shank3 mutant females. Front Behav Neurosci 15(October):735920

Deuster PA, Heled Y (2008) Testing for maximal aerobic power. In: The sports medicine resource manual. Elsevier, pp 520–528

Dunn TW, Marshall JD, Severson KS, Aldarondo DE, Hildebrand DGC, Chettih SN, Wang WL et al (2021) Geometric deep learning enables 3D kinematic profiling across species and environments. Nat Methods 18(5):564–573

Egnor SR, Seagraves KM (2016) The contribution of ultrasonic vocalizations to mouse courtship. Curr Opin Neurobiol 38(June):1–5

Eynaud A, Solomon J, Schoeman E, Wu Z, Amenyogbe N (2024) Adapting indirect calorimetry to measure metabolic status of healthy and septic neonatal mice. bioRxiv. https://doi.org/10.1101/2024.05.23.595520

Gaburro S (2011) A mouse model of high trait anxiety shows reduced heart rate variability that can be reversed by anxiolytic drug treatment. Int J Neuropsychopharmacol 14:1341–1355

Gaigé S (2014) Modification of energy balance induced by the food contaminant T-2 toxin: a multimodal gut-to-brain connection. Brain Behav Immun 37:54–72

Gallage S, Ali A, Avila JEB, Seymen N, Ramadori P, Joerke V, Zizmare L et al (2024) A 5:2 intermittent fasting regimen ameliorates NASH and fibrosis and blunts HCC development via hepatic PPARα and PCK1. Cell Metab 36(6):1371–93.e7

Gkrouzoudi A, Tsingotjidou A, Jirkof P (2023) A systematic review on reporting of refinement measures in mouse ECG telemetry implantation surgery. Lab Anim 57:9–25

Goulding EH, Schenk AK, Juneja P, MacKay AW, Wade JM, Tecott LH (2008) A robust automated system elucidates mouse home cage behavioral structure. Proc Natl Acad Sci USA 105(52):20575–20582

Granata LE, Valentine A, Hirsch JL, Brenhouse HC (2022) Infant ultrasonic vocalizations predict adolescent social behavior in rats: effects of early life adversity. Dev Psychobiol 64(3):e22260

Grieco F, Bernstein BJ, Biemans B, Lior Bikovski C, Burnett J, Cushman JD, van Dam EA et al (2021) Measuring behavior in the home cage: study design, applications, challenges, and perspectives. Front Behav Neurosci 15(September):735387

Guzman M, Geuther BQ, Sabnis GS, Kumar V (2024) Highly accurate and precise determination of mouse mass using computer vision. Patterns 5(9):101039

Habedank A, Urmersbach B, Kahnau P, Lewejohann L (2022) O mouse, where art thou? The mouse position surveillance system (MoPSS)—an RFID-based tracking system. Behav Res Methods 54(2):676–689

Hsu AI, Yttri EA (2021) B-SOiD, an open-source unsupervised algorithm for identification and fast prediction of Behaviors. Nat Commun 12(1):5188

Hu D, Tan M, Dongliang L, Kleiboeker B, Liu X, Park H, Kravitz AV et al (2023) TMEM135 links peroxisomes to the regulation of Brown fat mitochondrial fission and energy homeostasis. Nat Commun 14(1):6099

Huzard D, Ghosal S, Grosse J, Carnevali L, Sgoifo A, Sandi C (2019) Low vagal tone in two rat models of psychopathology involving high or low corticosterone stress responses. Psychoneuroendocrinology 101(March):101–110

Huzard D, Martin M, Maingret F, Chemin J, Jeanneteau F, Mery P-F, Fossat P, Bourinet E, François A (2022) The impact of C-tactile low-threshold mechanoreceptors on affective touch and social interactions in mice. Sci Adv 8(26):eabo7566

Huzard D, Marias M, Granat C, Oliva G, Soubeyre V, Grellier G, Negm A, Devaux J, Bourinet E, François A (2024) Primary sensory neuron dysfunction underlying mechanical itch hypersensitivity in a Shank3 mouse model of autism. bioRxiv. https://doi.org/10.1101/2024.12.29.630575

Iannello F (2019) Non-intrusive high throughput automated data collection from the home cage. Heliyon 5(4):e01454

Insafutdinov E, Pishchulin L, Andres B, Andriluka M, Schiele B (2016) DeeperCut: a deeper, stronger, and faster multi-person pose estimation model. arXiv [cs.CV]. http://arxiv.org/abs/1605.03170

Karashchuk P, Rupp KL, Dickinson ES, Walling-Bell S, Sanders E, Azim E, Brunton BW, Tuthill JC (2021) Anipose: a toolkit for robust markerless 3D pose estimation. Cell Rep 36(13):109730

Keenan BT, Galante RJ, Lian J, Simecek P, Gatti DM, Zhang L, Lim DC, Svenson KL, Churchill GA, Pack AI (2020) High-throughput sleep phenotyping produces robust and heritable traits in diversity outbred mice and their founder strains. Sleep 43(5):zsz278

Kelley AE (1993) Locomotor activity and exploration. In: Techniques in the behavioral and neural sciences. Elsevier, pp 499–518

Kinter LB (1996) Cardiovascular telemetry and laboratory animals welfare: New reduction and refinement alternatives (Abstract). In: General Pharmacology/Safety Pharmacology Meeting. Philadelphia, PA.

Kirillov A, Mintun E, Ravi N, Mao H, Rolland C, Gustafson L, Xiao T et al (2023) Segment anything. arXiv [cs.CV]. http://arxiv.org/abs/2304.02643

Klibaite U, Tianqing Li, Diego Aldarondo, Jumana F. Akoad, Bence P. Ölveczky, Timothy W. Dunn. 2025 Mapping the landscape of social behavior. Cell, 188(8):2249–2266. https://doi.org/10.1016/j.cell.2025.01.044.

Kramer K (2001) The use of radiotelemetry in small laboratory animals: recent advances. Contemp Top Immunobiol 40:9

Kramer K, Kinter LB (2003) Evaluation and applications of radiotelemetry in small laboratory animals. Physiol Genomics 13:197–205

Kramer K, Hachtman S, Girand M, Stiedl O (2021) Chapter 15: Applications of implantable radio telemetry in small laboratory animals. In: Handbook of laboratory animal science, 4th edn. CRC Press, Boca Raton

Lapp HE, Salazar MG, Champagne FA (2023) Automated maternal behavior during early life in rodents (AMBER) pipeline. Sci Rep 13(1):18277

Lauer J, Zhou M, Ye S, Menegas W, Schneider S, Nath T, Rahman MM et al (2022) Multi-animal pose estimation, identification and tracking with DeepLabCut. Nat Methods 19(4):496–504

Lefebvre E, Granon S, Chauveau F (2020) Social context increases ultrasonic vocalizations during restraint in adult mice. Anim Cogn 23(2):351–359

Lundt A (2016) EEG radiotelemetry in small laboratory rodents: a powerful state-of-the art approach in neuropsychiatric, neurodegenerative, and epilepsy research. Neural Plast 2016:1–19

Luxem K, Mocellin P, Fuhrmann F, Kürsch J, Miller SR, Palop JJ, Remy S, Bauer P (2022) Identifying Behavioral structure from deep variational embeddings of animal motion. Commun Biol 5(1):1267

Martin S (2024) Long-term, high-resolution telemetry monitoring of circadian rhythmicity of temperature and activity in socially housed mice. In: Australas Neurosci Soc Annu Sci Meet 21878. Australasian Neuroscience Society, Perth

Mathis A, Mamidanna P, Cury KM, Abe T, Murthy VN, Mathis MW, Bethge M (2018) DeepLabCut: markerless pose estimation of user-defined body parts with deep learning. Nat Neurosci 21(9):1281–1289

Matikainen-Ankney, Bridget A., Thomas Earnest, Mohamed Ali, Eric Casey, Justin G. Wang, Amy K. Sutton, Alex A. Legaria, et al 2021. “An open-source device for measuring food intake and

operant behavior in rodent home-cages." eLife 10 (March):e66173. https://doi.org/10.7554/eLife.66173.
Mattes A, Lemmer B (1991) Telemetric registrations on the effects of atenolol and amlodipine on circadian rhythms in blood pressure and heart rate of the rat. J Interdiscip Multidiscip Res 22:154
Meijer M (2006) The effect of routine experimental procedures on physiological parameters in mice kept under different husbandry conditions. Anim Welf 15:31–38
Mieske P, Diederich K, Lewejohann L (2021) Roaming in a land of milk and honey: life trajectories and metabolic rate of female inbred mice living in a semi naturalistic environment. Animals 11(10):3002
Mills PA (2000) A new method for measurement of blood pressure, heart rate, and activity in the mouse by radiotelemetry. J Appl Physiol 88:1537–1544
Nath T, Mathis A, Chen AC, Patel A, Bethge M, Mathis MW (2019) Using DeepLabCut for 3D markerless pose estimation across species and Behaviors. Nat Protoc 14(7):2152–2176
Ouyang W, Kilner KJ, Xavier RMP, Liu Y, Yinsheng L, Feller SM, Pitts KM et al (2024) An implantable device for wireless monitoring of diverse physio-behavioral characteristics in freely behaving small animals and interacting groups. Neuron 112(11):1764–77.e5
Pack AI, Galante RJ, Maislin G, Cater J, Metaxas D, Shan L, Zhang L et al (2007) Novel method for high-throughput phenotyping of sleep in mice. Physiol Genomics 28(2):232–238
Pedraza P, Velie T, Nichols K, Scott G (2025) Validation of the SoHoTM telemetry system for continuous body temperature monitoring in socially housed mice. Am Physiol Summit A 40(S1):2078.
Pennington ZT, Diego KS, Francisco TR, LaBanca AR, Lamsifer SI, Liobimova O, Shuman T, Cai DJ (2021) EzTrack-A step-by-step guide to behavior tracking. Curr Protoc 1(10):e255
Pereira TD, Tabris N, Matsliah A, Turner DM, Li J, Ravindranath S, Papadoyannis ES et al (2022) SLEAP: a deep learning system for multi-animal pose tracking. Nat Methods 19(4):486–495
Petersen N, Adank DN, Raghavan R, Winder DG, Doyle MA (2023) LIQ HD (lick instance quantifier home cage device): an open-source tool for recording undisturbed two-bottle drinking behavior in a home cage environment. eNeuro 10(4):ENEURO.0506-22.2023
Portfors CV (2007) Types and functions of ultrasonic vocalizations in laboratory rats and mice. J Am Assoc Lab Anim Sci 46(1):28–34
Premoli M, Pietropaolo S, Wöhr M, Simola N, Bonini SA (2023) Mouse and rat ultrasonic vocalizations in neuroscience and neuropharmacology: state of the art and future applications. Eur J Neurosci 57(12):2062–2096
Redmon J, Divvala S, Girshick R, Farhadi A (2015) You only look once: unified, real-time object detection. arXiv [cs.CV]. http://arxiv.org/abs/1506.02640
Rubio WB, Cortopassi MD, Banks AS (2023) Indirect calorimetry to assess energy balance in mice: measurement and data analysis. Methods Mol Biol (Clifton, NJ) 2662:103–115
Salem G, Cope N, Garmendia M, Alex P, Somenhalli A, Krynitsky J, Cubert N et al (2024) MouseVUER: video based open-source system for laboratory mouse home-cage monitoring. Sci Rep 14(1):2662
Sass F, Ma T, Ekberg JH, Kirigiti M, Ureña MG, Dollet L, Brown JM et al (2024) NK2R control of energy expenditure and feeding to treat metabolic diseases. Nature 635(8040):987–1000
Seibenhener, Michael L., Michael C. Wooten. 2015. "Use of the open field maze to measure locomotor and anxiety-like behavior in mice." J Vis Exp (96):52434. https://doi.org/10.3791/52434-v.
Sgoifo A, Stilli D, Medici D, Gallo P, Aimi B, Musso E (1996) Electrode positioning for reliable telemetry ECG recordings during social stress in unrestrained rats. Physiol Behav 60(6):1397–1401
Simola N (2015) Rat ultrasonic vocalizations and Behavioral neuropharmacology: from the screening of drugs to the study of disease. Curr Neuropharmacol 13(2):164–179
Škop V, Guo J, Liu N, Xiao C, Hall KD, Gavrilova O, Reitman ML (2020) Mouse thermoregulation: introducing the concept of the thermoneutral point. Cell Rep 31(2):107501

Škop V, Guo J, Liu N, Xiao C, Hall KD, Gavrilova O, Reitman ML (2023) The metabolic cost of physical activity in mice using a physiology-based model of energy expenditure. Mol Metab 71:101699

Sommer R (2005) Simultaneous collection of behavioural and physiological data in mice: integration of LABORAS with Dataquest. In: Measuring behavior. Laboras Publications

Speakman JR (2013) Measuring energy metabolism in the mouse—theoretical, practical, and analytical considerations. Front Physiol 4(March):34

Sulaiman MI, Ajabnoor MA, Al Khateeb T (1986) Effects of *Salvadora persica* extracts on mice exploratory locomotion activities. J Ethnopharmacol 17(3):263–268

Toth LA, Trammell RA, Ilsley-Woods M (2015) Interactions between housing density and ambient temperature in the cage environment:effects on mouse physiology and behavior. J Am Assoc Lab Anim Sci 54:708–717

Vaswani A, Shazeer N, Parmar N, Uszkoreit J, Jones L, Gomez AN, Kaiser L, Polosukhin I (2017) Attention is all you need. arXiv [cs.CL]. http://arxiv.org/abs/1706.03762

Venkatraman S, Jin X, Costa RM, Carmena JM (2010) Investigating neural correlates of behavior in freely behaving rodents using inertial sensors. J Neurophysiol 104(1):569–575

Venkatraman A, Bretl M, Kim S-I, Christensen L, Kelm-Nelson CA, Ciucci MR, Thibeault SL (2024) Stress-induced ultrasonic vocalization in laboratory rats and mice: a scoping review. Brain Sci 14(11):1109

Vidva R, Raza MA, Prabhakaran J, Sheikh A, Sharp A, Ott H, Moore A et al (2025) MyVivarium: a cloud-based lab animal colony management application with realtime ambient sensing. Comput Struct Biotechnol J 27(January):612–623

Virag D, Homolak J, Kodvanj I, Babic Perhoc A, Knezovic A, Osmanovic Barilar J, Salkovic-Petrisic M (2021) Repurposing a digital kitchen scale for neuroscience research: A complete hardware and software cookbook for PASTA. Sci Rep 11(1):2963

Virag D, Homolak J, Kodvanj I, Vargantolić A-M, Perhoč AB, Meglić P, Mužić PŠ et al (2024) My friend MIROSLAV: a hackable open-source hardware and software platform for high-throughput rodent activity monitoring in the home cage. bioRxiv. https://doi.org/https://doi.org/10.1101/2024.06.25.600592

Virag D, Homolak J, Kodvanj I, Virag A-M, Perhoč AB, Meglić P, Mužić PŠ et al (2025) My friend MIROSLAV: a hackable open-source hardware and software platform for high-throughput monitoring of rodent activity in the home cage. Behav Res Methods 57(7):1–19

Voikar V, Gaburro S (2020) Three pillars of automated home-cage phenotyping of mice: novel findings, refinement, and reproducibility based on literature and experience. Front Behav Neurosci 14(October):575434

von Ziegler LM, Roessler FK, Sturman O, Waag R, Privitera M, Duss SN, O'Connor EC, Bohacek J (2024) Analysis of behavioral flow resolves latent phenotypes. Nat Methods 21(12):2376–2387

Waidmann EN, Yang VHY, Doyle WC, Jarvis ED (2024) Mountable miniature microphones to identify and assign mouse ultrasonic vocalizations. bioRxiv. https://doi.org/https://doi.org/10.1101/2024.02.05.579003

Weinreb C, Pearl JE, Lin S, Osman MAM, Zhang L, Annapragada S, Conlin E et al (2024) Keypoint-MoSeq: parsing behavior by linking point tracking to pose dynamics. Nat Methods 21(7):1329–1339

Winn CB, Hwang S-K, Morin J, Bluette CT, Manickam B, Jiang ZK, Giddabasappa A, Liu C-N, Matthews K (2021) Automated monitoring of respiratory rate as a novel humane endpoint: a refinement in mouse metastatic lung cancer models. PLoS One 16(9):e0257694

Study Design and Data Analysis in Home Cage Monitoring Experiments

Reid D. Landes, Mara Rigamonti, and Steven R. Talbot

Abstract

Home cage monitoring (HCM) represents a paradigm shift in rodent behavioural research, replacing brief manual observations with continuous digital surveillance that captures animal behaviour in its natural context. This technological revolution generates vast amounts of data, offering both unprecedented opportunities and substantial analytical challenges. Effective HCM research depends on careful experimental design that often recognises the cage, rather than individual animals, as the fundamental experimental unit, with profound implications for statistical power. By adjusting cage density and employing randomised block designs, researchers can maximise statistical sensitivity while minimizing animal use.

Translating continuous behavioural streams into meaningful biological insights requires sophisticated yet transparent preprocessing. Moving averages reveal patterns obscured by moment-to-moment variability, while normalisation techniques enable comparisons across experiments and facilities. Heatmaps elegantly capture weeks of circadian rhythms and behavioural changes in single, interpretable displays. The statistical framework emphasises linear mixed-effects models that account for correlated

R. D. Landes (✉)
Department of Biostatistics, University of Arkansas for Medical Sciences, Little Rock, AR, USA
e-mail: rdlandes@uams.edu

M. Rigamonti
TECNIPLAST S.p.A, Buguggiate, VA, Italy
e-mail: mara.rigamonti@tecniplast.it

S. R. Talbot
Institute for Laboratory Animal Science, Hannover Medical School, Hannover, Germany
e-mail: talbot.steven@mh-hannover.de

S. Gaburro, S. Mandillo (eds.), *Home Cage Monitoring in Rodents: A Global Effort*,
https://doi.org/10.1007/978-3-032-19781-8_8

repeated measurements, alongside rhythmometric techniques extracting circadian parameters. A major strength of HCM is its capacity for continuous welfare assessment through composite indices that combine multiple physiological and behavioural streams, enabling early interventions and advancing refinement goals.

The chapter concludes by exploring how emerging machine learning approaches can enhance pattern detection while maintaining the statistical rigor and biological interpretability essential for translational research. Overall, HCM emerges not merely as a data collection technology but as a comprehensive framework for ethical, statistically robust behavioural phenotyping that advances all three Rs (Replacement, Reduction, and Refinement) of animal research through continuous digital biomarkers, proactive welfare monitoring, and efficient experimental designs.

Keywords

Longitudinal data analysis · Statistical validity · Continuous behavioural monitoring · Behavioural time series · Data aggregation

1 Introduction

Home cage monitoring (HCM) has shifted the centre of gravity of rodent research from brief, hands-on snapshots to continuous, hands-off observation. What used to be 5 min in a brightly lit arena is now days or weeks of rhythms, meals, naps, and social interactions recorded in situ. A single digital ventilated cage rack sampling floor capacitance at 4 Hz for 80 cages generates roughly a quarter of a gigabyte of raw traces per day (before any video or telemetry is added) (Fuochi et al. 2024). RFID (radio frequency identification) systems contribute tens of thousands of time-stamped visits and nose-pokes (Wilczyński et al. 2017). Though these torrents of numbers may overwhelm spreadsheets, they enable the 3Rs more so than traditional experiments. By reading behaviour as it naturally unfolds, we refine our welfare insights and reduce handling (Refinement), can reduce animal numbers for certain study types (Reduction), and, in some contexts, replace acute assays with continuous digital biomarkers (Fuochi et al. 2024; Grieco et al. 2021; Kahnau et al. 2023).

This chapter is a guided walk-through of what to do with all those data. We keep the structure simple: first, how to design an HCM experiment so that the statistics work with you; second, how to turn streams of raw signals into clean, analyzable measures; third, how to test ideas without violating assumptions; and fourth, how to describe rhythms and irregularities. We finish with a look ahead at AI-enabled analysis. Along the way, we provide realistic examples and figure ideas that biologists and veterinarians can use immediately (Grieco et al. 2021; Golini et al. 2020; Kahnau et al. 2023; Stephenson and Brown 2012; Moore et al. 2024; Nelson et al. 1979; Cornelissen 2014).

2 Design First, Then Analyse

The most consequential step is correctly recognizing the experimental unit (EU). The EU is the unit to which experimental conditions, including control conditions, are randomly assigned. The EU allows us to estimate experimental variability. Experimental variability is what allows us to make valid statistical inferences. In digital ventilated cages, sensors aggregate at the cage level, making the cage the EU, even though we can randomise experimental conditions to individual animals. Importantly, increasing the number of EU increases power. For example, if we have 24 mice to split between 2 groups, 12 cages with 2 mice per cage make a statistically more powerful design than 6 cages with 4 mice per cage (Fig. 1a, b).

In radio frequency identification (RFID) or video tracking of individual animals, individual animals can be the EU. However, the shared cage context may induce a correlation among data coming from cage mates (Grieco et al. 2021; Golini et al. 2020; Kahnau et al. 2023; Landes 2025). In this situation, treating each mouse as independent would be a type of pseudoreplication (Lazic 2010; Festing and Altman 2002). We must include unique cage identifiers in the dataset and add the cage identifier variable as a cluster random factor in the statistical model.

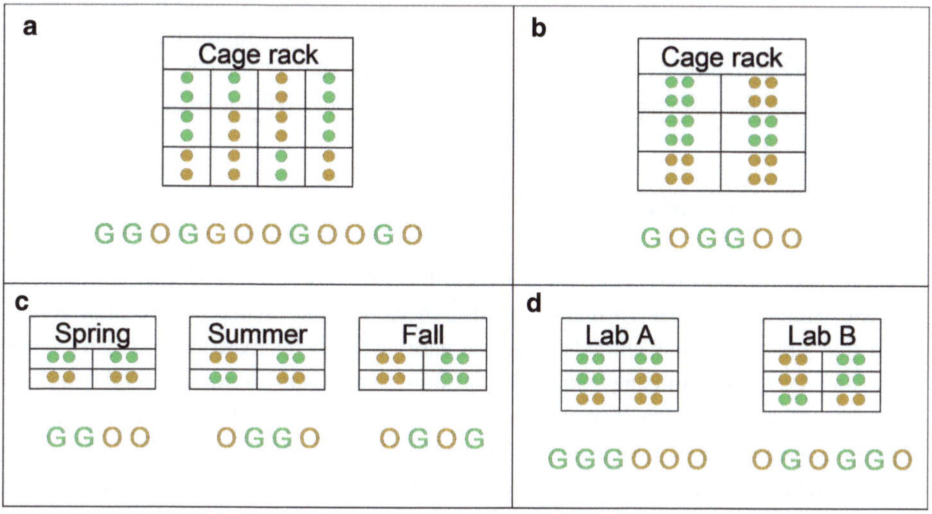

Fig. 1 Four designs with 24 mice (represented with filled circles). Cages were randomised equally between the blind-coded Green and Orange groups on a cage rack. Cage is the EU. We randomised a list of *G*s and *O*s for the number of cages to be used on the rack and filled them in, reading left to right and top to bottom. (**a**) Completely randomised design with 2 mice/cage gives 12 EU. (**b**) Completely randomised design 4 mice/cage gives 6 EU. (**c**) Randomised block design with seasonal cohorts as blocks; randomisations within each cohort. (**d**) Randomised block design with different laboratories as blocks; randomisations within each laboratory

Randomisation is important. When experimental conditions or treatments are administered to individual animals, randomizing the treatments ensures independence both among groups and within groups—two key assumptions of both parametric and non-parametric analyses. In HCM experiments, since cages are most often the EU, treatments should be randomised to cages (and, when the treatment is administered to individual animals, the mice therein). Sometimes experimental conditions cannot be randomised, like when comparing a wildtype (WT) genotype to a knock-out (KO) genotype. But randomisation is still needed in these situations: randomisation of cages on a cage rack and the order in which observations are made is also important, as it reduces or eliminates bias from unknown factors like temperature and light gradients or human errors. Randomisation can be documented and is not generally a process that "just happens," like grabbing mice out of a box and administering treatments or placing cages in a "mixed up" order in a cage rack. Planning randomisation before it happens improves reproducibility (Percie du Sert et al. 2020); see Fig. 1. Blinding is also important in removing bias. Though some of those working with the animals will know which cages are in which experimental groups, concealing the names of experimental conditions in the HCM data is one way to reduce bias; see Fig. 1. Verhave et al. (2024) provide methods for applying blinding and randomisation in animal experiments.

Sometimes it is necessary to run your experiment in cohorts or different spaces, or you may need to replicate your experiment, or there may be some other factor that introduces heterogeneity into your experiment; see Fig. 1c and d. This heterogeneity factor (or blocking factor in statistical jargon) can increase the power and help with the reproducibility of your experiment, but that factor must be included in the statistical analysis (Richter et al. 2011; Festing 2020; Frommlet and Heinze 2021; Voelkl and Würbel 2024).

3 The Power of Design

In HCM experiments, the cage is usually the EU. Increasing EU in HCM experiments increases statistical power for detecting differences, but increasing EU does not always mean that the number of animals must increase: we can decrease cage density while increasing the number of cages. Suppose you want to compare an experimental condition to a control condition, with 24 mice available for each group, totaling 48 mice. Consider four housing densities: 4 mice/cage, 3 mice/cage, 2 mice/cage, and single housing. For a 0.05 significance level, to detect a difference in means (or Cohen's *d*) of size 1 SD, where SD is the within-group standard deviation of the cages, the power would be 0.35 with 12 cages holding 4 mice each, 0.46 with 16 cages holding 3 mice each, 0.64 with 24 cages holding 2 mice each, and 0.92 with 48 singly housed mice. Of course, there must be a scientific rationale to justify housing social laboratory animals singly. (The fact that single housing gives more power is not a valid reason to jeopardise the welfare of the animals.) This example assumes that the experimental and control cages are completely randomised to the experimental conditions and randomised on one HCM rack—*a* completely randomised design; see Fig. 1a and b for example (Festing 2020). Analyses appropriate for completely randomised designs are independent group *t*-tests and one-way ANOVAs, along with non-parametric analogues, Mann-Whitney (or Wilcoxon) tests and Kruskal-Wallis tests. If the design is not completely randomised, then these analyses may not be appropriate.

Sometimes it is not possible to have all the cages planned for an HCM experiment starting at the same time and place. Some researchers feel they must analyse the data from different times or places (like replications of an experiment within a lab or among labs) separately *because* of these differences; see Fig. 1c and d, for example. Or they can plainly see variability among the data from different times and/or places and don't want to pool the data. But we can and should pool the data; it's just a matter of how to do so appropriately. Appropriately pooling data across different times and/or places increases power by combining all the data into a single analysis instead of spreading it out among several analyses. ANOVA makes appropriate pooling possible. ANOVA, or "analysis of variance," is fundamentally about partitioning out the different sources of variability (Altman and Krzywinski 2015). These blocking factors (e.g. different times and/or places) are part of the experimental design, and such designs are called randomised block designs. Importantly, within each block, experimental conditions are randomised to EU (Festing 2020); see Fig. 1c and d. Because blocks are part of the experimental design, we need to record unique identifiers for the different blocks and include these identifiers as data; these identifiers become a blocking variable (or blocking factor) in the ANOVA. Indeed, in multi-site clinical trials in humans, including site as a factor in the analysis has been the standard for decades (Fleiss 1986). Some may consider including an interaction of the blocking factor (e.g. time or place) with the treatment factor in the ANOVA. There are philosophical considerations regarding what an interaction means; see Littell et al. (2006) and Mead (1990) for discussion. Usually, many researchers hypothesise that the direction and magnitudes of experimental effects will be the same, regardless of which block the EUs are in; hence, excluding the block×treatment interaction is consistent with such hypotheses. Appropriate analyses of a randomised block design are an additive two-way ANOVA having blocks and treatments as the two factors, without adding the interaction of these two factors, or the Friedman's test (a non-parametric analogue to the additive two-way ANOVA).

Though adding more cages (or EU) to an HCM experiment will boost power, repeatedly measuring the cages can also increase power by reducing measurement error. This is true when comparing *within* a group, such as before and after treatment, and also when comparing *between* groups, like a treated and a control group. The number of times we plan to collect measurements for analysis and the spacing of those time points are part of the experimental design. For within- and among-group comparisons, the more we measure an individual cage, the more precisely we know the average value for that cage. When the cage's average value over time is of interest, the repeated measures reduce the measurement error of that average. For example, suppose we consider measuring a cage 1, 4, or 9 times under a particular experimental condition, such as after treatment or in the control group. When we measure a cage one time, the variability in that measure is made up from both experimental error (variability among different cages in the same group) and measurement error. (It is like measuring your heart rate once during the day and using that as your average heart rate versus measuring it multiple times during the day and using the mean of those measures as your average heart rate.) The measurement error of a 4-observation mean from a single cage will be half ($\sqrt{1/4}$) as variable as that from a single observation from a cage. The 9-observation mean from that single cage will be 2/3 ($\sqrt{4/9}$) less variable than the 4-observation mean. However, the group sample size is also important; you cannot expect to measure a minimal number of cages repeatedly and hope these repeated measures will substantially increase your power. (Just like having the average heart rate from a few adults from the same population would not give a precise estimate of the average heart rate for the entire population.) Finally, when analyzing the data, including time as a (quantitative) covariate instead of as a (categorical) factor can increase power, reduce the number of multiple comparisons, and allow for a more straightforward explanation of time effects (Gelman and Hill 2007; Littell et al. 2006; Hedeker et al. 1999).

4 From Data Streams to Analyzable Measures

HCM collects data 24/7. However, for many studies, the focus is on a behavioural or physiological parameter averaged over a time window, such as 12 h a day or even a week. Though the usual summary of the 24/7 data is a mean, other summary statistics can be useful, like the median to define the point where the cage's distribution of values is split in half, or a standard deviation to define how variable a cage's values are over the window of time. These summary statistics are computed at the cage level (assuming individual monitoring of animals in a cage is not possible). The values of the summary statistics become the variable to analyse statistically.

A few points about these summary statistics are as follows: (Point 1) When the number of observations in the window is large, for example, in the hundreds, then the distribution of the summarizing statistic (e.g. mean, median, standard deviation) tends to be unimodal and approximately normal or at least easily transformed to a normal distribution; see Fig. 2. Usual transformation functions used are square root or logarithm. Box-Cox transformations are a type of transformation that uses the data to determine an appropriate transformation. Most statistical softwares have functions that allow the user to pick a suitable Box-Cox transformation. Additionally, the square root and logarithm transformations are special cases of the Box-Cox transformation. (Point 2) It is always a good idea to record the number of animals in a cage when gathering the summarised data for statistical analysis. When the number of animals in a cage differs among the cages, then the variability of the summarised data will also vary. That is, if some cages have, for whatever reason, only 1 animal in them, and others have 2 animals, then the variability of the summary statistic from the 2-animal cages will be about $\sqrt{1/2}$ of that from the 1-animal cages. Figure 3 illustrates how the variability of cage observations depends on the number

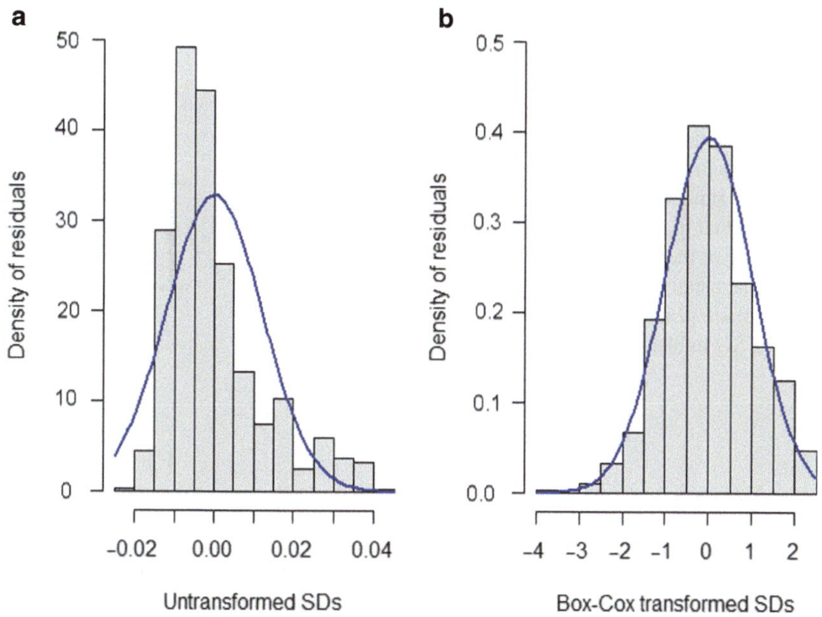

Fig. 2 Standard deviations (SDs) were used to summarise the variability of activity in 12 h of light (720 min) for 11 cages over 30 days. (**a**) After fitting a linear model accounting for day, the histogram of residuals from the raw SDs is unimodal with moderate skew. (**b**) After a Box-Cox transformation of the SDs, the residuals are approximately normal

of animals in the cage. The number of animals in a cage can be used as a weighting variable in the statistical analysis to better ensure homogeneous or constant variance assumptions are satisfied (Johnson et al. 2015). (Point 3) The time windows from the cages being summarised should all have analogous start and end times. For example, for cages at two different locations with different start times for the light hours, the time windows should be in terms of time from the same reference point, like the first minute of the light cycle being defined as Minute 0, regardless of what time of day it is at the location. (Point 4) Normalizing the summarised data will shift and scale the values to lie between 0 and 1. A common normalisation algorithm is the min-max normalisation (subtracting the data minimum from each data point, then dividing by the data range). The minimum and maximum values should be taken from all the data under consideration. It would be a mistake to normalise the data from one group within itself and then another group, as doing so would remove any differences between groups. Normalisation does not transform the data into a normal distribution; it simply places the data points on a standardised scale so that the distribution can be compared to other normalised distributions. For example, normalised activity data from one disease model can be compared to those from another disease model in a different experiment.

An example: We want to summarise the variability in nighttime activity to evaluate whether it changes over 7 weeks. Activity was measured every minute over the 7 weeks.

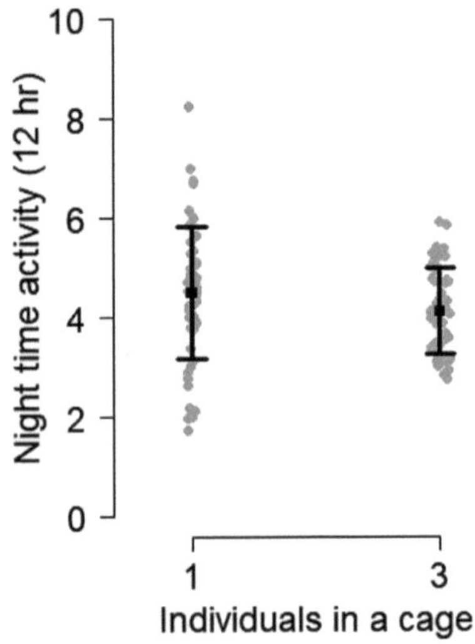

Fig. 3 Variability of cage-level measures decreases as the number of animals in the cage increases. We were able to record the nighttime activity for 3 individuals in a cage. Activity from a randomly selected individual in the cage and the average of the 3 individuals (the usual cage-level measure) are plotted in gray, mean ± SD in black

We use only the 720 min (12 h) of nighttime. First, we find the maximum and minimum nighttime activity values across all 7 weeks and all cages and use these to perform a min--max normalisation of nighttime activity. The trace for normalised activity for a randomly selected cage is displayed in the bottom third of Fig. 4. For each cage, we then computed the standard deviation (SD) of the 720 nighttime minutes in each of the 49 days; see the middle third of Fig. 4. Finally, we took the median of the 7 SDs in each week; see the top third of Fig. 4. We would then use these weekly median SDs of nighttime activity as data for a statistical analysis.

An example: We want to compare 12-h rest-time activity between a wild-type (WT) mouse strain and a strain for which a gene under investigation has been knocked out (KO). Because rest-time activity may change over time, we also want to evaluate whether change occurs within each population, and whether those changes are different between WT and KO mice. We had 11 cages of WT mice and 9 cages of KO mice, tracking their minute-by-minute activity over 20 weeks with an HCM system. (All cages had 3 female mice.) Mice were considered fully matured adults at 14 weeks into the experiment. We decided to use the rest-time activity from week 14 and week 20. For each cage, we took the mean activity over the 12 light hours for each day in week 14 and in week 20. Then, we calculated the average of the 7 days of light-hour means for week 14 and for week 20; thus, there were two values for a cage: mean rest-time activity at week 14 and week 20. Finally, we normalised these values across both strains and weeks with the min-max normalisation. We analysed these normalised values with a repeated measures ANOVA that had strain (an among-cage factor), week, and the strain×week interaction (within-cage factors) as the fixed effects. To account for the repeated measures nature of the data, we included cage (each with a unique identifier) as a random intercept in this model. This model assumes the standard deviation is the same between both strains and also between both time points; it also implicitly assumes the within-cage correlation between the pair of

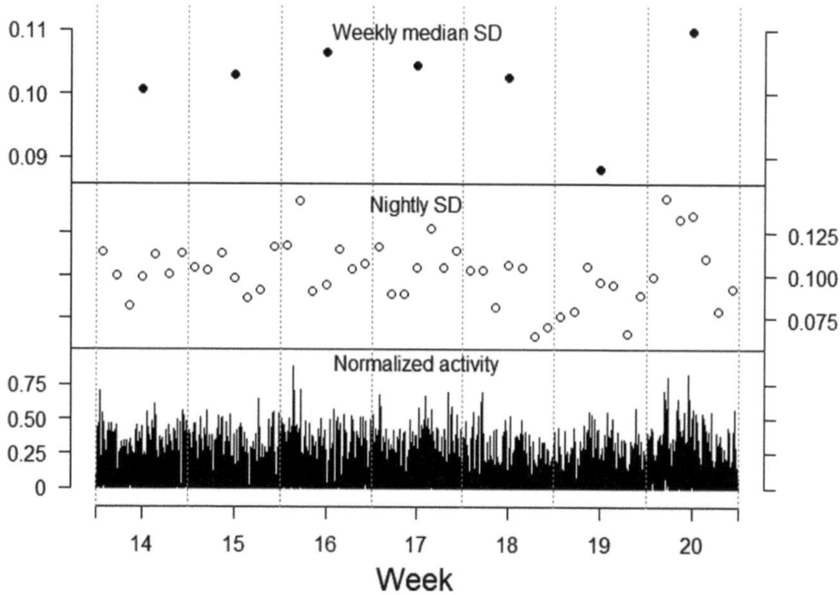

Fig. 4 Steps of summarizing data streams into analyzable measures for one cage. Normalised nighttime activity over 7 weeks is on the bottom; nightly SDs are in the middle, and the medians of the SD over each week are in the top

values from weeks 14 and 20 is the same between the two strains (sometimes referred to as an exchangeable or compound symmetric structure). We plot the individual cage values at both time points with a spaghetti plot to illustrate the repeated measures nature of the data, as shown in Fig. 5a. Figure 5b shows the strain-specific change over time and compares these changes between the strains. Though not illustrated in Fig. 5, when averaged over the weeks, KO mice exhibited higher rest-time activity than WT mice (the main effect of strain). Similarly, when averaged over strains, rest-time activity increased from Week 14 levels by Week 20 (the main effect of time).

An example: We want to determine whether the variability in 12-h nighttime activity changes as mice age, and whether those changes depend on mouse strain, specifically comparing the WT and KO mouse strains from the earlier example. For each cage, we computed the weekly median SD (Fig. 4). We analysed these in a repeated measures analysis of covariance (rmANCOVA), having strain as an among-cage factor and week as a within-cage covariate; we also included the interaction of strain and week—a within-cage covariate. We included cage (each with a unique identifier) as a random intercept in this model. This model assumes the standard deviation is the same between both strains and across the weeks. It also implicitly assumes that the within-cage correlation between time points is the same for any two time points and between strains. This is called an exchangeable or compound symmetric correlation.

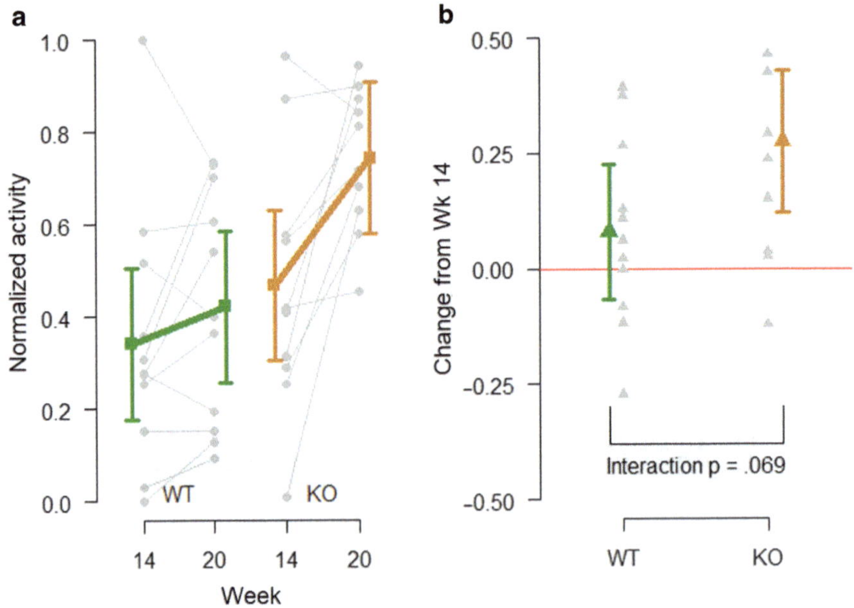

Fig. 5 Normalised rest-time activity was summarised per cage at weeks 14 and 20. (**a**) Pairs of Weeks 14 and 20 values are plotted for each cage, and the strain means at each time point, along with the estimated SD (root mean square error from the statistical model), appear. (**b**) Changes within a strain are compared to 0 with 95% confidence intervals, and the changes in WT are compared to those in KO with the strain×time interaction

Though analysed in the same statistical model, for clarity's sake, we plot the profiles of individual cages separately for each strain across the 7 weeks (weeks 14–20) in Fig. 6, along with the model-estimated regression lines. For the WT strain, the SD of nighttime activity was estimated to be 0.113 at week 14. By week 20, the estimate was 0.117; that is a slope of +0.0006 per week (95% confidence interval: −0.0005, +0.0016; $p = 0.276$). However, for the KO strain, variability in nighttime activity significantly decreased from 0.115 at week 14 to 0.104 by week 20; a slope of −0.0017 per week (95% CI: −0.0027, −0.0006; $p = 0.003$). To correctly determine whether the change in variability for the KO cages differed from the same change for WT cages, we look to the interaction of the week covariate and strain: The difference in slopes between the two strains was 0.0006—(−0.0017) = 0.0022; this was a significant difference (95% CI: +0.0007, +0.0037; $p = 0.004$).

This rmANCOVA example assumed a simple within-cage correlation structure across time—an exchangeable correlation. Another sensible correlation structure to consider is a first-order autoregressive correlation, where the correlation between two observations diminishes as their time separation increases. How do we know which correlation structure is better than others? The correlation structure is part of the statistical model. We can compare the fit of two sensible statistical models by looking at the corrected Akaike

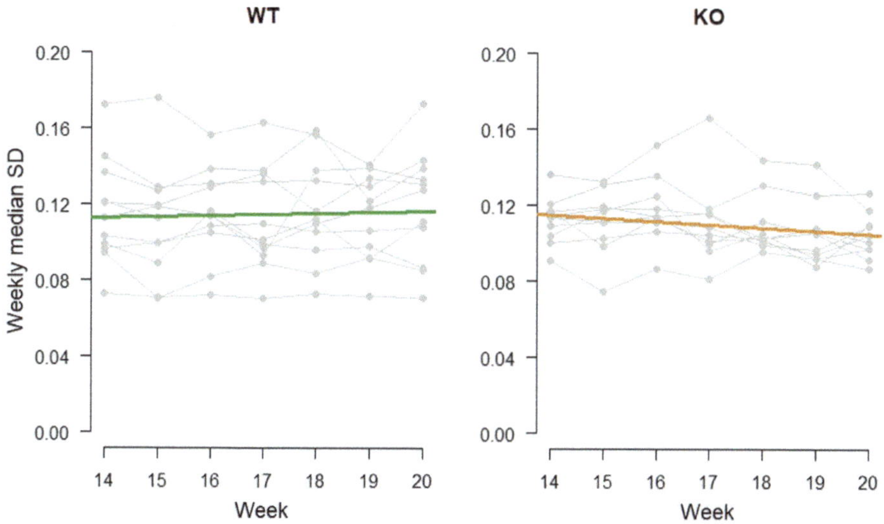

Fig. 6 Weekly median SD plotted over the 7 weeks for individual cages (gray profiles), and the fitted regression lines for the wildtype (WT) and knock-out (KO) strains analysed in the same repeated measures ANCOVA

Information Criterion (AICc for AIC-corrected) based on REML estimation: The correlation structure associated with the lower AICc tends to be better at describing the correlation among within-cage observations (Littell et al. 2006).

5 Moving Averages in Practice

A brief, transparent smoothing step often stabilises noisy data streams. However, smoothing is typically performed for display purposes and is conceptually distinct from any aggregation used for analysis. It is treated separately (Grieco et al. 2021; Golini et al. 2020; Kahnau et al. 2023; Stephenson and Brown 2012). Simple moving averages (MAs) are a routine smoothing procedure that enhance the legibility of plots. Still, MAs are generally confined to presentation rather than incorporated into daily totals or other analytical summaries.

Minute-resolution traces of a monitored outcome from home cage systems are famously "jittery." Brief bursts, pauses, and sensor idiosyncrasies create a ragged line that obscures the overall pattern scientists may care about (see, for example, the bottom portion of Fig. 4). A moving average (MA) replaces each point with the average of its neighbors so the underlying structure (bouts, waves, and day–night drift) emerges. A simple MA with a trailing window of length L minutes computes the mean of the last L observations and uses that as the value "now." For a 5-min MA, the point at 09:00 summarizes 08:56–09:00. In Fig. 7, the raw minute signal is shown in a faint gray, while MAs with windows of length 5-, 15-, and 60-min provide progressively smoother views of the same behavior. An MA

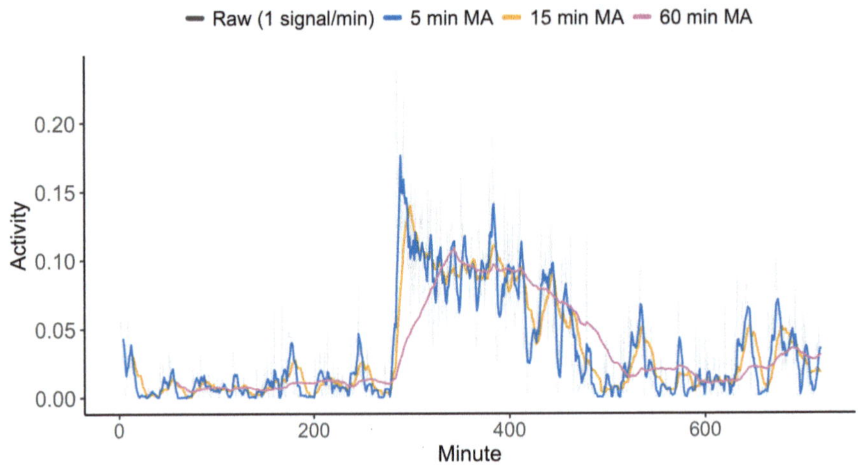

Fig. 7 Minute-by-minute aggregated activity of a single cage with 2 mice (Raw (*1 signal/min*), gray) overlaid with *trailing* moving averages (5, 15, and 60 min; coloured). The moving averages clarify trends at different time scales by reducing high-frequency noise, but they also introduce a ~L/2 lag and attenuate short peaks

with a centered window computes the mean of about L/2 minutes in the "past" and the other half in the "future;" for example, the 5-min MA at 09:00 summarizes 08:58–09:02. Centered window MAs can only be made after all times of interest have been observed and are impossible for live monitoring. Only trailing window MAs are appropriate for live monitoring.

The concept of MA has the unavoidable consequence of blunting: short spikes are lowered and broadened, and sharp steps become ramps. Readability improves, but fast, brief events are attenuated or even lost. Another consequence relevant for trailing window MAs is lag: because the MA looks backward in time, peaks and drops appear later than they truly occurred. With a trailing window (the only type suitable for live monitoring), the information is effectively centred about $L/2$ minutes in the past, so a rapid increase at 10:00 may reach the smoothed curve around 10:02–10:03 with a 5-min window and much later with a 60-min window.

The choice of the moving-average window L should be anchored in the shortest behaviour that needs to be distinguished. When activity and rest bouts typically last about 3–10 min, a window of 5 min preserves that structure while reducing high-frequency noise. A 15-min window tends to reveal short-term trends such as feeding waves, and a 60-min window makes the circadian envelope apparent. As a rule of thumb, L should be chosen so that fluctuations faster than roughly $L/3$ to $L/2$ are muted, while patterns slower than L remain visible. Over-smoothing should be avoided, meaning the window should not exceed the duration of the events of interest. Edge effects should also be considered. The first L minus 1 min lacks a full window and is less reliable unless partial windows are allowed, in which case the bias should be noted.

MAs can be used for monitoring individual cages, as shown in Fig. 7, and for HCM *experiments*, they can also summarise the outcome of interest for experimental groups. The MAs from different groups are typically plotted together to visualise potential differences (or similarities) between groups. In Fig. 8, activity after a cage change is compared between a WT and KO mouse strain. When computing MAs for a group, the time periods to be summarised with the MA must be aligned among the cages within the group. For example, when taking activity after a cage change, if a few cages in the group are changed at 09:00 and the remaining ones at 12:00, the time 0 for both sets of cages is set at the time the cage change started.

Sampling is not always uniform at one sample per minute. When exact time stamps contain irregular gaps or bursts, the target scale is defined before smoothing. One route aggregates to a regular grid. For continuous measures such as accelerometry, the minute-wise mean is appropriate. For counts such as beam breaks, the minute-wise sum is natural. The same moving-average logic then applies. A second route retains irregular sampling and applies time-based rolling windows that span the last 5, 15, or 60 min of real time rather than a fixed number of samples. Missing minutes are handled deliberately. They can be left as explicit gaps, filled by carrying the last value forward, or imputed with care. Each choice alters the shape of the smoothed curve and should be reported.

Why use MAs in home cage monitoring at all? They make dense, noisy traces legible to both specialists and non-specialists, damp down single-sample glitches, and provide a consistent "lens" for comparing cages or sessions. They are also easy to explain (e.g. the "average of the last few minutes"), which makes them ideal for figures and dashboards. But the same properties that improve clarity introduce caveats. Detection is delayed by about $L/2$ minutes with trailing windows, so onsets at lights-on or after dosing will appear

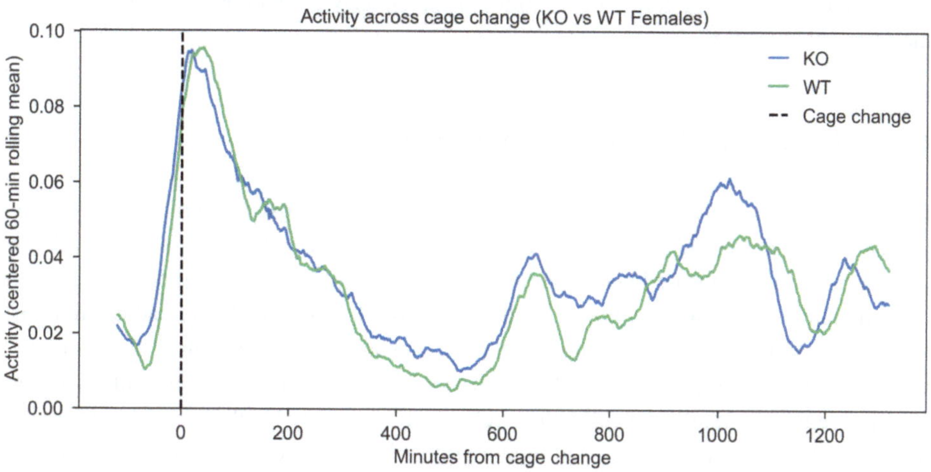

Fig. 8 Moving average of activity with a centred 60-min window for two strains of female mice on the day of a cage change (during light hours). The WT moving average is based on 11 cages, and the KO on 10 cages. All cages had 2 mice

late. Short bouts may be smeared into broader humps, peak amplitudes are reduced, and bout durations can be overestimated. Long gaps followed by resumed sampling can create artificial ramps. Hour-scale windows can cross zeitgeber boundaries, softening transitions at lights on/off. Variance is mechanically reduced, so quantitative comparisons between smoothed series (or between different windows) can shift simply because of the filter, not because the animal changed. For these reasons, MAs are best treated as visual summaries. Statistical analyses should be conducted on appropriately preprocessed raw data or with time-series models designed for the task.

There are alternatives when the trade-offs of a simple MA are too limiting. Exponential moving averages weigh the most recent data more heavily and can reduce apparent lag for a similar degree of smoothing. Median filters suppress isolated spikes without blurring edges as much, though they can distort plateaus. LOESS (locally estimated scatterplot smoothing) or spline smoothers adapt to local structure and produce elegant presentation curves, but introduce their own tuning choices and are less transparent than, say, a "5-min window MA." For inference about latent states (sleep/wake, active/inactive), state-space or hidden Markov models move beyond smoothing to classification, often avoiding some artifacts at the cost of complexity.

Clarity and honesty can coexist. Plotting a raw trace behind a smoothed curve shows what has been attenuated. The window length and its alignment should be reported, for example, as a "trailing 5-min moving average." Interventions, zeitgeber changes, and gaps in the record should be annotated. The figure is revisited with a somewhat shorter and a somewhat longer window to confirm that qualitative conclusions do not depend on an arbitrary choice of *L*. In the minute-sampled example here, a five-minute moving average is a sensible default. It reveals bout-level structure without erasing sharp transitions, and longer windows provide complementary context. The moving average is treated as a lens: useful and transparent, but not a substitute for the underlying data or for models suited to the scientific question.

6 Heat Maps That Answer Questions

High-dimensional behaviour data collected by HCM are most interpretable when displayed in compact visual summaries. Actogram-style heat maps have become a workhorse because they align repeated behavioural trajectories over long recording periods, providing a detailed overview of activity, as shown in Fig. 9. They display circadian rhythms, long-term trends, short-term changes, or anomalies all at once. A matrix is constructed where each row corresponds to a full day of recording, each column corresponds to a short time bin (e.g. a minute), and cell colour reflects the intensity level of activity or another behavioural metric. A superimposed light–dark bar helps the reader locate zeitgeber transitions. The underlying data should be raw or pre-binned rather than smoothed so that irregular day lengths produced by interventions can be padded with missing values and the light–dark bar remains accurate. Colour scales require special attention: for intra-unit

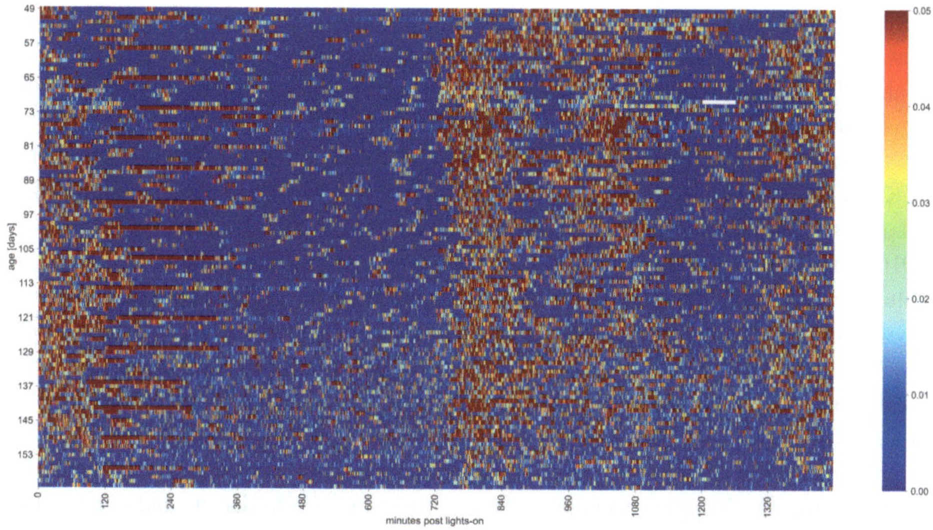

Fig. 9 Heatmap of minute-by-minute activity across 24 h from 7 to 24 weeks of age in a cage of KO male mice ($n = 2$ per cage)

comparisons, one can standardise each row (subtracting the mean and dividing by the standard deviation of the baseline day) to highlight deviations from that animal's baseline, whereas group comparisons benefit from a global scale derived from percentile ranges across all cages to avoid interpreting colour differences as biological effects. Light smoothing applied only for display, for example, a centred three-bin moving average, reduces pixel noise without altering raw values and should be clearly annotated. Marginal summaries add a dashboard-like quality: a strip beside the heat map displays total activity for each day, and a top panel displays the average 24-h profile. Similar principles extend to time-budget matrices, where behaviours classified from video are plotted against time of day, and to occupancy maps that show how animals explore multi-zone cages. These heat maps also benefit from consistent bin widths, carefully chosen colour palettes, and clear legends.

7 Quantifying Rhythms and Irregularity

After visual inspection, quantify rhythmicity and irregularity with models that match the circadian structure of HCM data (Cornelissen 2014; Refinetti 2016). Cosinor analysis fits a sine curve and reports a rhythm-adjusted mean called the MESOR (Midline Estimating Statistic of Rhythm), which is the average level around which the curve oscillates, an amplitude that captures the size of the oscillation, and an acrophase that locates the time of the peak (Nelson et al. 1979; Cornelissen 2014). Significance is assessed with an F-test, and confidence intervals convey uncertainty for the estimated amplitude and timing.

Periodogram analysis provides a complementary frequency-domain view, estimating the power of oscillations at different periods to reveal dominant rhythmic components (Tir et al. 2025). When sampling is uneven or has gaps, the Lomb–Scargle periodogram extends Fourier methods to irregular series and is widely used in circadian work (Scargle 1982; Nelson et al. 1979; Cornelissen 2014; Wu et al. 2016; Refinetti 2016). The non-parametric JTK_CYCLE procedure (based on the Jonckheere-Terpstra-Kendall algorithm) offers robustness to waveform shape under the assumption of a roughly periodic signal (Wu et al. 2016). Inter-daily variability and intra-daily stability quantify the consistency of activity patterns across and within days and can reveal changes of circadian structure even when rhythmicity remains detectable (Tir et al. 2025). MetaCycle then integrates Lomb–Scargle, ARSER, and JTK_CYCLE by combining *p* values and averaging period and phase and recalculates amplitude by ordinary least squares to stabilise the rhythm estimates (Wu et al. 2016).

Irregularity of activity pattern can also be summarised with the Regularity Disruption Index (RDI), which applies sample entropy (a measure of disorder or randomness) to a filtered activity series and rises when activity becomes more erratic (Golini et al. 2020). In a disease model, RDI increased with fragmented activity. The accompanying analyses used non-parametric repeated measures methods, the ANOVA-type statistic, and the Sankoh–Huque–Dubey adjustment to control error rates with correlated endpoints (Brunner et al. 2002; Noguchi et al. 2012; Sankoh et al. 1997). Whatever the method, define analysis windows such as light and dark in advance and keep binning consistent across conditions so that numerical summaries match the heat-map displays (Grieco et al. 2021; Golini et al. 2020; Kahnau et al. 2023; Stephenson and Brown 2012).

8 Testing Hypotheses with Appropriate Statistical Models

HCM generates longitudinal observations and replication at the cage or animal level, requiring statistical models that account for within-subject correlation. Linear mixed-effects models are well-suited to this structure. They treat cages or animals as random intercepts and can include random slopes for time when trajectories differ between subjects. Fixed effects represent biological factors such as genotype, treatment, or sex. When residuals deviate from normality or variances are heterogeneous, rank-based methods like the ANOVA-type statistic provide robust inference for repeated measures (Brunner et al. 2002; Noguchi et al. 2012). When multiple endpoints are analysed simultaneously, controlling the false discovery rate via the Benjamini–Hochberg procedure and using correlation-aware adjustments such as the Sankoh–Huque–Dubey method reduce type-I errors (Benjamini and Hochberg 1995; Sankoh et al. 1997). In studies exploring numerous time points or behavioural features, researchers should report effect sizes with confidence intervals and relate them to biological meaning, thereby linking statistical significance to welfare or clinical relevance (Percie du Sert et al. 2020; Festing and Altman 2002).

9 Integrating Multiple Signals into Composite Indices

Automated monitoring records diverse streams like body weight, burrowing, temperature, heart rate, activity, and more, each reflecting different aspects of welfare. Composite indices condense these streams into a single trajectory and enhance sensitivity to subtle changes. Simple approaches standardise each variable to z-scores and average them, whereas principal component analysis summarises correlated variables into orthogonal components. More advanced schemes, such as the Relative Severity Assessment (RELSA), derive severity scores by weighting physiological and behavioural measures. RELSA combines body weight, burrowing performance, heart rate, heart rate variability, body temperature, and activity to produce a dimensionless severity score with thresholds that classify animals into severity levels. This method distinguishes between models like sepsis, surgery, restraint stress, and colitis and yields bootstrapped confidence intervals for reliability (Talbot et al. 2022). A broader comparative severity assessment used a similar composite measure scheme to integrate behavioural and biochemical parameters, reporting that these composite scores allowed for direct comparison of welfare across models and provided an objective, reproducible metric (Kahnau et al. 2023). Composite indices should be used as a high-level signal to flag when and how much welfare deviates. Researchers can then return to the raw contributors for biological interpretation. Effective visualisations include radar plots at peak severity and overlaid line plots ("spaghetti plots"), showing group means and confidence intervals across time (Grieco et al. 2021; Golini et al. 2020; Kahnau et al. 2023; Stephenson and Brown 2012).

10 Long-Term Welfare Monitoring

Continuous monitoring over weeks or months reveals slow changes in health or circadian organisation that would be missed in endpoint assessments. Actogram-style heat maps allow researchers to visualise how day–night rhythms evolve, whether free-running patterns emerge, and whether interventions cause phase shifts or fragmentation (Grieco et al. 2021; Golini et al. 2020; Kahnau et al. 2023; Stephenson and Brown 2012). The Regularity Disruption Index provides a quantitative measure of irregularity and has been used to identify disease-related fragmentation (Golini et al. 2020). Composite indices like RELSA integrate multiple physiological streams to produce a holistic welfare trajectory and can alert caregivers when the trajectory exceeds a severity threshold (Talbot et al. 2022). In long-term studies, mixed-effects models can test whether trajectories differ by genotype or treatment while accounting for cage-level variation (Pinheiro and Bates 2000; Bates et al. 2015; Gelman and Hill 2007). Together, these tools permit early detection of chronic welfare issues and inform refinements in husbandry. In ageing studies, where observations can span a year or more, continuous monitoring can reveal how activity patterns evolve with age across genotypes or experimental conditions, while individual longitudinal profiles show major periodic oscillations of activity over months (Pernold et al. 2021; Santin et al. 2024).

11 Severity Assessment During Experimental Procedures

HCM can objectively quantify distress during surgeries, disease induction, or pharmacological manipulations. The RELSA score, developed for post-operative monitoring, combines body weight, burrowing, heart rate, heart rate variability, temperature, and activity and provides thresholds corresponding to mild, moderate, and severe distress (Talbot et al. 2022). Comparative studies demonstrate that composite scores differentiate severity across procedures: sepsis models elicit the highest scores, followed by surgical wounds, restraint stress, and colitis (Talbot et al. 2022). Heat maps and 24-h profiles reveal how interventions alter circadian activity patterns and how quickly animals recover (Grieco et al. 2021; Golini et al. 2020; Kahnau et al. 2023; Stephenson and Brown 2012). Statistical analyses using mixed-effects models detect differences between treatment groups while controlling for repeated measures (Pinheiro and Bates 2000; Bates et al. 2015; Gelman and Hill 2007), and rank-based methods provide robust alternatives when assumptions are violated (Brunner et al. 2002; Noguchi et al. 2012). Reporting effect sizes and confidence intervals helps translate numerical scores into welfare decisions (Percie du Sert et al. 2020; Festing and Altman 2002).

12 Experiments and Group Comparisons

When HCM is used as a primary readout in experiments, the analytical pipeline must support hypothesis testing and reproducibility. Actogram heat maps and time-budget matrices display group differences in activity and behaviour across the light–dark cycle (Grieco et al. 2021; Golini et al. 2020; Kahnau et al. 2023; Stephenson and Brown 2012). Cosinor or MetaCycle analyses compare rhythmic parameters such as amplitude and acrophase between genotypes or treatments (Stephenson and Brown 2012; Wu et al. 2016). Lomb–Scargle periodograms handle uneven sampling and missing data, ensuring that group comparisons are not biased by variable recording schedules (Scargle 1982; Nelson et al. 1979; Cornelissen 2014; Wu et al. 2016; Refinetti 2016). Linear mixed-effects models test for group differences while accounting for cage-level correlation, and multiple comparison procedures control the false discovery rate (Pinheiro and Bates 2000; Bates et al. 2015; Gelman and Hill 2007; Benjamini and Hochberg 1995; Sankoh et al. 1997). Combined with composite indices, these analyses provide a robust framework for detecting treatment effects and distinguishing biological signal from noise.

13 Transitioning to Advanced Analytics and Artificial Intelligence

The next generation of HCM will harness machine learning and sensor fusion to provide more granular and proactive welfare monitoring. Deep learning has already transformed pose estimation: DeepLabCut allows markerless tracking of individual body parts with accuracy comparable to human annotation and can be combined with supervised classifiers to score complex behaviours. SLEAP extends this approach to multi-animal tracking and supports both top-down and bottom-up identity tracking, providing real-time pose estimation with latencies below 3 ms and throughput exceeding eight hundred frames per second (Mathis et al. 2018; Pereira et al. 2020). Unsupervised approaches such as the autoregressive hidden Markov model (AR-HMM) infer latent behavioural modules and transition probabilities from continuous time series; Wiltschko and colleagues showed that the AR-HMM can discover behavioural consequences of experimental manipulations without observer bias, because the model is fully specified and the only tuning parameter controls timescale selection (Wiltschko et al. 2015). Integration of multiple sensors further enriches the data stream: the SmartCage combines floor vibration sensors and infrared matrices to monitor movement and sleep–wake states across up to 16 cages simultaneously, and a recent smart home cage concept uses near-infrared and thermal cameras to derive heart rate, respiratory rate, body temperature, and activity without implants. Multimodal models that combine facial expressions, body posture, and movement trajectories via attention-based networks yield improved accuracy for emotion recognition and allow real-time monitoring of fear states. Bayesian hierarchical models implemented in packages such as brms extend mixed-effects analyses by estimating full posterior distributions, allowing researchers to incorporate prior knowledge and model non-linear relationships (Bürkner 2017). Rhythm toolkits such as MetaCycle combine multiple detectors to enhance robustness (Wu et al. 2016). As these approaches mature, HCM will move from retrospective data mining to closed-loop systems that detect anomalies and trigger interventions in real time, integrate uncertainty across cages and cohorts, and maintain generalisability across strains, facilities, and seasons. Interpretability will be equally important, ensuring that AI outcomes can be traced to understandable features of the data and that researchers can verify the biological plausibility of detected patterns. Validation across diverse conditions remains essential to ensure that AI-driven alerts genuinely reflect animal welfare and do not embed hidden biases (Grieco et al. 2021; Golini et al. 2020; Kahnau et al. 2023; Stephenson and Brown 2012; Moore et al. 2024; Percie du Sert et al. 2020).

14 The Path Forward: From Rich Description to Ethically Grounded Action

Automated home cage monitoring has moved behavioural science from episodic tests toward the sustained analysis of life in situ. The central claim of this chapter has been that the strongest results arise when statistical validity is built into the design and preserved through every step from sensors to inference. Design determines what can be learned, preprocessing determines what is measurable, and modelling determines how convincingly those measurements speak to the biological question. The intention has not been to catalogue every technique but to lay out a disciplined route that many studies can follow and to show where principled alternatives fit.

The design layer begins with a clear statement of the experimental unit. Where sensors aggregate at the cage level, the cage carries the randomisation and the inference. Where individuals are tracked through RFID or video, animal-level analyses become possible, but the shared cage context is still present and must be modelled rather than ignored. Randomisation and blinding remove structure that would otherwise masquerade as effect. Cohorts, seasons, and laboratories are not nuisances to be swept aside. Treated as blocks in the design, they can be pooled in analysis in ways that preserve their identity and increase power. Repeated measurement is not a complication so much as a source of precision, provided the correlation it induces is represented in the model rather than pushed into the residuals.

From signals to measures, the guiding principle is consistency. Windows are aligned to a common reference, such as lights on. The number of animals per cage is recorded to allow for unequal cage density when variances differ. Transformations are introduced only where they stabilise variance or regularise distributions. Normalisation is used to place streams on a comparable scale without erasing genuine differences between groups, which requires that its parameters be defined across the dataset to be compared. Smoothing serves presentation, not inference. Moving averages and related filters help readers see the structure of bouts and rhythms. At the same time, the statistical analysis works on appropriately preprocessed values or on models that respect the native time scale. Missingness, clock drift, and device resets are declared and, where possible, corrected by procedures that leave an audit trail.

The modelling is chosen to match the question. Linear and generalised mixed-effects models estimate group differences while accounting for the dependence produced by repeated measures. When the scientific interest lies in diurnal organisation, rhythmometry provides compact parameters for amplitude, phase, and level, which allows direct comparison between conditions. When the question is the evolution of a measure across weeks, a repeated measures analysis with time treated as a quantitative covariate reduces unnecessary multiplicity and sharpens the estimate of the trend. Where distributional assumptions are doubtful, rank-based longitudinal methods preserve type I error and retain acceptable power. Correlation structures are not an arcane detail, but a model of temporal memory. First-order autoregressive and exchangeable forms are pragmatic starting points and can be compared with information criteria under restricted maximum likelihood estimation (REML). Communication follows the same logic. Figures show raw traces behind any smoothed curve. Contrasts are reported with interval estimates rather than dichotomous decisions. Decisions about alignment, transformation, weighting, and exclusion are made explicit so that the work is reconstructible.

Several issues remain open and deserve coordinated attention. Synchronisation across modalities and devices would benefit from shared standards and routine reporting. The handling of unequal cage density should move beyond ad hoc rules to agreed weighting strategies with sensitivity analyses. Composite severity metrics need validation across sites using data and code that can be transferred. Device heterogeneity, firmware updates, and sensor drift call for calibration records that accompany the data. None of these are administrative niceties: they determine whether conclusions generalise beyond a single rack and a single experimenter.

The near future promises a deeper integration of modelling and measurement. Artificial intelligence will extend rather than replace the statistical toolkit. Representation learning can translate long multivariate streams into low-dimensional embeddings that preserve circadian structure, bout statistics, and coordination across animals. Such representations can support clustering of behavioural regimes, alignment across devices, and change-point detection under realistic noise. Supervised and weakly supervised models will fuse RFID, video, and environmental signals to identify difficult behaviours at scale while passing uncertainty forward into cage-level summaries and group contrasts. Sequence models can forecast expected trajectories over days and weeks, flagging departures from baseline early for welfare interventions. State-space and hidden Markov models can provide interpretable latent states that bridge raw signals and ethological categories, which are essential for clinical translation and for communication with animal care staff. Generative models calibrated to real data can simulate entire experiments to study design choices under realistic variability, missingness, and drift. Federated learning will enable cross-laboratory models without centralising sensitive data, while drift detection and recalibration will maintain performance as colonies age and hardware evolves. Causal modelling will help separate correlation from effect by formalising interventions in time, clarifying the role of confounding, and aligning estimates with the intended biological contrast. Throughout, interpretability and uncertainty quantification remain non-negotiable. Explanations, posterior checks, and simulation-based validation help ensure that models explain rather than obscure.

The destination is a research programme in which design, transparency, and biological meaning work together. Automated home cage monitoring will support the 3Rs in practice by replacing acute assays with validated digital biomarkers, refining welfare through early detection, and reducing numbers through efficient designs and principled pooling. The methods presented here outline one workable path. Many alternatives will be appropriate for particular aims, and new approaches will arrive as devices, algorithms, and standards mature. What matters is that conclusions rest on designs that support them, on measures that are defined with care, and on models that reflect dependence, rhythm, and scale. With these foundations, HCM can move from rich description to robust prediction and, in time, to ethically grounded action.

Acknowledgements We thank the authors of Golini et al. (2020) for providing the data that we used to generate many of the example figures. RDL received support during the preparation of this manuscript from the Center for Childhood Obesity's Scholarly Writing Program (funded under grant P20 GM109096 from the National Institute of General Medical Sciences/National Institutes of Health).

References

Altman N, Krzywinski M (2015) Sources of variation. Nat Methods 12:5–6. https://doi.org/10.1038/nmeth.3224

Bates D, Mächler M, Bolker B, Walker S (2015) Fitting linear mixed-effects models using lme4. J Stat Softw 67(1):1–48

Benjamini Y, Hochberg Y (1995) Controlling the false discovery rate: a practical and powerful approach to multiple testing. J R Stat Soc B 57(1):289–300

Brunner E, Domhof S, Langer F (2002) Nonparametric analysis of longitudinal data in factorial experiments. Wiley

Bürkner P-C (2017) brms: an R package for Bayesian multilevel models using Stan. J Open Source Softw 2(13):e326

Cornelissen G (2014) Cosinor-based rhythmometry. Stat Methods Med Res 23(1):46–65

Festing MF (2020) The "completely randomised" and the "randomised block" are the only experimental designs suitable for widespread use in pre-clinical research. Sci Rep 10(1):17577

Festing MFW, Altman DG (2002) Guidelines for the design and statistical analysis of experiments using laboratory animals. ILAR J 43(4):244–258

Fleiss JL (1986) Analysis of data from multiclinic trials. Control Clin Trials 7(4):267–275

Frommlet F, Heinze G (2021) Experimental replications in animal trials. Lab Anim 55(1):65–75

Fuochi S, Rigamonti M, O'Connor EC, De Girolamo P, D'Angelo L (2024) Big data and its impact on the 3Rs: a home cage monitoring oriented review. Front Big Data 7:1390467

Gelman A, Hill J (2007) Data analysis using regression and multilevel/hierarchical models. Cambridge University Press

Golini E, Rigamonti M, Iannello F et al (2020) A non-invasive digital biomarker for the detection of rest disturbances in the SOD1G93A mouse model of ALS. Front Neurosci 14:896

Grieco F, Bernstein BJ, Biemans B et al (2021) Measuring behavior in the home cage: study design, applications, challenges, and perspectives. Front Behav Neurosci 15:735387

Hedeker D, Gibbons RD, Waternaux C (1999) Sample size estimation for longitudinal designs with attrition: comparing time-related contrasts between two groups. J Educ Behav Stat 24(1):70–93

Johnson JL, Kreidler SM, Catellier DJ, Murray DM, Muller KE, Glueck DH (2015) Recommendations for choosing an analysis method that controls type I error for unbalanced cluster sample designs with gaussian outcomes. Stat Med 34(27):3531–3545

Kahnau P, Mieske P, Wilzopolski J et al (2023) A systematic review of home-cage monitoring in laboratory mice and rats. BMC Biol 21:256

Landes RD (2025) More power for less money: statistical, power, and cost analyses that account for Intracluster correlation in experiments with same-group cage mates. J Am Assoc Lab Anim Sci 1(aop):1–3

Lazic SE (2010) The problem of pseudoreplication in neuroscientific studies: is it affecting your analysis? BMC Neurosci 11:5. https://doi.org/10.1186/1471-2202-11-5

Littell RC, Milliken GA, Stroup WW, Wolfinger RD, Schabenberger O (2006) SAS® for mixed models, 2nd edn. SAS Institute Inc

Mathis A, Mamidanna P, Cury KM et al (2018) DeepLabCut: markerless pose estimation of user-defined body parts with deep learning. Nat Neurosci 21:1281–1289

Mead R (1990) The design of experiments: statistical principles for practical applications. Cambridge University Press

Moore JL, Kennedy J, Hassan AA (2024) Automated home cage monitoring of an aging colony of mice—implications for welfare monitoring and experimentation. Front Neurosci 18:1489308

Nelson W, Tong YL, Lee JK, Halberg F (1979) Methods for cosinor-rhythmometry. Chronobiologia 6(4):305–323

Noguchi K, Gel YR, Brunner E, Konietschke F (2012) nparLD: an R software package for nonparametric analysis of longitudinal data in factorial experiments. J Stat Softw 50(12):1–23

Percie du Sert N, Hurst V, Ahluwalia A et al (2020) The ARRIVE guidelines 2.0: updated guidelines for reporting animal research. PLoS Biol 18:e3000410

Pereira TD, Shaevitz JW, Murthy M (2020) Quantifying behavior to understand the brain. Nat Methods 17:1215–1228

Pernold K, Rullman E, Ulfhake B (2021) Major oscillations in spontaneous home-cage activity in C57BL/6 mice housed under constant conditions. Sci Rep 11:4961. https://doi.org/10.1038/s41598-021-84141-9

Pinheiro JC, Bates DM (2000) Mixed-effects models in S and S-PLUS. Springer

Refinetti R (2016) Circadian physiology, 3rd edn. CRC Press

Richter SH, Garner JP, Zipser B, Lewejohann L, Sachser N, Touma C, Schindler B, Chourbaji S, Brandwein C, Gass P, van Stipdonk N (2011) Effect of population heterogenization on the reproducibility of mouse behavior: a multi-laboratory study. PLoS One 6(1):e16461

Sankoh AJ, Huque MF, Dubey SD (1997) Some comments on frequently used multiple endpoint adjustment methods in clinical trials. Stat Med 16(22):2529–2542

Santin Y et al (2024) Computational and digital analyses in the INSPIRE mouse cohort to define sex-specific functional determinants of biological aging. Sci Adv 10:eadt1670. https://doi.org/10.1126/sciadv.adt1670

Scargle JD (1982) Statistical aspects of spectral analysis of unevenly spaced data. Astrophys J 263:835–853

Stephenson R, Brown RE (2012) Circadian rhythms in cage activity and body temperature in two strains of mice. J Exp Biol 215(1):36–44

Talbot SR, Struve B, Wassermann L et al (2022) RELSA—a multidimensional procedure for the comparative assessment of Well-being and the quantitative determination of severity in experimental procedures. Front Vet Sci 9:937711

Tir S, Foster RG, Peirson SN (2025) Evaluation of the digital ventilated cage® system for circadian phenotyping. Sci Rep 15:3674

Verhave PS, van Eenige R, Tiebosch IA (2024) Methods for applying blinding and randomisation in animal experiments. Lab Anim 58(5):419–426

Voelkl B, Würbel H (2024) Heterogeneity of animal experiments and how to deal with it. Lab Anim 58(5):493–497. https://doi.org/10.1177/00236772241260173. Epub 2024 Sep 24

Wilczyński P, Kaczmarek J, Mazur A et al (2017) PyMICE: a python library for analysis of IntelliCage data. Behav Res Methods 49(4):1341–1359

Wiltschko AB, Johnson MJ, Iurilli G et al (2015) Mapping sub-second structure in mouse behavior. Neuron 88(6):1121–1135

Wu G, Anafi RC, Hughes ME, Kornacker K, Hogenesch JB (2016) MetaCycle: an integrated R package to evaluate periodicity in large-scale data. PLoS Comput Biol 12(6):e100495

Achieving Independence and Precision—A Guide for Do-It-Yourself (DIY) Home Cage Monitoring

Daniela Duarte-Domingues, Paul Mieske, Pia Kahnau, Lars Lewejohann, Marion Rivalan, and Davor Virag

Abstract

Do-It-Yourself (DIY) systems offer cost-effective and customizable solutions for researchers who require specialized equipment that is not readily available or affordable commercially. In fact, there are a number of systems for home cage monitoring (HCM) behavior that have been built independently. This concept is supported by new trends in the development of software and electronic hardware. By combining off-the-shelf hardware with open-source software, DIY systems enable the creation of prototypes that can be scaled into robust, mature systems for long-term experiments. The chapter explores the advantages and challenges of DIY systems compared to commercial solutions, emphasizing the importance of detailed documentation, modular

D. Duarte-Domingues and P. Mieske contributed equally as first authors to this chapter.

D. Duarte-Domingues
Paris Brain Institute – ICM, Sorbonne Université, Inserm U1127, CNRS UMR 7225, Paris, France

Lyon Neuroscience Research Center – CRNL, Université Claude Bernard Lyon 1, INSERM UMRS 1028, CNRS UMR 5292, Bron, France
e-mail: daniela.domingues@inserm.fr

P. Mieske · L. Lewejohann (✉)
German Federal Institute for Risk Assessment (BfR), Berlin, Germany, German Centre for the Protection of Laboratory Animals and Experimental Toxicology (Bf3R), Berlin, Germany

Institute of Animal Welfare, Animal Behavior and Laboratory Animal Science, School of Veterinary Medicine, Freie Universität Berlin, Berlin, Germany
e-mail: Lars.Lewejohann@fu-berlin.de

S. Gaburro, S. Mandillo (eds.), *Home Cage Monitoring in Rodents: A Global Effort*,
https://doi.org/10.1007/978-3-032-19781-8_9

design, and adherence to animal welfare standards. Key considerations include system design, housing conditions, enrichment tools, activity tracking, individual vs. group tracking, synchronization, and data processing. Strategies for minimizing single points of failure (SPOFs) and ensuring reliable power and data infrastructure are discussed. The chapter also highlights the significance of sharing DIY systems and data in open-source repositories to promote transparency, reproducibility, and collaboration within the scientific community. By following best practices, researchers can develop effective and scalable DIY HCM systems that enhance the quality and reproducibility of animal research while reducing costs.

Keywords

DIY · Tracking · Open-source · Microcontroller · Requirements

1 Introduction

Researchers often face the challenge of needing specialized technical equipment for their experiments that is either not commercially available or only available at a high cost. In this context, we refer to Do-It-Yourself (DIY) systems as devices developed in laboratories, usually by scientists, to reduce costs and adapt animal experiments to their specific experimental requirements. Self-developed systems usually blend off-the-shelf hardware with custom and open-source software. In this chapter, we will illustrate the concept using a few selected examples, mostly from our own work and/or user experience.

Most DIY systems start out as simple prototypes. Creating a functional prototype can be done quickly and inexpensively, making it an excellent way to gather preliminary data. This helps, for example, to gain insights into further research directions or to strengthen a grant application, making such prototypes extremely valuable. In terms of technical expertise, this chapter can provide a better understanding of the strengths and limitations of using preexisting or creating new technology to meet your specific experimental needs. It thus serves as a decision-making guide as to whether further investments in such systems, whether commercial or DIY (ideally open source), should be made.

With the increasing growth of the open-source community, the amount of shared DIY resources has also expanded exponentially. That said, before starting your own DIY

P. Kahnau
German Federal Institute for Risk Assessment (BfR), Berlin, Germany, German Centre for the Protection of Laboratory Animals and Experimental Toxicology (Bf3R), Berlin, Germany

M. Rivalan
Institute of Neuroscience Paris-Saclay, CNRS, University of Paris-Saclay, Saclay, France

D. Virag
Department of Pharmacology and Croatian Institute for Brain Research, University of Zagreb School of Medicine, Zagreb, Croatia

system, we recommend doing literature and web research to check whether there is already a developed system that meets the required specifications of your experiment (chapter "Commercializing Home Cage Monitoring: From Prototype to Global Access"). This chapter provides a valuable list of resources you are invited to visit before heating up the soldering iron yourself. In addition, we provide an overview of best practices, pros and cons and examples of DIY technologies, namely, focusing on home cage monitoring (HCM) systems for rodents as well as devices that can improve or contribute to observing animals in their home environment. Nonetheless, if there is no existing solution for your specific problem or the current options are too expensive, it is good to consider the development of a new system. In this chapter, we guide the reader from the conceptual phase to the data collection and analyses phases. We end the chapter with some DIY tips, recommendations and examples related to the sharing of newly developed systems with the community, with an emphasis on open-source practices.

Engaging in a DIY system has advantages and disadvantages, namely, in terms of costs, time and the type and quantity of data acquired. In Table 1, we summarize the most important aspects to take into account.

2 Experimental Setup/Design

The best system for your experiment is the one that allows you to collect the data you need to answer your research question. Given this context, it is especially important to identify which variables need to be extracted and how precisely they need to be measured. Sometimes, even while setting up the device, it becomes apparent that the data being collected are much more powerful than expected, allowing previously unconsidered questions to be addressed *en passant*. Depending on your hypothesis, developing a new system (from design through validation to implementation) can be simple or complicated, quick or lengthy, and inexpensive or costly. Therefore, before you start a new project, we recommend the following:

- Research on existing solutions (i.e., literature, web search, www.thebehaviourforum.org) and their suitability. It is generally better to build on existing solutions if possible to reduce time, effort, and ecosystem fragmentation (Fig. 1).
- Identify the variables you want to extract (individual metrics vs. group dynamics, location- and movement-related variables vs. fine, detailed behaviors).
- Determine the specific features (geometry, partitions, dark/light areas?) of the system that are likely to influence the behavior to be measured. Depending on the research question and experimental design, more or less consideration needs to be given to the size, shape and color of the materials used. The overall design of the system needs to meet the requirements of the experiment as well as to comply with animal welfare standards.

Table 1 Summary of the advantages and disadvantages of implementing existing commercial systems or DIY systems (open-source systems or new systems)

	DIY systems	Commercial solutions
Costs	Cost-effective when implementing an existing open-source system. More costly when setting up a new DIY system since it usually requires trial and error (note: Your own time is also a cost that is often overlooked).	Due to the commercial nature of company-based solutions, commercial systems are usually much more expensive than DIY systems. In addition to the price of the product itself, other additional costs include the replacement of parts and technical help as a service.
Time	The experimenters have control over how much time they can and are willing to spend. However, this is usually not predictable.	Especially at the beginning, if you can rely on customer service, commercial solutions are usually implemented more quickly. Nevertheless, you are dependent on the company's availability.
Necessary expertise	It is usually the intention that nonexperts should be able to implement DIY systems. However, this can be tricky, e.g., if new hard and software versions are necessary. Additional help is usually provided by the original developers and an online community of users, through forums. You are dependent on their time and expertise so it is important to check if the community is still active.	Using sophisticated commercial products might also require expert knowledge in how the system works. The use of the full potential of a system might not be clear at the beginning. The risk of the product being discontinued and professional service stop being available exits.
Data access	Full access to the data acquired. Control on the type and format of the data. With this power comes the responsibility to consider a data format that can be used effectively in the long term, ideally according to the FAIR principles.	Data formats and type of data provided will be decided by the company. Some even use proprietary data formats that only can be analyzed using their software.
Data quality	The user is primarily responsible to handle and preprocess the data.	Risk of relying on proprietary, nonstandard data formats.
Equipment	In theory, you know exactly how the system is made since all the detailed information should be published and publicly available. In practice, not everyone respects it.	You might need to team up with technical experts for personalized setups or analyses.
Connectivity	You can implement interfaces to connect with other devices if needed.	Interfaces have to be provided and often are only compatible with other devices of the same company.

Note that nonopen source DIY systems sold by companies are closer to commercial solutions in this regard

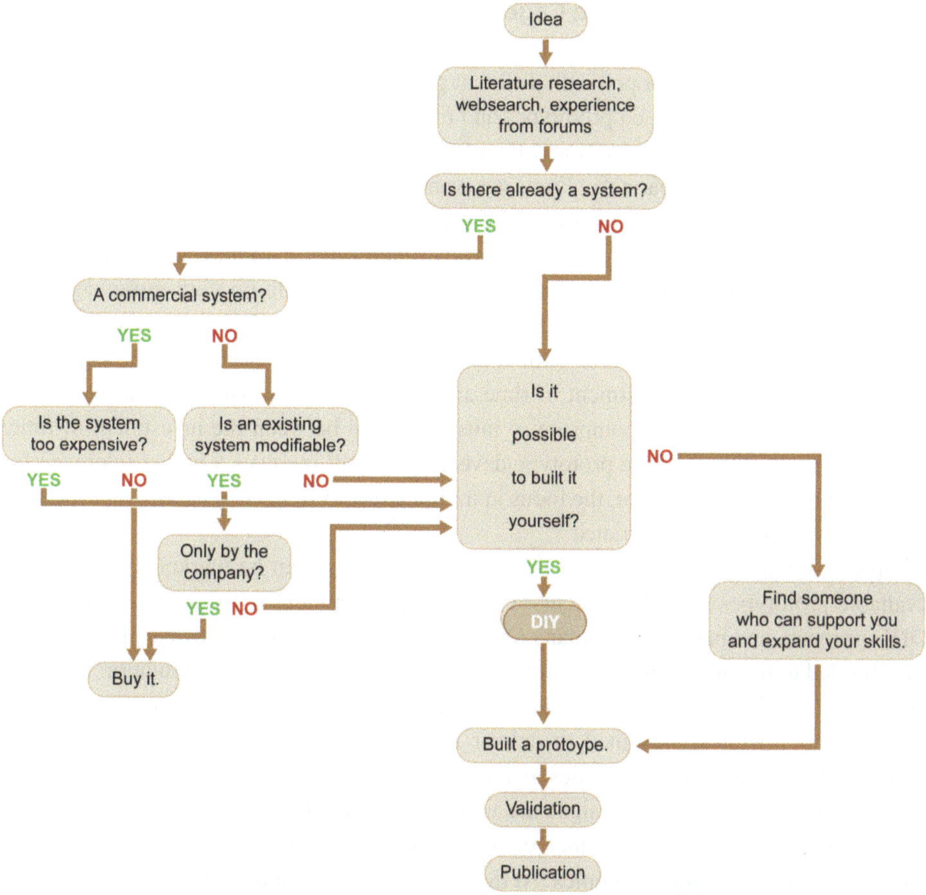

Fig. 1 Decision tree. Guidance for the decision-making process regarding when a test system can or should be developed on its own. First, it is advisable to research whether there is already a system available that can answer your specific question. If so, you need to clarify whether it is commercially available at an affordable cost, or if it can be replicated. Consider whether you can replicate the system yourself or if you need to find someone to help you create the prototype

- Space! How large and suitable is your animal housing? This is important to decide cage size, which must be sufficient to actually measure the desired behaviors. It is also important to note that the system itself requires space (e.g., for camera-based systems, a viewing angle-dependent distance, cable routing, and housing for electronics).
- Feedback. We strongly recommend discussing the project with all parties involved, especially the animal care staff, at an early stage.

2.1 Approaches to Home Cage System Design

HCM systems can be developed with different goals in mind, and one possible categorization is the distinction between prototypes and mature systems. These two approaches pursue different (intermediate) goals and therefore have advantages and disadvantages that should be considered separately. First, we want to emphasize that the ability to create prototypes is a major advantage of the DIY approach. Prototypes make it possible to provide proof of concept without having to invest much time or money. Once these initial questions have been answered, researchers often want to scale up with more cages and longer, more complex experiments. The focus in development shifts to robustness, scalability, and the ability to work well with other systems or local conditions at the same time. At this point, a greater investment of time and money is often justified to achieve these goals. In this framework, a compromise must be found between the investment of time/money and robustness. While prototype development still involves a higher tolerance for errors and much trial and error, the focus in more mature systems is on good, robust reproducibility with low error tolerance.

Since commercial systems must be mature before they can be marketed, all publicly available prototypes are DIY systems. Prototype development is an essential part of the DIY approach, and in that sense, many DIY systems are more or less advanced prototypes. This has led to the unfortunate situation in which DIY systems have a reputation for being more fragile and less robust. In fact, however, this is a characteristic of prototype systems, which are deliberately designed to deliver usable data quickly and cost-effectively in return. In fact, the problem often lies in unclear expectations of a device. This can become problematic when prototype designs are used for investigations in which robustness and scalability are of crucial importance or when prototypes continue to be used as experiments become increasingly complex. At the same time, it is not clear for all available DIY equipment what stage of development it is at. This is particularly true since the current stage is unlikely to be the same fit for all planned experiments. Although there are mature and robust DIY systems, both the user and the system developer must clearly define their goals and expectations to find a suitable design.

2.2 Home Cage Designs

2.2.1 Dimensions

Like all housing systems, home cage systems for observing animals must comply with animal welfare standards (i.e., EU directive 2010/63/EU; for more information about animal welfare, see chapter "Enhancing Animal Welfare Through Home Cage Monitoring Systems"). These are partly regulated by law and usually relate to the stocking density, i.e., how many animals may be kept per housing area. However, it should be noted that the maximum stocking density is not necessarily the best for the animals but rather reflects a minimum mandatory requirement. In addition, it must be ensured that animals are not prevented from displaying species-specific behavior. For example, a rodent must be able to rear itself within the enclosure. However, any ceiling or cage openings should be small enough or out of reach to prevent animals from escaping.

What exactly constitutes a home cage can be interpreted differently (chapter "Home Cage Monitoring: Where We Are and What We Need?") depending on varying needs, resources and scientific objectives. Moreover, the ideal size also depends on the context. In terms of dimensions, homemade cage systems have the advantage that they can be optimally adapted to the test setup and the user's spatial conditions. Beyond the legal minimum requirements, the height, width, and depth of the cage can be adapted to the location where the cage will actually be set up (e.g., cage rack, a table in the room). The dimensions of a cage should always take accessibility into account. It is advisable to be able to reach every corner of a cage with an average arm length (i.e., the experimenter's and the animal caretakers' arm). This is crucial to avoid unnecessary "chasing" of animals if they need to be caught regularly.

It is important to ensure that the animals have enough space and enrichment tools (see Sect. 2.3) to comply with animal welfare standards. However, this applies to all experiments involving animals, not just DIY systems. The more space there is, the greater the freedom to design cages that allow the animals to express their natural behaviors. In fact, it has been shown that animals in a DIY system that offers them more freedom of movement express a significantly broader range of behaviors (Mieske et al. 2021). Therefore, a larger space not only better meets animal welfare requirements but also enables better data collection (Mandillo et al. 2008).

2.2.2 Materials

When building a DIY system, it is also necessary to consider the materials to be used. All materials used should either be safe for direct contact and possible ingestion by the animal or not accessible to the animal. If there is regular contact with certain materials, these materials should meet the corresponding hygiene requirements of the experimental environment and allow some form of disinfection (e.g., heat-resistant, liquid-resistant) as well as safety requirements (e.g., isolated cables from animals).

Polycarbonate is probably the most commonly used material in animal husbandry. Cages, housing and enrichment items are made from this material. It has the advantage of being very heat resistant, dimensionally stable, impact-resistant and appears to be harmless to animal health. However, it is not always possible to produce polycarbonate items in your own facility. It is therefore a good idea to produce 3D printed objects from polylactic acid (PLA), especially for prototypes. 3D printers and filaments are relatively inexpensive. In addition, any necessary adjustments can be made quickly. PLA objects have already been used in the development of HCM systems (Habedank et al. 2022). PLA enrichment items and lockboxes (to investigate learning behavior) have also been used within the home cage (Hobbiesiefken et al. 2021; Hohlbaum et al. 2024). A pathological examination revealed no evidence of toxicological-pathological effects associated with PLA (Hohlbaum et al. 2024).

It is also recommended that the color of the setup contrasts with the animal's fur color (e.g., light setup for black mice; dark setup for white mice) since video tracking systems usually require optical contrast. It is also important to ensure that there are no (or only necessary, such as nests and shelters) opaque hiding places within the setup, especially for video recording, to allow for continuous data tracking. One way of surpassing the need to use opaque objects is to use red transparent material, as mice are significantly less sensitive to red light than humans (Peirson et al. 2018). It is therefore assumed that red is perceived as dark by rodents. Cameras that record in the IR range (most video cameras do this; sometimes an IR filter must be removed) see very well through the transparent red.

2.2.3 Design

It is always advantageous to maintain a certain degree of flexibility when creating a new DIY system. By dividing a system into modules that can be exchanged and worked on individually, one can quickly adjust the system to new requirements without compromising the entire setup. It is important to remember that optimizations are never complete and that there is an 'opportunity sweet spot' where the system is good enough for the research hypothesis in question—it is important not to miss this spot! By understanding common points and modes of failure, builders can implement safeguards in their systems, and users can better manage their systems on their own. Furthermore, technology and system architecture, which 20 years ago were accessible only to a few trained specialists, are now easily accessible to researchers and developers with little or no technical background.

2.2.4 Inclusion

When operating a housing cage and handling the laboratory animals on a daily basis, you should not rely solely on your own judgment. As a rule, most of the work with animals is carried out by animal caretakers. It is therefore advisable to incorporate their perspective and expertise into the development of a possible design from the outset. It should be equally easy for everyone involved to take care of the animals and operate the equipment. In fact, animal caretakers often bring experience that goes far beyond that of an experimenter (Abelson et al. 2023). When introducing the system to all those who will be working with it, it is also important to give them the opportunity to ask questions about using the system. A good presentation and briefing, as well as detailed technical manuals, will reduce any fear of contact and promote positive communication. In turn, this dialog is extremely helpful in improving the system and moving it out of the pure prototype stage. Particularly in the early stages of development, it is important to detect even the smallest errors in the system so that they can be corrected.

2.3 Enrichment Tools and Space

2.3.1 Space

To maximize the available space inside a cage, it is a useful strategy to place various objects inside it that are suitable for enlarging the surface area. Depending on the design of the home cage, it can be possible to provide a second floor level. The animals then have shelter below and can use the enclosure area by climbing up to the second level. This allows them to engage in their natural climbing behavior. Other climbing options include ropes (e.g., made of hemp) that can be attached to the grid cover. If there is no grid cover, ladders or other frames can be set up instead. However, if the cage is not covered (e.g., in the Live Mouse Tracker (de Chaumont et al. 2019), automated visual burrow system Rivalan et al. 2024), it is important to ensure that the mice cannot climb too high and escape. Transparent, perforated ceiling partitions can be installed on some structures to prevent escape while still allowing video recording or visual checks, as well as air to flow into the cage.

2.3.2 Nesting and Sheltering

The natural behaviors of rodents include nest building and sheltering. When working with mice, different nesting materials, such as paper, cotton wool or wood wool, should be provided. The amount of nesting material supplied should be appropriate for the size of the group. One way of determining whether sufficient material is available is to assess the structure of the nests built by the animals. As mice are prey animals, they tend to avoid open, unprotected areas. Therefore, it is necessary to provide them with shelter. A well-known example is the 'triangular house' (Fig. 2). Due to its relatively small size, it can be

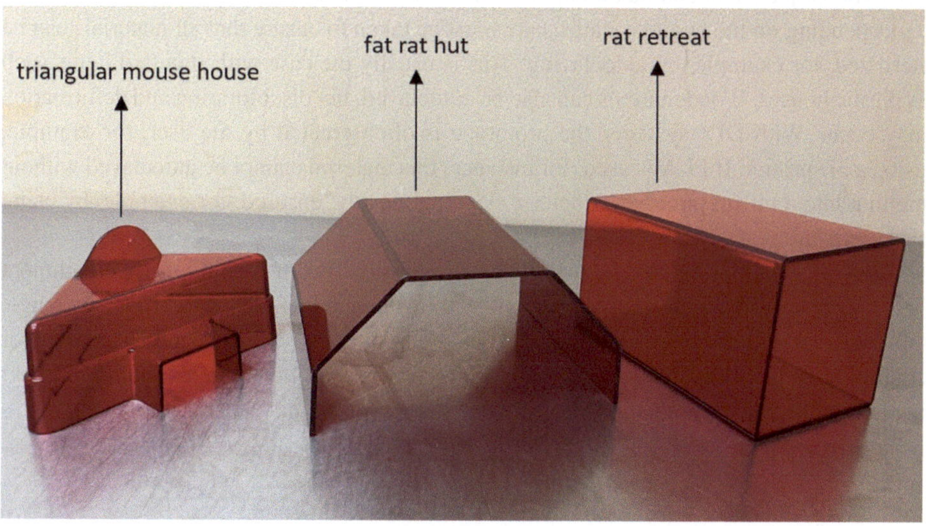

Fig. 2 Shelters. Shelter options made of red polycarbonate that are transparent to humans but appear dark to mice

incorporated into all housing systems. It is transparent to humans for visual inspection. However, as mice largely lack cone cells for perceiving red color, they perceived these houses as a dark shelter. Nevertheless, this option does not offer enough space for larger groups. Depending on the available room, 'fat rat huts' can be an alternative (Fig. 2).

Wooden shelters and climbing structures are ideal for allowing mice to additionally engage in their natural gnawing behavior. However, opaque wooden objects are only suitable if continuous observation, for example, by cameras, is not necessary (due to the risk of occlusion). It should also be noted that climbing structures can prevent animals from being within the reading range of RFID (radio frequency identification) antennas, in case this is the tracking method selected. In general, it is important to consider how tracking can be reconciled with animal welfare.

2.3.3 Enrichment Tools

There are many different ways to design the home cage to allow the animals to express their natural behavior. However, depending on the design of the DIY system, only certain items may be suitable. Often, there is a lack of experience in handling enrichment materials, and it can be unclear how the animals use them. When introducing new items, it is advisable to observe the animals first to determine the usefulness of the enrichment items to the animals and the system. Of course, it is also possible to draw on existing experience (Hobbiesiefken et al. 2021, 2023).

In groups of male mice in particular, care should be taken to create escape routes and avoid dead-end situations, as these can encourage aggressive and/or overly defensive behaviors. There are also various ways of providing escape options. One possibility is to attach swings or open tubes to the grid. Weber et al. (2023) also recommend providing mice with nesting material or other manipulable enrichment items to minimize aggressive behavior. Objects that can be monopolized by individual animals should be avoided.

Depending on the hygiene status, care must be taken to ensure that all materials can be sterilized, for example, by autoclaving. This is usually the case with standard items such as plastic houses. Wooden items can also be autoclaved, but discoloration and deformation may occur. With DIY systems, the prototype is often created by the user, for example, using a 3D printer. If PLA is used, for instance, this material cannot be autoclaved without melting into a pitiful pile. Nevertheless, cleaning must be ensured, for example, by using surface disinfectants.

As with shelters and nesting materials, care must be taken with all other enrichment items to ensure that the animals remain within the field of vision or tracking range. Otherwise, it will not be possible to track and consequently record the animals' behavior continuously, resulting in data loss. Although the use of enrichment items can make tracking more difficult, enrichment should not be omitted for animal welfare reasons.

2.4 Food and Water Delivery

One of the main advantages of using HCM systems is the ability to test animals without withholding food or water and therefore be able to incorporate water deprivation (or targeted feeding) short-term tasks into long-term experiments. Having access to the behavioral setups 24/7 allows animals to engage in the behavioral paradigm "self-motivated", without a forced time constraint or a stressful human interaction. Currently, there are multiple open-source devices with these functions. As an example, the FED3 is an open-source rodent feeding and training device that is now used by more than 100 research labs around the world and can be easily placed in home cage systems (Matikainen-Ankney et al. 2021). PiDose is an open-source system for accurate and automated oral drug administration to group-housed mice (Woodard et al. 2020). FreiBox is an open-source system controlled by a custom Python interface that integrates a lickometer, allowing the tracking of mouse licking behavior in real time and consequent control of task events on a submillisecond scale (Crompe et al. 2023). These are just three great examples of open source DIY systems that already take into account the importance of measuring and automatically delivering food and water to animals.

2.5 Prototype Testing

Once we consider all the design constraints, a prototype of the experimental setup can be built. The conditions should be as similar as possible to those of the actual experiment. This step is particularly important because we can only develop this prototype from a human perspective; it will then have to be tested by the animals. It is at this stage that they show us what we have not thought of. For example, access to areas that the animals should not be able to reach, fear of unknown objects/materials, or destruction of objects through excessive gnawing, possibly exacerbated by boredom (Mieske et al. 2022). Again, it is helpful to talk to others, as it is often surprising to discover that experiences are quite similar. It is also crucial to check that the system does not produce any disturbing noise or vibration or that light sources are not present in such a way as to affect the tracking or welfare of the animals. In some systems, especially when using continuously running electronics, it may be advisable to check the heat development with a simple thermal imaging camera (e.g., a top-down IR camera). This is important to prevent overheating but also to prevent the animals from being affected by an additional heat source.

3 Data Collection

Once it is clear which variables are needed to extract to answer a specific question, you need to consider how the data will be collected. Depending on the research question, different devices and methods may be used. For example, there are cameras with different resolutions that can be used to record animal behaviors, each with its own unique pros and cons.

Both when testing the prototype and during the actual experiment, it is advisable to check the data for errors or inconsistencies. On the one hand, it is essential to ensure that data are recorded as intended. For example, a common problem is that timestamps are not stored correctly or become desynchronized between systems due to clock drift. On the other hand, animals may not behave as expected, and adjustments to the system (both software and hardware) may be necessary, which may introduce incompatibilities against older data recordings. Finally, it is important to check that the recorded data can be easily analyzed and interpreted.

Today, the open source ecosystem enables relatively easy, affordable, and rapid construction of a setup that can produce useful scientific data. The very first question is the choice of electronic platform, which will largely determine a DIY device's characteristics, features, and limitations, as shown in Table 2.

On one side of the spectrum, the purpose of microcontroller boards is to provide a simple connection to electronic components such as sensors, actuators (e.g., a motor), and LEDs. Although some electronics and programming knowledge is needed, the data obtained are usually a time series of discrete values that are relatively easy to analyze.

On the other end, a PC with a directly attached camera can be used. Such a setup is practically plug-and-play, but data storage and analysis of hours, days, or weeks of video presents a significant obstacle. Full computers also usually require active cooling and fans, making them ill-suited to the environment of an animal habitat (due to potential heat and ultrasonic sound emissions). An example of a software architecture that facilitates PC-based setups is Open Balena (open balena – github, 2025).

Table 2 HCM electronic platforms. The electronic platform determines a DIY HCM device's range of recording modalities, as well as tradeoffs in different aspects of the device's technical operation and data output

		Technical operation		Data output	
Electronic platform	What can I attach? Monitoring modalities	Setup difficulty	Robust-ness	Processing power	Output data complexity
A microcontroller (e.g. Arduino board)	Sensors and actuators	High	High	Low	Low
A single-board computer (e.g. Raspberry Pi)	Sensors, actuators, low-quality cameras	Moderate	Moderate	Moderate	Moderate
A personal computer	Sensors, actuators, low- and high-quality cameras, high quality audio such as USV recording	Low	Low	High	High

Single-board computers (SBCs) run a full operating system, which is usually Linux-based, affording the benefits of using a full computer, such as easier data storage and network operation (an example is Raspberry Pi). SBCs can easily interface with the entire spectrum of electronic and electromechanical components, similar to microcontroller boards, and can interface with lower-quality cameras (e.g., webcams). Their limitation is that they usually cannot perform high-throughput data acquisition (e.g., high-quality video and audio) due to limited processing power. SBCs are more resilient to the animal habitat environment, although they are generally less robust than microcontroller boards.

3.1 A Microcontroller-Based System

To introduce the fundamental principles of data acquisition as the translation of physical phenomena to raw scientific data, we will start a simple microcontroller-based use case, as the microcontroller platform is the one most involved in the fundamentals of the process. Later, more complex variants and their benefits will be described.

For data acquisition, the three main components are (i) a sensor, which records natural phenomena as electric signals (e.g., a light sensor), (ii) a microcontroller, which reads sensor signals as data (e.g., an arduino), and (iii) a means of data logging, either to a wired or networked computer or to an attached data storage (e.g., an SD card). Aside from sensing, interaction with the animal is possible using LED lights as cues and actuators as gates or reward dispensers. Video recording usually requires a more powerful device than a microcontroller—a single-board computer (e.g., a Raspberry pi) or a PC.

3.1.1 Sensors

The most commonly employed technologies in DIY systems are radio-frequency identification (RFID), passive infrared sensors (PIR), and beam-break sensors due to the existence of easy-to-use sensor modules, low complexity of recorded data, and affordability. Video recording offers the most comprehensive data, but at the cost of large storage needs and high complexity. The main characteristics of these technologies are briefly described in Table 3. More information can also be found in chapter "Study Design and Data Analysis in Home Cage Monitoring Experiments". Members of the TEATIME COST Action CA20135 have also compiled a comprehensive summary of home cage systems (both commercial and DIY). This catalog contains numerous examples of how the various sensors are used (COST Action TEATIME – HCM Technologies Catalog at www.thebehaviourforum.org, COST (2025).

3.1.2 Microcontrollers

The most commonly used way to transfer and save data from sensors to a computer is through a USB connection. A microcontroller can be programmed to interface with different types of sensors and even perform basic preprocessing (e.g., averaging multiple readings as a means of denoising) before sending data to a computer.

Table 3 Commonly used sensing technologies in DIY systems

Technology	What does it do?	What does it record?	How is it used?
Video recording 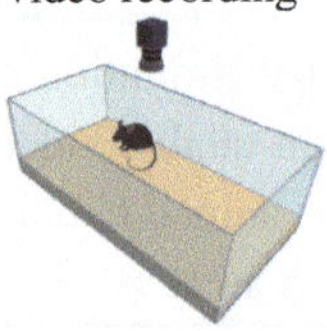	One or multiple cameras recording videos for automatic, video acquisition, processing and analysis.	Image series over time, in the visible or visible+infrared spectrum (for night vision).	*Full cage area* or *points of interest.* *Multiple cameras* may be used for: Redundancy, or 3D pose estimation
Example: Alonso et al. (2023)			
Radio-Frequency identification (RFID) 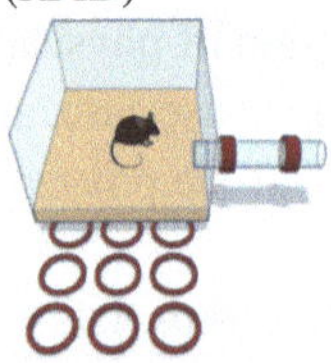	Reading identification data from a batteryless implanted transponder (tag) when in vicinity of an antenna/reader.	All of: Static tag data (e.g. animal ID) Dynamic tag data (e.g. temperature) Timestamp when the tag entered/exited the vicinity of the antenna.	Either: 1. Continuous positional monitoring of multiple animals individually (unique tags) using a grid of readers spanning the *full cage area,* Or: 2. Monitoring access to *points of interest* (e.g. tunnels, gates) using strategically placed readers.
Example: Lewejohann et al. (2009); Habedank et al. (2022)			
Passive infrared (PIR) sensor modules 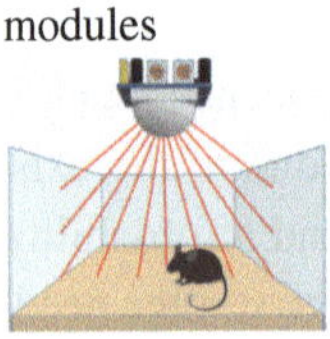	Animal infrared radiation is sensed. The sensor module changes its state from 0 to 1 when the detected movement crosses a predefined threshold.	Binary sensor state (logical 0 or 1) continuously, at a fixed sampling rate (e.g. every second)	Circadian activity measurement by monitoring the *full cage area* *(more common usage)*
		Timestamp when the sensor detected movement.	Detecting the presence at a *point of interest* using a focused field of view.
Example: Brown et al. 2017			
Beam-break sensors 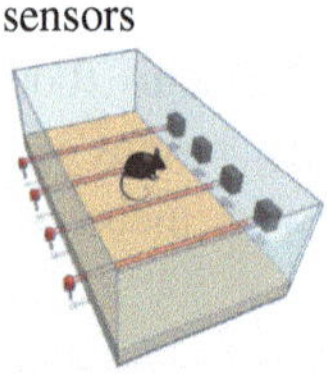	An infrared LED transmitter/receiver pair form a beam. Occlusion (and reestablishment) of the beam by the animal is detected by the receiver.	Timestamp when the beam was broken and reestablished	Detecting presence and loitering at *points of interest*, e.g. specific area, platform, or nosepoke opening *(more common usage).*
		Number of beam-break events over a time interval (e.g. every hour).	At one or multiple points to monitor circadian activity across the *full cage area.*
Example: FED3 2025; Alexxai Kravitz (2025), Med Associates Inc. – Operant Conditioning + General Behavior (2025)			

At the forefront of DIY electronics used in research is the Arduino platform. When talking about "Arduino", the term encompasses both Arduino-branded microcontroller boards and the Arduino programming framework, which is supported by many other boards as well. While Arduino-branded boards are not a requirement for DIY (and, indeed, other manufacturers can sometimes offer Arduino-compatible boards additional functionality at a competitive price), the Arduino framework is highly recommended. With this framework, it is possible to obtain valuable data using a device programmed with approximately 15 lines of code—Box 1 shows minimal operational code for a simple device utilizing a passive infrared sensor (PIR; a motion detector as it is commonly used to control outdoor, automatic lights) to monitor locomotor activity. For example, a PIR-based device, termed "PIROSLAV" (Prototype InfraRed Open Source Locomotor Activity eValuator), was built by attendees of the Second COST-TEATIME Advanced Training School in Berlin, 2024, with a manual composed by attendees available here: Domingues and Melloni 2025.

Furthermore, the code works with little to no modifications across most Arduino-compatible microcontroller boards. Finally, with the large ecosystem that has grown around the platform, there is a high chance that an open source code library can be found for most commercially available sensors or sensor modules. In a similar manner to the framework itself, libraries simplify the code necessary to interact with sensors and often come with useful example codes. In addition, the open source community is currently also doing video tutorials that truly facilitate the process of understanding this platform.

Box 1 A Complete Arduino Programme to Record Movement Data Using a Passive-Infrared (PIR) Sensor

```
int pin = 27; //this is the number of the physical pin where the sensor is attached to
int reading;

void setup() {
  // put your setup code here, to run once:
  pinMode(pin, INPUT); // set the mode of pin to INPUT
  Serial.begin(115200); // initialise communication with the PC over USB
}

void loop() {
  // put your main code here, to run repeatedly:
  reading = digitalRead(pin); // measure the pin state and store its state
                              // (0 or 1) into the `reading` variable
  Serial.println(reading); // send the value of reading to the PC
  delay(100); // pause for 100 ms to not overwhelm the PC/me with readings
}
```

Box 2 A Complete Python Programme to Log Arduino Data to a File

```
from datetime import datetime
import serial

arduino = serial.Serial("COM3", 115200) //this is the COM number of the connection between your computer and arduino
log_file = open("log.csv", "w")

try:
    while True:
        line = arduino.readline()
        line = datetime.now().isoformat()+";"+line+"\n"
        log_file.write(line)
        print(line)
except KeyboardInterrupt:
    arduino.close()
    log_file.close()
```

Data Logging with Arduino The most common way of receiving and logging Arduino data is via the same USB connection used to program the microcontroller board. The raw data can be viewed in Arduino's Serial Monitor and plotted with Arduino's Serial Plotter in real time. For quick prototyping, data can be copied from the Serial Monitor to a CSV file. For home cage monitoring, a simple Python script (Box 2) is often sufficient to complement previous Arduino code, totalling approximately 30 lines of code for a device capable of recording and extracting to a csv file locomotor activity.

The Single-Board Computer (SBC) A basic setup with a single-board computer such as a Raspberry Pi usually includes one or more sensors as described above and/or a USB-attached webcam. In the aforementioned microcontroller-based prototype PIR-based HCM device, the microcontroller can be substituted by an SBC running appropriate code, which stores data directly to a storage medium (e.g., an SD card) instead of sending it to a PC.

Personal Computer At a high level, a personal computer offers unparalleled flexibility in terms of processing power, storage options, networking, and user-friendly tools for high-level peripherals and interfaces. A use case where a PC is absolutely necessary is the acquisition of large volumes of data, such as high-resolution, uncompressed video and/or audio (especially ultrasonic, useful for monitoring rodent vocalizations). The high bitrate requires greater processing power than microcontrollers or SBCs can currently offer. In these situations, a PC will be the best option. The PC can also interface with simple sensors and actuators by attaching microcontroller boards via USB to act as bridges, as described previously.

3.2 Motion Capture

There are various options and camera devices available to capture motion. It is important to decide in advance whether group or individual animals will be recorded and what level of behavioral detail needs to be captured.

There are a few things to consider when deciding where and how to install cameras for home cage monitoring to minimize occlusions as much as possible. Moreover, it is also important to carefully consider which camera you want to use in advance, as the camera you use will affect the video quality. In addition, the amount of time recorded (if continuously or not) is positively correlated with the amount of data produced and, as importantly, with the amount of data that needs to be stored and analyzed. Therefore, it is necessary to consider whether 24/7 recording is required to answer the scientific question. Since rats and mice are nocturnal, recording only during this phase may be sufficient. As this is the dark phase, cameras equipped for this purpose, i.e., with infrared capabilities, must be used.

3.2.1 Cameras

Most commercially available web cameras have a 30 Hz frame rate, which is sufficient to capture bulk locomotion activity, usually by tracking the center of mass of the animal. With only this information, one can quantify, for example, animals' speed and space occupancy. Regular security cameras used for controls outside of (human) homes can sometimes recapitulate the need for night vision with embedded IR (infrared) lighting, satisfying the quality of images and relatively low storage needs. For catching finer behaviors such as whisker movements or grooming fine sequences, a high-speed camera might be necessary (Roy et al. 2011).

Researchers have also been using 3D depth cameras to capture the full spectrum of behaviors in rodents (Weinreb et al. 2024). They used multiple cameras to estimate keypoints in 3D (including keypoints that were not visible in the overhead-camera 2D data set) and confirmed that the 3D keypoints had higher intrinsic dimensionality than 2D keypoints.

Overall, it is quite easy to record animal movements. However, there are many alternatives, so it is sometimes difficult to decide on a system. The most important factor is the frame rate required for your camera, which depends on the behavior you want to record and the amount of data to be captured (continuous or not). Another important point is the selection of video software that allows you to record and save the desired type (quality and size) of videos and that can start and stop recording automatically according to a schedule (e.g., using Bonsai, Lopes et al. 2015) or through manual operation (e.g., OBS Studio, 2025).

3.2.2 Alternatives: LEDs and RFIDs

In addition to using video tracking, there are other alternatives to capture animal bulk behavior:

- Light barriers comprising infrared light-emitting diodes (LEDs). Infrared LEDs allow animal behavior to be captured easily and lightly in terms of data. Using a pair of light barriers is enough to obtain information on movement (e.g., speed) and on the direction of movement. However, to obtain data, the animals must be kept individually. For refinement reasons, this should always be reconsidered.
- Radio frequency identification (RFID). RFIDs under the base of the cage or between different compartments of the cage are a good alternative to "passively" capture animal motion. Researchers have used RFID data to measure an index of distance traveled, place preference and entropy within different areas of the cage (Freund et al. 2013). RFID technology can also be used to collect individual data from animals that are kept in groups.
- Passive infrared sensor (PIR). PIR sensors react to changes in infrared heat radiation. More information can be found in chapter "Technologies for Home Cage Monitoring in Preclinical Research".

Animal motion capturing allows overall quantification of locomotion metrics that are key measures in many animal behavioral studies. In Table 4, we describe the pros and cons of the 3 most commonly used approaches: video tracking with a camera, LEDs and RFIDs.

3.3 Individual Tracking in a Group Setting

RFID tags are used in animal research to automatically identify and track animals in a group setting. In addition to existing commercial systems (e.g., TSE Systems – Phenoworld, 2025; see also chapter "Commercializing Home Cage Monitoring: From Prototype to Global Access" of this book), the simplicity of RFID technology offers the possibility for

Table 4 Comparison of activity tracking devices

Device	Pros	Cons
Camera (for video tracking)	Different types (infrared, stereo, time-of-flight…)	The need for a clear view restricts the number and type of enrichment tools
	Can capture most of the behavioral repertoire	Needs space for careful placement
	Produces rich, extensive data	Depending on the frame rate and continuous vs. triggered recording, gigabytes to terabytes of storage may be needed, with high processing requirements
Beam-break sensor (LEDs)	Simple data which is easy to process	No individual tracking
	Cheap, many pairs can be used for better spatial accuracy	Animals or bedding can block the sensor
RFID	Simple data which is easy to process	Poor spatial accuracy
	Individual animal identification	Missed readings possible due to animals moving too fast or out of the reading range of the sensors (e.g. on elevated surfaces)

customization and DIY projects. As RFID readers can be equipped with a ring coil, they are usually placed on connecting tubes between different sections (e.g., home cages, tubular entrances) to track the lab animals being held (Puścian et al. 2016; Habedank et al. 2022). This allows quantification of individual preference areas and resource monopolization (e.g., food, water). In combination with "doors", RFID can also be used to control access to different areas of an experimental setup (commercially: (Winter and Schaefers 2011; Rivalan et al. 2017; Mei et al. 2020; Kahnau et al. 2023a)).

Another option to track animal motion is to arrange the coils of the RFID readers as a grid under a housing area (micecraft – LMT, 2025). This allows the recording of the movement of many individual animals in their home cage environment. Moreover, the RFID data can be synchronized with video recording for direct and visual identification of individual animals.

Finally, multianimal pose estimation, identification and tracking are now possible with open-source tools such as DeepLabCut (Mathis et al. 2018) and Bonsai (Lopes et al. 2015). DeepLabCut allows the identification of individual animals in a group setting by applying deep learning methods to the analysis of the video recording (Lauer et al. 2022).

There are multiple advantages of tracking in a home cage setting: (1) animal self-engage in the task, at their own pace, not pressured by time constraints or human interactions; (2) increased collection of data more reproducible since conditions are the same over time; and (3) possibility of validation of a battery of tests in the testing chamber, enhancing results comparability (Rivalan et al. 2017).

3.4 Synchronization

Aside from experimental logs, precise timekeeping on the order of <1 second is particularly important with multiple concurrent recording modalities (e.g., video with USVs or RFID logs). It is essential to decide on the accuracy required since different strategies will need to be employed for <1 s offset as opposed to <1 ms. In the example of synchronizing video and ultrasonic vocalizations, good synchronization would require, roughly estimated, a difference of no more than a quarter to half of the period between individual video frames. For example, if the video is recorded at 30 frames per second, a frame is recorded every 33 milliseconds; therefore, ideally, the audio recording would be offset by less than ±8.25 ms to match audio events to each video frame precisely. For other combinations, e.g., RFID with video to keep track of identities, synchronization within a few hundred milliseconds would likely allow good identity matching between video and RFID logs.

Time synchronization between multiple devices with separate clock sources can be done by synchronizing devices against a Network Time Protocol (NTP) server via the internet (~10 ms accuracy) or on the local network (~1 ms accuracy)—The Secure Network Time Protocol (NTPsec, 2025) Distribution. Due to drift (usually a few seconds of accumulated offset per day), automatic periodic resynchronization is a common feature in many NTP tools and libraries.

However, desynchronization can also occur while using only one device (i.e., physical clock source) for concurrent recordings from multiple sensing modalities. Consumer operating systems are not "real time"—most tasks, from recording data to drawing out the user interface, can be shuffled and slightly delayed to prioritize another task, generally with the intent of making the system user interface (UI) smooth and responsive. Practically speaking, after a software command, there is a delay before data acquisition actually begins on a hardware level. With an unpredictable timing from microseconds to hundreds of milliseconds, this delay cannot be compensated for. The effects of this limitation on data acquisition can be seen in practice in a non-HCM DIY device (see Supplementary Material 2 of Virag et al. 2021).

While software approaches exist (e.g., low-latency and real-time kernels), a definite solution is to stimulate both recording modalities at once with a tightly coupled multimodal stimulus. Similar to a movie set, a clapperboard is used at the beginning of a scene to give an acoustic and visual signal for synchronization. Furthermore, microcontrollers can produce signals within tens of nanoseconds. This feature can be employed in two ways. First, a single device can produce a light and a sound with an LED and a speaker, respectively, at the same time. Second, many professional recording devices have special connectors precisely for this purpose—hardware triggering. BeDSy (Virag 2024), a DIY platform, was thus used to simultaneously send a signal to start audio recording to a USV microphone amplifier and to continuously send signals to a number of cameras every time a frame needs to be recorded. In this way, the audio start signal is tightly coupled with the first frame record signal.

3.5 The SPOF Protocol

To minimize the risk of data loss, a good way to assess the architecture of the workflow is to follow the path of the data and pinpoint single points of failure (SPOF), i.e., critical components that could take down the whole system and/or might cause data loss upon failure. SPOFs should ideally be removed or designed to be as failure-proof as possible. Importantly, SPOFs can be analyzed at different levels. For example, the home cage-attached device is a SPOF as a singular device, but we can analyze each of its components separately as well. Usually, components include a microcontroller with sensors and/or actuators, each of which can also cause data loss upon failure. Therefore, each component is also considered a possible SPOF.

3.5.1 Examples of SPOFs: The Cage-Attached Device

DIY animal cages usually have microcontrollers (e.g., Arduino) as the basis of their platform. The microcontroller is a necessary SPOF, and its failure is usually due to errors in code (firmware bugs), which can be mitigated with sufficient testing. Sensors can be redundant to increase the robustness of the device (Virag et al. 2025), and actuators can be fitted with sensors of their own, monitoring their operation.

3.5.2 Examples of SPOFs: The PC as a Control and Data Storage Device

The most common setup is a home cage-attached embedded electronic device communicating with a PC directly via USB (Table 4). The attached PC is the only device that can acquire data from the HCM device, and as such, it is a Single Point Of Failure (SPOF). In continuous operations, the PC is less reliable than microcontrollers and single-board computers (SBCs). This is due to PCs being composed of a large number of complex components, where the failure of any one of them can be critical and possibly stop the operations. Second, writable memory can become corrupt and thereby destroy data retroactively. Third, PCs are often dependent on fan cooling, which produces noise and can be hindered by dust over time. Finally, HCM designs using PCs often need manual intervention to restart software components in case of power failures or even automatically restart due to improper out-of-box configuration (e.g., automatic system updates during an experiment).

While the high processing power of PCs is necessary in some applications (e.g., recording video), it is advised to design systems where the SPOF potential of PCs is reduced as much as possible (e.g., use an autostart protocol, disable automatic software updates or use specialized operating systems, use industrial computers with redundant hardware or implement redundant arrays of independent disks (RAID) for storage, duplicate power supplies, etc.).

3.5.3 Alternatives to PC as a SPOF: Direct Storage

One of the ways to avoid using the PC as a storage device is to directly save the data on a physical component. One example is the FED3 home cage operant conditioning device, which saves the data directly to an SD card (Table 4). In this case, the SPOF is the SD card as a single component. Even if SD cards can become corrupted after a large number of writes, there are high endurance options available at low cost. In this configuration, the loss of data risk due to crashing or component failure is greatly reduced compared to a PC.

3.5.4 Alternatives to the PC as a SPOF: Networking

As a further step, the embedded cage-attached device can be equipped with networking capability. An example of such architecture is the MIROSLAV system (Virag et al. 2025). A standard Wi-Fi network is used to propagate data to multiple computers simultaneously (e.g., via the MQTT protocol (Andrew Banks et al. 2019)). Since the computers connect through Wi-Fi, they do not need to be in the same room as the experimental HCM devices. To ensure precise timekeeping, which is especially important while using multiple HCM systems concurrently, the HCM devices synchronize time from a local or online NTP (network time protocol) server. In this way, redundant timestamps are recorded, which can be cross-checked: one of the local times recorded by the HCM device and another recorded by the receiving computer.

In this configuration, the SPOF is now moved from the computer to the router, which establishes the local area network. However, like the HCM device itself, the router is also an embedded device designed for unattended operation over extended periods of time and without maintenance under a variety of conditions that would be unsuitable for a PC. In this way, the router is a "safer"/more prepared and robust SPOF than the computer itself.

3.5.5 Balancing SPOFs and Practicality

In an ideal system, there are no SPOFs, but how could this be achieved? Let us take the data collection infrastructure as an example, where using an SD card connected to the device in combination with an uninterruptible power supply (UPS)-protected network would be an option. In practice, however, this approach can be cumbersome for the infrastructure used and is often infeasible for embedded devices that are attached to a cage.

A good approach is to minimize the number of SPOFs to reduce the risk of data loss as much as possible. The developer of a DIY device must decide what failure rate is "acceptable" in the worst case based on the specific conditions and requirements of their experiment. Very quick and practical measures, such as introducing a UPS, can significantly reduce the risk of data loss. To support the process of developing a reliable and practical design, Table 5 provides an overview of various devices, such as SPOFs, and options for increasing their robustness.

3.6 Power and Data Infrastructure

Physical connections between components of a home cage system need to take into account (i) power and (ii) data integrity.

An inadequate power supply can lead to the oddest of failures—brownouts. These are small voltage drops that are insufficient to cause a full device crash but corrupt the running device's working memory (RAM), which can lead to unpredictable behavior. In any DIY system, the power supply should be the first suspect when errors occur that are inconsistent and/or difficult to reproduce.

For power supplies, the voltage needs to be matched, while the current/power needs to be sufficient (at least the wattage required by all attached components). It is prudent to "overrate" the power supply. For example, in the case of a 10 W expected load, a 50 W power supply is preferred over a 15 W one, even though the latter should be sufficient.

For power, wires need to be thick enough to not drop voltage and heat up. For data transmission, protocol standards usually specify the maximum cable length.

3.7 Upgrading the HCM System

As described in Sect. 2.1, when a prototype proves its usefulness, requirements tend to shift from proof-of-concept to sustained use in complex experiments. Therefore,

Table 5 Overview of devices found in HCM architectures as single points of failure (SPOF)

Potential SPOF	Failure mechanisms or susceptibility	Mitigation strategies
Cage-attached device 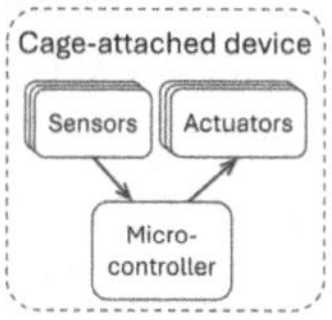	Microcontroller failure Very rare Usually, user/builder errors (e.g. firmware bugs)	Extensive, creative testing: Multitude of conditions With additional diagnostics (e.g. camera)
	Sensor failure	Redundant sensors Real-time data validation
	Actuator failure	Diagnostic sensors Actuators with feedback
PC 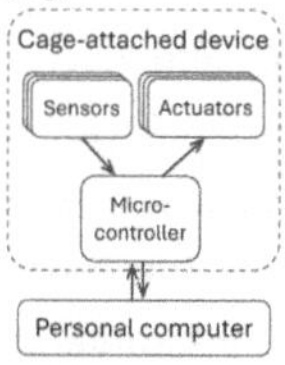	Large number of complex components, each a SPOF Writable memory susceptible to corruption Dependent on fan cooling—produces noise and can be hindered by dust over time	Configuration selection: Hard drives can be made redundant by using mirrored RAID to read and write data to both in parallel RAM with built-in error checking and correction (ECC) memory
SD card 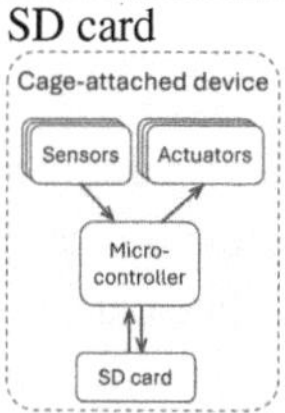	Data corruption or automatically locked into read-only mode after exceeding the rated number of writes	Brand-name cards High endurance variants Avoids frequent writes of small amounts of data
Router 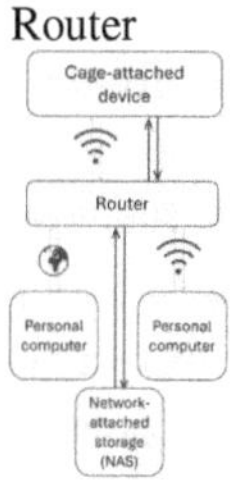	Extremely rare (embedded system designed for continuous operation)	Industrial/business variants with redundant power supplies Complex infrastructures where routers can take over for each other in case of failure (e.g. virtual router redundancy protocol).

researchers may decide to continue developing their prototypes into mature solutions. These systems are usually not created as such from scratch, but in an iterative process where prototype shortcomings are assessed, possible solutions are tested until one is decided upon and implemented. The process is repeated until the design is satisfactory overall, and the solution is usually published as such. Based on information previously described, we will illustrate the process by taking a closer look at the rationale behind some crucial design decisions in two mature systems developed by the authors of this chapter: the MoPSS, a mouse position tracker using RFID (Habedank et al. 2022; (Refinement Reference Center – github 2025), and MIROSLAV (Virag et al. 2025), a rodent circadian locomotor activity tracker using PIR sensors, much like the prototype (described in Sect. 3.1.)

Both systems focused on reliability in long-term operation to acquire specific data for a well-defined purpose. As such, video recording was not needed, greatly simplifying the required architecture in terms of data transmission, storage, and computing requirements. RFID and PIR sensors generate simple, low-bitrate data, where a microcontroller is sufficient, and the data could be stored to an SD card directly (MoPSS) or transmitted via Wi-Fi in real time (MIROSLAV). Removing the PC as a SPOF (Sect. 3.5) increases reliability in long-term use. Furthermore, both systems keep track of real time and can periodically resynchronize via the network, enabling precise synchronization (Sect. 3.4) with other HCM systems.

To have a system that can be part of the lab's regular experimental toolkit, the prototype needs to become flexible enough to support various experimental designs, which goes beyond purely supporting a large number of sensors. Both solutions were developed to easily allow for additional circuit boards that can include more sensors and new functionalities. The systems can be as extensive or compact as the experiment requires. For example, MIROSLAV can even be stripped off of all HCM functionality and used as a standalone Wi-Fi environmental monitor for recording temperature, humidity and light intensity in the habitat.

To provide quick feedback for an overview of system operation, the MoPSS is equipped with a small display that provides all technical information needed for daily maintenance and calibration. MIROSLAV achieves this goal by continuously transmitting data via Wi-Fi, where the feed can be accessed from any device (including a smartphone) connected to the network.

It is important to note that "the solution" to a particular design problem arises from the circumstances under which the device is being developed, which are usually specific to the laboratory to some extent. In these examples, MIROSLAV provides much of its functionality through heavy reliance on Wi-Fi connectivity, which may not be easily available in all facilities. Both systems are open-source, which enables other researchers to recreate them as a mature system, adapt it to their needs, and even contribute to their development, enhancing the system's modularity and customizability.

4 Data Processing and Storage

Once all the relevant data have been recorded after an experiment, data processing comes into play. The first step of data processing would be the "cleaning" of your data. Get rid of errors you noticed and remove duplicates or inconsistencies. The second step was the data conversion. On the one hand, this can be the conversion of proprietary data from a DIY setup into common data formats to make the data generally accessible and further processable or the conversion of the collected data to use in special analysis software. After conversion, the data are analyzed, and the last step is the long-term storage of the experimental data. Lossless compression into other data formats can save storage space and therefore resources.

There are a range of applications for data conversion and data analysis. In DIY projects, however, it is not uncommon for data to be recorded in the format in which they will be further processed. Basic programming languages for data processing (e.g., Python) are suitable. All these programming languages are established and extensively documented. Moreover, the use of AI tools and your own research can help achieve the desired data processing pipeline.

An important aspect of data processing is the documentation of the steps taken. Even if you carry out a project on your own, other researchers may use your script for data transformation or analysis at some point. This is when a well-commented script pays off. In general, codes and scripts should be clearly commented on and provided with a timestamp so that the individual steps can also be traced in the next project. It is easier to fall back on code that has already been written than to write new code—as long as you can understand it.

Once the data processing is complete, its result should be saved in a suitable format. The most commonly used format for exchanging scientific data is the.csv format. The comma-separated-values format saves tabular data in a simple text file in which every line is a row of tabular data. Within each line, the commas indicate individual values—or columns—of tabular data. This uncompressed, textual data format is easy to integrate into various applications and can be compressed easily (e.g., zipped) for storage efficiency but can become unwieldy with large amounts of data. Other columnar formats have been developed with specialized encoding and built-in compression for faster and more storage-efficient handling of large amounts of data commonly found in HCM. An example is the open source Apache Parquet format. Although not textual, data can be read from or written into Parquet files with a single line of Python or R code.

Good scientific practice is to follow rule 3 when storing experimental data. There should always be three (3) separate copies of a data set. The copies should be stored on two (2) different types of storage media, and one (1) of the copies should be in a physically separate location (different offices, different buildings, online databases).

When naming the saved data sets, the same applies as for the analysis scripts—it should be clearly recognisable when the data set was collected. It is good to pay attention to a sorted folder structure from the very beginning and to document this for other users of the data (readme files). For further insights into storing large data sets derived from HCM, we recommend reading a recent article by members of the TEATIME consortium (Bains et al. 2025).

5 Sharing your DIY System

5.1 The Importance of Documented Information

Any system that cannot be operated is worthless, and poorly documented DIY systems are no exception. It is therefore extremely important to document the entire operation process in detail (including errors and potential pitfalls!) to provide other users with a verifiably useful system. The UCLA miniscope (Miniscope 2014) is a good example of an open-source, well-documented tool that is highly used by the neuroscience community. They provide online courses on all the steps of the process of using their miniscope: from the construction to the surgery and the analysis pipeline. They have a webpage with all the information and an active forum to ask/answer questions. The publication of a methods-like paper on the construction or development of a new setup or software can also be a great way to document a DIY project for the community. This can be based on commercial systems (Kahnau et al. 2023b) or open-source projects such as DeepLabCut (Mathis et al. 2018).

The Behavior Forum (The Behaviour Forum 2025) is an online forum developed as part of the EU COST Action TEATIME (COST (2025) for the animal behavior community, with a particular focus on automated HCM of rodents in biomedical research. In the Behavior Forum, one can find webinars, conferences and training advertisements, job opportunities, questions and answers (Q&As) on diverse topics as well as guides and protocols.

The development of a new DIY system usually requires animal testing. We recommend that such pilot studies also be subject to preregistration (i.e., Animal Study Registry 2025). Preregistration raises scientific standards because it requires thorough advance planning. When individual steps are described in as much detail as possible, the results obtained are reproducible. Any deviations from the plan can also be noted and justified. This makes adjustments to the DIY system transparent, enabling complete documentation. For further information, please see Bert et al. (2019) and Heinl et al. (2022).

In sum, DIY systems need to be extremely well documented to ensure reproducibility within and across labs and reduction of time and costs on preventable errors by other users.

5.2 From an Idea to a Robust Product

The development of a DIY system has different hidden costs, both in terms of time and money. Own working hours are usually not considered part of the costs. Systems that are not well maintained may be working with parts that no longer exist in the market or with software packages that are not updated. This requires additional time and expertise from the user to adapt the solution to their needs.

Additionally, creating a system that works in a lab is just a proof of concept. Making that system reliably scalable and industry-ready requires an additional level of work at the hardware and software levels. For example, at the hardware level, prototypes with jumper wires can be replaced by Ethernet or BNC cables before commercialization to ensure more robustness. At the software level, it is recommended to create a graphical user interface (GUI) to increase the pool of users (with a GUI, even nonprogramming researchers can use and interact with the software) or even develop protocols using a visual programming language (Lopes et al. 2015).

Moreover, it is important to test the setup in conditions as similar as possible to those of the experiment per se. In a multidimensional study, (Alonso et al. 2023) tested classical and HCM approaches to evaluate the effects of brain serotonin deficiency on the expression of cognitive and social functions in different contexts in the same animals. Surprisingly, no function evaluated in the classical testing appeared altered by the absence of brain serotonin. However, in the day-to-day context of the home cage, the absence of brain serotonin most strikingly affected the animals' sexual behavior, maintenance (eating, drinking, grooming), and defensive behaviors as well as levels of home cage activity, weight, and corticosterone. These findings highlight the importance of studying everyday life functions within the dynamic social living environment to model the full spectrum of complexity of animal models.

In particular, HCM systems improve animal research by allowing the experiments to be conducted in the familiar environment and during the natural activity period of the animals (e.g., the dark period in rodents) since they can be automated and therefore performed in the home cage. DIY systems also have the potential to improve the reproducibility of scientific results. As many DIY solutions are open-source, they can be easily developed and replicated by other researchers. This contributes to transparency in science and facilitates the exchange of methods and results if detailed documentation is provided (Wenzel 2023).

5.3 Sharing Data from DIY Systems

Exchanging knowledge lies at the heart of scientific research. For others to be able to make use of the data we share, some principles should be kept in mind from the very beginning of the data generation process (chapter "Data Sharing and Metadata").

Any data are inevitably, almost by definition, an inaccurate representation of real-world phenomena to a greater or lesser degree. To start to gain insight, first, the inaccuracies need to be compensated for, and subsequently, the information of interest is extracted and brought to the forefront. The inaccuracies are largely determined by the sensor technology used (different sensor types produce different types of artifacts), which in turn determines data preprocessing steps, starting with filtering and thresholding on a hardware level of the electrical signal, and continues in software (chapter "Technologies for Home Cage Monitoring in Preclinical Research"). Eventually, as processing steps start to heavily depend on the desired parameter, other information becomes noise, and the data necessarily becomes less accurate or impossible to use for other parameters that are not in focus. For example, with locomotor activity monitoring, we might want to fit a 24-hour sinusoid to the data to analyze circadian rhythm parameters; however, other parameters (e.g., immediate response to personnel entrances) cannot be extracted from sinusoid parameters. For this reason, it is important to (i) thoroughly document every processing step and (ii) share data in its rawest form possible, especially for DIY HCM devices, where all of these steps are under our direct control.

As a rule, even with simple sensors, the longitudinal nature of HCM yields rich, complex data, and there are a myriad of ways of doing so in DIY systems. With more complex data, it is increasingly likely that we, or someone else, will identify a novel, interesting behavioral parameter that can be extracted from the raw data. It is unreasonable to expect that we can extract everything that will ever be of interest, rendering raw data useless. Furthermore, to be able to use raw data in a meta-analytical approach, data from different systems need to be standardized, which can only be done with thorough documentation of all processing steps, from the sensor to the uploaded data set (Bains et al. 2025). Due to the variety of possible system designs, the aforementioned recommendations are fairly general, but all the more important to adhere to—the DIY builder needs to judge the best way of doing so for their specific system.

5.4 Disseminate Your System

To share your system within the scientific community, you need to guarantee that all data and information are sharable. There are different ways to do so, and here, we provide some recommendations, namely, those focused on open-source policies.

By following this process, detailed documentation of all process steps can be guaranteed, from printed circuit board (PCB) design to the actual publication of the article. That said, during the development of your system, prefer the use of open-source tools: from the design of your PCBs (e.g., KiCad 2025) to the analysis software pipeline (e.g., Python, R) so that your research is not locked behind paywalls.

In general, we recommend sharing your (meta)data in a FAIR-compliant (Findable, Accessible, Interoperable, and Reusable) repository (Bains et al. 2025) and your code in a public repository such as GitHub (GitHub 2025). Detailed protocols can be published in protocols.io (protocols.io 2025) and your entire paper can be available on a preprint server (e.g. biorXiv). Moreover, currently, there are great alternatives to share your data within the community, for example, on PeerComunityIn (Peer Community In 2025), which is a nonprofit organization of researchers offering peer review, recommendation and publication of scientific articles in open access for free.

6 Summary and Conclusion

Do-it-yourself home cage systems, especially open-source systems, have provided the community with new tools that are accessible to everyone at reduced costs. Developing such a system has advantages and disadvantages, namely, advantages in terms of personalization but also costs in terms of money and time.

In this chapter, we summarized the main pros and cons of engaging in the development of a DIY system. We commented on the importance of available detailed information and how to go from an idea to a robust market-ready product. We shared advice to guide new potential developers to decide on key features for their own system, namely, (1) food and water delivery, (2) enrichment tools and space and (3) overall design. We explained the importance and provided tips about the SPOF protocol and the advantages of prototype testing.

In the last two sections, we focused on more detailed information regarding data collection (e.g., motion capture, individual tracking in a group setting, power and data infrastructures) and data processing (e.g., data formats and storage).

One of the most important messages in this chapter is that DIY systems must be extremely well documented to ensure reproducibility and dissemination in different laboratories and to reduce time and costs due to avoidable mistakes made by other users. This is the only way to ensure that your system is used and shared in the best possible way.

References

Abelson KS, Chambers C, De La Cueva T et al (2023) Harmonisation of education, training and continuing professional development for laboratory animal caretakers, technicians and technologists: report of the FELASA-EFAT Working Group. Lab Anim 57:599–610. https://doi.org/10.1177/00236772231175550

Alonso L, Peeva P, Stasko S et al (2023) Constitutive depletion of brain serotonin differentially affects rats' social and cognitive abilities. iScience 26:105998. https://doi.org/10.1016/j.isci.2023.105998

Animal Study Registry (2025) In: AnimalStudyRegistry. https://www.animalstudyregistry.org/asr_web/index.action

Bains RS, Huzard D, McCutcheon JE et al (2025) Too big to lose – a FAIR repository for biomedical data derived from home-cage monitoring

Banks A, Briggs E, Borgendale K, Gupta R (2019) MQTT Version 5.0. In: MQTT Version 5.0. https://docs.oasis-open.org/mqtt/mqtt/v5.0/os/mqtt-v5.0-os.html. Accessed 7 Nov 2025

Bert B, Heinl C, Chmielewska J et al (2019) Refining animal research: the animal study registry. PLoS Biol 17:e3000463. https://doi.org/10.1371/journal.pbio.3000463

Brown L, Hasan S, Foster R, Peirson S (2017) COMPASS: continuous open mouse phenotyping of activity and sleep status [version 2; peer review: 4 approved]. Wellcome Open Res 1. https://doi.org/10.12688/wellcomeopenres.9892.2

COST Action TEATIME – HCM technologies catalog. In: Home Cage Monitoring Technologies Catalog https://www.cost-teatime.org/about/technologies/. Accessed 6 Nov 2025

Crompe BDL, Schneck M, Steenbergen F et al (2023) FreiBox: a versatile open-source behavioral setup for investigating the neuronal correlates of behavioral flexibility via 1-photon imaging in freely moving mice. eNeuro 10. https://doi.org/10.1523/ENEURO.0469-22.2023

de Chaumont F, Ey E, Torquet N et al (2019) Real-time analysis of the behaviour of groups of mice via a depth-sensing camera and machine learning. Nat Biomed Eng 3:930–942. https://doi.org/10.1038/s41551-019-0396-1

Domingues D, Melloni A (2025) In: Workshop "Design and Print a Home Cage System". https://zenodo.org/records/17550425. Accessed 7 Nov 2025

FED3 (2025) Alexxai Kravitz Kravitz Lab. In: FED3, Kravitz Lab. https://kravitzlab.com/fed3

Freund J, Brandmaier AM, Lewejohann L et al (2013) Emergence of individuality in genetically identical mice. Science 340:756–759. https://doi.org/10.1126/science.1235294

GitHub (2025) In: GitHub Change is constant. GitHub keeps you ahead. https://github.com/
Habedank A, Urmersbach B, Kahnau P, Lewejohann L (2022) O mouse, where art thou? The Mouse Position Surveillance System (MoPSS)—an RFID-based tracking system. Behav Res 54:676–689. https://doi.org/10.3758/s13428-021-01593-7
Heinl C, Scholman-Végh AMD, Mellor D et al (2022) Declaration of common standards for the preregistration of animal research—speeding up the scientific progress. PNAS Nexus 1:pgac016. https://doi.org/10.1093/pnasnexus/pgac016
Hobbiesiefken U, Mieske P, Lewejohann L, Diederich K (2021) Evaluation of different types of enrichment – their usage and effect on home cage behavior in female mice. PLoS One 16:e0261876. https://doi.org/10.1371/journal.pone.0261876
Hobbiesiefken U, Urmersbach B, Jaap A et al (2023) Rating enrichment items by female group-housed laboratory mice in multiple binary choice tests using an RFID-based tracking system. PLoS One 18:e0278709. https://doi.org/10.1371/journal.pone.0278709
Hohlbaum K, Andresen N, Mieske P et al (2024) Lockbox enrichment facilitates manipulative and cognitive activities for mice [version 2; peer review: 2 approved]. Open Res Europe 4. https://doi.org/10.12688/openreseurope.17624.2
Kahnau P, Jaap A, Diederich K et al (2023a) Determining the value of preferred goods based on consumer demand in a home-cage based test for mice. Behav Res 55:751–766. https://doi.org/10.3758/s13428-022-01813-8
Kahnau P, Jaap A, Urmersbach B et al (2023b) Development of an IntelliCage-based cognitive bias test for mice [version 2; peer review: 2 approved]. Open Res Europe 2. https://doi.org/10.12688/openreseurope.15294.2
KiCad (2025) In: KiCad a cross platform and open source PCB design suite. https://www.kicad.org/
Lauer J, Zhou M, Ye S et al (2022) Multi-animal pose estimation, identification and tracking with DeepLabCut. Nat Methods 19:496–504. https://doi.org/10.1038/s41592-022-01443-0
Lewejohann L, Hoppmann AM, Kegel P et al (2009) Behavioral phenotyping of a murine model of Alzheimer's disease in a seminaturalistic environment using RFID tracking. Behav Res Methods 41:850–856. https://doi.org/10.3758/BRM.41.3.850
Lopes G, Bonacchi N, Frazão J et al (2015) Bonsai: an event-based framework for processing and controlling data streams. Front Neuroinform 9. https://doi.org/10.3389/fninf.2015.00007
Mandillo S, Tucci V, Hölter SM et al (2008) Reliability, robustness, and reproducibility in mouse behavioral phenotyping: a cross-laboratory study. Physiol Genomics 34:243–255. https://doi.org/10.1152/physiolgenomics.90207.2008
Mathis A, Mamidanna P, Cury KM et al (2018) DeepLabCut: markerless pose estimation of user-defined body parts with deep learning. Nat Neurosci 21:1281–1289. https://doi.org/10.1038/s41593-018-0209-y
Matikainen-Ankney BA, Earnest T, Ali M et al (2021) An open-source device for measuring food intake and operant behavior in rodent home-cages. eLife 10:e66173. https://doi.org/10.7554/eLife.66173
Med Associates Inc. – Operant Conditioning + General Behavior. In: Med Associates Inc. https://med-associates.com/product-category/operant-conditioning-general-behavior/. Accessed 7 Nov 2025
Mei J, Kohler J, Winter Y et al (2020) Automated radial 8-arm maze: a voluntary and stress-free behavior test to assess spatial learning and memory in mice. Behav Brain Res 381:112352. https://doi.org/10.1016/j.bbr.2019.112352
micecraft – LMT. In: Live Mouse Tracker – MiceCraft. https://micecraft.org/lmt/. Accessed 29 Oct 2025

Mieske P, Diederich K, Lewejohann L (2021) Roaming in a land of Milk and honey: life trajectories and metabolic rate of female inbred mice living in a semi naturalistic environment. Animals (Basel) 11:3002. https://doi.org/10.3390/ani11103002

Mieske P, Hobbiesiefken U, Fischer-Tenhagen C et al (2022) Bored at home?—a systematic review on the effect of environmental enrichment on the welfare of laboratory rats and mice. Front Vet Sci 9. https://doi.org/10.3389/fvets.2022.899219

Miniscope (2014) In: Miniscope Wiki. http://miniscope.org/index.php/Main_Page. Accessed 7 Nov 2025

OBS Studio. In: OBS – Open Broadcaster Studio. https://obsproject.com/. Accessed 7 Nov 2025

open balena – github. In: balena-io/open-balena. https://github.com/balena-io/open-balena. Accessed 29 Oct 2025

Peer Community In. In: Peer Community In – free peer review & validation of preprints of articles. https://peercommunityin.org/. Accessed 29 Oct 2025

Peirson SN, Brown LA, Pothecary CA et al (2018) Light and the laboratory mouse. J Neurosci Methods 300:26–36. https://doi.org/10.1016/j.jneumeth.2017.04.007

protocols.io. In: ptotocols.io – bring structure to your research. https://www.protocols.io. Accessed 29 Oct 2025

Puścian A, Łęski S, Kasprowicz G et al (2016) Eco-HAB as a fully automated and ecologically relevant assessment of social impairments in mouse models of autism. eLife 5:e19532. https://doi.org/10.7554/eLife.19532

Refinement Reference Center – github. In: Refinement Reference Center. https://github.com/RefinementReferenceCenter. Accessed 29 Oct 2025

Rivalan M, Munawar H, Fuchs A, Winter Y (2017) An automated, experimenter-free method for the standardised, operant cognitive testing of rats. PLoS One 12:e0169476. https://doi.org/10.1371/journal.pone.0169476

Rivalan M, Alonso L, Mosienko V et al (2024) Serotonin drives aggression and social behaviors of laboratory male mice in a semi-natural environment. Front Behav Neurosci 18. https://doi.org/10.3389/fnbeh.2024.1450540

Roy S, Bryant JL, Cao Y, Heck DH (2011) High-precision, three-dimensional tracking of mouse whisker movements with optical motion capture technology. Front Behav Neurosci 5. https://doi.org/10.3389/fnbeh.2011.00027

The Behaviour Forum. In: COST Action TEATIME – The Behaviour Forum. https://www.thebehaviourforum.org/login. Accessed 29 Oct 2025

The Secure Network Time Protocol (NTPsec) Distribution. In: The Secure Network Time Protocol (NTPsec) Distribution. https://docs.ntpsec.org/latest/. Accessed 29 Oct 2025

TSE Systems – Phenoworld. In: TSE Systems. https://www.tse-systems.com/products/phenoworld/. Accessed 29 Oct 2025

Virag D (2024) davorvr/bedsy. https://github.com/davorvr/bedsy. Accessed 29 Oct 2025

Virag D, Homolak J, Kodvanj I et al (2021) Repurposing a digital kitchen scale for neuroscience research: a complete hardware and software cookbook for PASTA. Sci Rep 11:2963. https://doi.org/10.1038/s41598-021-82710-6

Virag D, Homolak J, Kodvanj I et al (2025) My friend MIROSLAV: a hackable open-source hardware and software platform for high-throughput monitoring of rodent activity in the home cage. Behav Res 57:198. https://doi.org/10.3758/s13428-025-02719-x

Weber EM, Zidar J, Ewaldsson B et al (2023) Aggression in group-housed male mice: a systematic review. Animals 13:143. https://doi.org/10.3390/ani13010143

Weinreb C, Pearl JE, Lin S et al (2024) Keypoint-MoSeq: parsing behavior by linking point tracking to pose dynamics. Nat Methods 21:1329–1339. https://doi.org/10.1038/s41592-024-02318-2

Wenzel T (2023) Open hardware: from DIY trend to global transformation in access to laboratory equipment. PLoS Biol 21:e3001931. https://doi.org/10.1371/journal.pbio.3001931

Winter Y, Schaefers ATU (2011) A sorting system with automated gates permits individual operant experiments with mice from a social home cage. J Neurosci Methods 196:276–280. https://doi.org/10.1016/j.jneumeth.2011.01.017

Woodard CL, Nasrallah WB, Samiei BV et al (2020) PiDose: an open-source system for accurate and automated oral drug administration to group-housed mice. Sci Rep 10:11584. https://doi.org/10.1038/s41598-020-68477-2

Data Sharing and Metadata

Hamish Forrest, Damien Huzard, Leonardo Restivo,
Szczepan W. Baran, and Benoit Petit-Demoulière

Abstract

This chapter explores the critical role of data sharing and standardised metadata in advancing home cage monitoring (HCM) research. It examines the scientific, ethical, and computational advantages of sharing HCM data, particularly in the context of enhanced research quality in accordance with the 3Rs principles (Replacement, Reduction, Refinement). Challenges hindering widespread data sharing, including cultural, incentive, technical, and governance issues, are discussed. Strategies for effective data sharing, such as data storage solutions, FAIR (Findable, Accessible, Interoperable,

H. Forrest (✉)
Mary Lyon Centre at MRC Harwell, Oxfordshire, UK

UK Research and Innovation, London, UK

D. Huzard
Neuronautix, Montpellier, France

Metadatapp, Montpellier, France

L. Restivo
Department of Fundamental Neuroscience, Faculty of Biology & Medicine, University of Lausanne, Lausanne, Switzerland

S. W. Baran
Baran.Cafe, Cambridge, MA, USA

Tech4Pets.Healthcare, Cambridge, MA, USA

B. Petit-Demoulière
Université de Strasbourg, CNRS UAR 2062 PHEN-ICS, INSERM US66, CELPHEDIA, Illkirch-Graffenstaden, France

S. Gaburro, S. Mandillo (eds.), *Home Cage Monitoring in Rodents: A Global Effort*,
https://doi.org/10.1007/978-3-032-19781-8_10

and Reusable) data principles, and the use of controlled vocabularies and ontologies, are presented. The chapter envisions a future where federated networks of interoperable HCM platforms enable advanced data/metadata integration and analysis powered by advanced computational tools. These systems would yield valuable insights into biomedical research, animal behaviour, and welfare in an AI-ready field.

Keywords

Metadata · FAIR · Ontologies · Knowledge graphs · Data sharing

1 Introduction

HCM systems significantly advance nonclinical research. They offer continuous, minimally invasive observations that enhance animal welfare and provide opportunities to quantify behaviour and physiology more precisely.

HCM systems continuously record gigabytes of video, sensor readings, and behavioural metrics. Researchers realise HCM's potential by sharing and pooling these datasets across labs. However, researchers willing to rely on data sharing currently face significant technical and cultural hurdles. Cultural resistance, governance gaps, and infrastructural limitations restrict open data sharing in HCM research. Communities must adopt agreed standards and FAIR practices to integrate datasets from different HCM platforms (Wilkinson et al. 2016). Researchers can use standardised ethograms and formal ontologies (like Mouse Behaviour Ontology, MBO) to define behaviours uniformly (Beck et al. 2009). The HCM community must prepare its data infrastructure for artificial intelligence (AI) if it is to leverage emerging technology.

2 Why Share HCM Data and Metadata?

Three interconnected motivations support sharing HCM data and metadata: ethical imperatives, scientific advantages, and computational opportunities.

2.1 Data and Metadata Reuse in the Context of the 3Rs

When researchers use HCM data and metadata across studies, they enhance animal welfare and reproducibility, directly supporting the 3Rs mission (Zentrich et al. 2021). This is because in collecting and analysing extensive datasets over time, they reduce their reliance on multiple animals and minimise the number of animals needed for research purposes (Baran et al. 2022).

For example, researchers introduced a novel approach for Reduction of animal numbers by leveraging historical control data to enhance statistical power (RELACS Consortium et al. 2021). This statistical method can reduce the minimum required sample size whilst maintaining power. The authors validated this approach using seven independent rodent studies. Their work shows how welfare, reduction, and scientific progress interconnect through data sharing.

Replacing animal models completely remains difficult for behavioural and physiological research because comprehensive alternatives do not yet exist. However, data and metadata sharing and reuse can support partial replacement or reduction strategies. For example, the pharmaceutical industry is developing and validating Virtual Control Groups that repurpose historical control data to serve as "virtual" control cohorts, replacing the need for live animals in concurrent control groups (Steger-Hartmann et al. 2025).

Researchers also refine experiments through data reuse. Mining large behavioural and physiological datasets, like continuous HCM data, scientists identify patterns that optimise husbandry and minimise animal distress (Baran et al. 2021). These insights enable researchers and veterinary staff to improve experimental procedures and housing conditions.

The research community can achieve reduction, replacement, and refinement simultaneously by using modern data management and sharing principles, such as the FAIR principles, shown in Fig. 1 and expanded on later in the chapter.

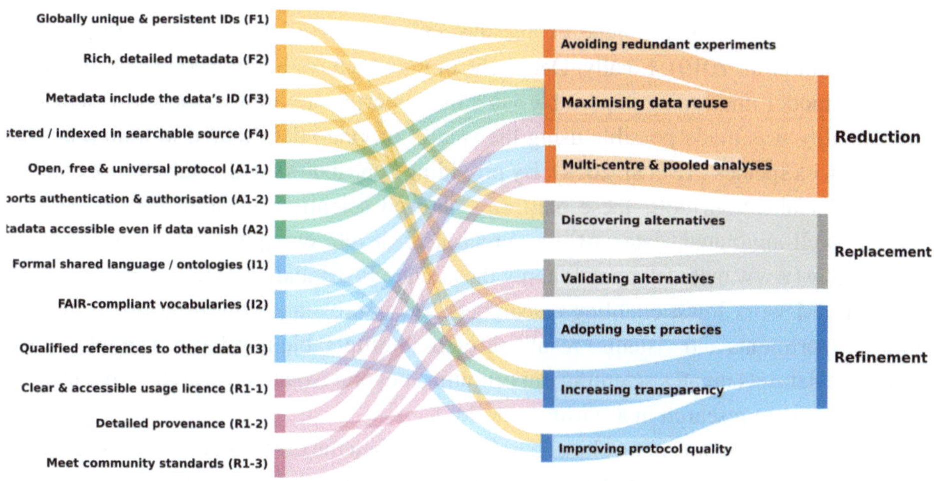

Fig. 1 the welfare motivation for FAIR data. Sankey representation of how each FAIR data subprinciple (left) supports concrete data-sharing practices (centre) that, in turn, contribute to the implementation of the 3Rs in animal research (right). Rich metadata, persistent identifiers, and open indexing enable data reuse and multi-Centre analyses that reduce unnecessary experiments (reduction, green). Shared ontologies, FAIR vocabularies, and robust cross-referencing support the discovery and validation of non-animal models (replacement, red). Transparent licensing, provenance tracking, and adherence to standards improve protocol quality and reproducibility (refinement, blue). (Image generated with the SankeyMatic.com online tool)

2.2 Scientific Advantages: Enhanced Research Quality and Discovery

Beyond ethical imperatives, data sharing delivers concrete scientific benefits. Neurophysiology and genomics communities demonstrate the impact of successful data sharing. The Allen Brain Observatory facilitates community-wide research and collaboration by providing standardised, openly accessible neurophysiological datasets (De Vries et al. 2023). Similarly, the International Mouse Phenotyping Consortium (IMPC) has characterised thousands of genes through consistent workflows implemented at scale across multiple countries, demonstrating the power of coordinated data generation and sharing (Groza et al. 2023).

Aggregating data from diverse animal studies enhances external validity and generalisability across experiments, strains, and institutions. This approach improves research quality through broader biological representation while providing more reliable control group baselines (Von Kortzfleisch et al. 2020).

Established data-sharing platforms demonstrate how standardisation and integration create practical value for contributors. The Mouse Phenome Database (MPD) transformed contributor experience by implementing specialised analysis tools for standardised data formats. These tools delivered immediate benefits, including enhanced quality control capabilities and ontology-based data browsing (Bogue et al. 2019). Similarly, the Jackson Laboratory's Mouse Genome Database deployed advanced visualisation interfaces allowing researchers to compare gene expression and phenotypic annotations across mouse studies (Bult et al. 2019). Finally, DeepLabCut now features automated pose estimation, although model fine-tuning is possible via a user interface to improve performance. This functionality was made possible using the wealth of video data shared to train a unified model across species (Ye et al. 2024). By providing contributors with ready-to-use analytical and visualisation tools, these platforms showed scientists an immediate payoff for sharing well-annotated data. At the preclinical level, emerging platforms such as Metadatapp (www.metadatapp.net) apply these same FAIR and ontology-based principles within HCM workflows, enabling researchers to capture standardised metadata directly during experiments and visualise results through interoperable interfaces. The integration of diverse datasets creates scientific opportunities beyond isolated research, while sharing tools to facilitate research in a 'virtuous cycle'.

Recent advancements in machine learning strengthen the case for HCM data sharing. A 2025 study on deep behavioural phenotyping describes novel algorithms for extracting complex behavioural signatures from continuous HCM data, paired with visualisation tools for non-technical users (Sabnis et al. 2025). Critically, these methods require far larger datasets for training and validation than any single laboratory can produce. By contributing to shared repositories, individual researchers gain access to enhanced data and tools to use in their investigations.

2.3 Emerging Computational Opportunities: Enabling the Next Generation of HCM Analysis

By annotating and aggregating behavioural data, we make HCM datasets machine-readable (i.e. structured so that software can automatically process, search, and analyse the data), transforming them into computational resources for discovery and analysis. This work will be essential to leverage emerging capabilities of data science, AI, and data management technologies.

2.3.1 Modern Data Management and Data Linking

Knowledge graphs offer the potential to generate robust insights from the large, multidimensional datasets collected in HCM systems. These data structures are defined as directed, labelled graphs, wherein nodes denote domain-specific entities and edges represent the relationships between the nodes. A semantic model defines the conceptual structure: which entities exist, their properties, and relationships. Knowledge graphs implement the semantic model as machine-readable, linked data structures with actual instances. For example, a semantic model might specify that 'behaviours have temporal relationships,' while a knowledge graph would store specific instances like 'grooming precedes rearing in mouse A'.

In clinical medicine, knowledge graphs support personalised treatment by linking patient characteristics with outcomes across large databases, even enabling prediction of disease onset in at-risk individuals (Al Khatib et al. 2024). In drug discovery, knowledge graph analyses have revealed unexpected therapeutic effects by analysing networks of molecular interactions, gene expression changes, and phenotypic outcomes. (Sudhahar et al. 2024). The power of such semantic integration has also been recognised in industry. Roche undertook an ontology-based data management initiative to enhance drug discovery (Tan et al. 2025). Semantic integration is now being applied in preclinical research through platforms such as *Metadatapp*, which uses ontology-driven metadata integration to enable FAIR and AI-ready data sharing in HCM. At the publication level, initiatives like *FAIR²* (www.fair2.ai) aim to extend semantic rigour to research outputs, promoting machine-actionable data citations and structured provenance. Together, these successes illustrate how knowledge graph–driven approaches are becoming an essential tool in the use of complex data.

2.3.2 Integrating Highly Annotated HCM Datasets with Emerging Computational Tools

Recent work in computational modelling opens the door to combining HCM data with simulations and analyses. Researchers have created an anatomically detailed Drosophila model with a realistic range of movement, which can be used with deep reinforcement learning to recreate behaviour in a virtual space (Vaxenburg et al. 2024). This virtual organism can serve as a testing ground for behavioural hypotheses or for validating algorithms that track behaviour. The potential of integrating these models with empirical data was further shown by another team who built a "virtual rat" animated by deep reinforcement learning to exhibit naturalistic behaviour and integrated it with repositories of neural activity data (Aldarondo et al. 2024).

2.3.3 Federated Learning to Facilitate Collaboration Between HCM and ML

Emerging data-sharing technologies are now addressing many of the technical and ethical challenges the HCM community will eventually need to solve. Federated learning enables model training on data in situ. In a federated learning architecture, each site keeps its sensitive data in-house during model training. Federated learning has already shown practical value in the HCM field when researchers improved the performance of a deep learning model for detecting specific animal activities in home cage videos (Mao et al. 2022). However, to scale federated learning architecture, the HCM community will need to offer tightly curated, well-annotated datasets. This underscores the importance of standardised data and ontologies such as the MBO as this chapter will explore.

Researchers will generate highly annotated HCM data with integrated knowledge graphs as standards mature. External machine learning engineers might deploy a federated algorithm across dozens of facilities collecting these annotated data sets or use a secure virtual environment termed a Trusted Research Environment (UK Health Data Research Alliance and NHSX 2021; Kavianpour et al. 2022). With highly annotated behavioural and physiological HCM data feeding into complex simulations, emerging AI systems may detect more subtle phenotypes than with any single dataset in isolation.

2.4 Benefits Across Key Stakeholders

HCM data and metadata reuse deliver concrete benefits to key stakeholders in animal research:

- *Researchers and data sharers* gain access to larger tightly annotated datasets that improve experimental design and statistical power, yielding more robust and reproducible findings. They also benefit from value added to their data through collaboration in a 'virtuous cycle'.
- *Collaborators (particularly machine learning engineers)* develop their tools and add value to complex datasets without spending time on running experiments and developing HCM expertise.
- *Institutions* save costs and labour by avoiding unnecessary duplicative experiments and demonstrate compliance with 3Rs principles and open-science mandates (thereby increasing operational efficiency).
- *Public and regulators* observe greater transparency in research practices and a stronger commitment to minimizing animal use, which foster public trust and confidence in the ethical conduct of science.

3 Why Don't We Realise the Potential of Data and Metadata Sharing?

Despite these ethical, scientific, and computational advantages, the HCM field has not fully realised data and metadata sharing. While HCM data have been shared previously across groups to investigate welfare (Ulfhake et al. 2022), this initiative is driven by a specific scientific purpose, rather than a community-wide shift towards openness and interoperability. Challenges to data and metadata sharing in HCM span cultural practices, governance, and technical barriers.

3.1 Cultural and Incentive Challenges

3.1.1 Credit and Attribution

The academic community relies on credit assignment, so ensuring that datasets and their authors receive recognition is critical to open data sharing. Scientific communities have developed mechanisms ensuring proper credit for shared resources. Research Resource Identifiers (RRIDs) successfully link scientific tools to their creators in databases like Mouse Genome Informatics (MGI). The HCM community could adapt this model for their own data attribution. Repositories assign persistent identifiers such as Open Researcher and Contributor ID (ORCIDs) and Digital Object Identifiers (DOIs) to provide unique, trackable references for datasets. Citations are likely to continue being used for credit and studies show a strong correlation between citation counts and funding success for scientists (Wilson et al. 2021; Mosleh et al. 2022). Surveyed researchers understand this link and view increased citations as a key benefit of data sharing (Colavizza et al. 2020). In short, academia has a long-established credit system that can encourage data sharing, although is not necessarily optimised for it.

Industry data sharing attribution operates under fundamentally different constraints, prioritising intellectual property protection and competitive advantages over open attribution. Large pharmaceutical companies use specialised platforms like Vivli providing DOI-based attribution for clinical trial data while maintaining strict access controls (Li et al. 2022) working against open, data sharing standards (Miller et al. 2019). Unlike academia's citation-based approach that encourages broad sharing, industry attribution mechanisms often employ tiered access models, embargo periods, and selective collaboration agreements that limit recognition to trusted partners, creating challenges for establishing comprehensive credit systems that accommodate both commercial imperatives and proper attribution.

3.1.2 How to Reward Data and Metadata Sharing in Science?

Creating effective incentives for researchers to share HCM datasets challenges both academia and industry to balance immediate reward with long-term career benefit. For data sharing to become widespread, the incentive structure must deliver near-term benefits that justify researchers' time investment while also providing meaningful career advancement for scientists who depend on grants and publications (Woods and Pinfield 2022; Hendriks et al. 2022). Research shows that only 11% of senior researchers respond positively to data sharing requests compared to 72% of early career scientists, suggesting established researchers perceive minimal personal benefit from sharing their valuable datasets (Campbell et al. 2019). Moreover, senior researchers often have control over whether data are shared, dampening the enthusiasm of early career scientists and data sharers. Successful data-sharing initiatives must provide both immediate recognition and lasting professional impact.

As the HCM community matures, more researchers will deliberately build datasets as community resources, following the model established by institutions like the Allen Institute. To include academic laboratories and individual scientists, the community needs metrics that value data-sharing contributions. The proposed "data-index" represents one such approach, designed to elevate data sharing from an afterthought to a prioritised research activity. The data-index balances both the number of datasets shared with impact (number of data-index citations) to prioritise both generation and sharing. The data-index has been designed to complement other metrics of scientific output and notes that one credit system alone does not capture the diversity of success in science (Hood and Sutherland 2021). These metrics (such as DOIs and citation credits) transform data sharing from invisible work into measurable career achievements, with researchers reporting 25–40% higher citation rates for publications associated with shared datasets (Christensen et al. 2019; Colavizza et al. 2020). Recognizing this need for new incentive metrics, in 2024 the U.S. National Institutes of Health (NIH) launched the S-Index Challenge to develop novel measurements quantifying and incentivizing data sharing (Challenge.gov 2025). These initiatives create measures to reward and prioritise data-sharing beyond traditional citation counts.

In addition, sharing negative results could bring additional controls and discarded hypotheses to the community, while getting credit for these experiments. Case studies demonstrate the potential for career advancement through data sharing: researchers from Memorial Sloan Kettering leveraged crowdsourced data from Project Data Sphere to discover breakthrough biomarkers for prostate cancer treatment monitoring, resulting in high-impact publications and establishing him as a leader in collaborative cancer research (Guinney et al. 2017). Currently, cultural barriers directly undermine the scientific advantages of sharing data and metadata. Without proper incentives, the ethical imperative to maximise animal welfare through data reuse remains unrealised.

3.1.3 Data Quality and Risk of Misinterpretation

Neuroscience researchers report risking misinterpretation when they share data without proper context (Hendriks et al. 2022). Misinterpretation concerns are particularly relevant for HCM research, where multiple disciplines intersect within unique methodologies, terminologies, and analytical frameworks. Researchers can capture expert knowledge and experimental context in ontologies and knowledge graphs, provided it is diligently recorded. The more diverse our collaborations become, the more structured context will be required to prevent misunderstanding. As HCM datasets grow larger and analyses become more automated, the risk of misinterpretation can be amplified if data are divorced from the conditions under which they were generated.

To address misinterpretation concerns, researchers should implement robust data provenance tracking in shared datasets. Provenance systems document the complete history of a dataset including its origin, the transformations it has undergone, and the experimental conditions under which it has been generated. The Virtual Fly Brain (VFB) platform exemplifies effective data integration through its provenance system, linking all entries to original sources with machine-readable metadata. VFB's workflow explicitly captures knowledge about data sources and transformations, with machine-readable metadata describing key experimental conditions. This ensures that when integrating across data types and disciplines datasets maintain their experimental context and reduce misinterpretation risk (Osumi-Sutherland et al. 2012, 2014; Court et al. 2023).

3.2 Governance and Policy Issues

3.2.1 Funder and Publisher Requirements

Funding agencies and journals are shifting requirements from voluntary sharing to mandatory compliance by implementing formal data-sharing requirements. These top-down policies have become powerful drivers of behaviour, complementing traditional incentives like citations. For researchers, understanding and meeting these evolving requirements is now essential not only for maximizing impact, but also for securing and maintaining funding.

In the United States, federally funded research requires data sharing at the point of publication as of 2025, marking a significant policy shift. The NIH already mandates that all grant applications include a detailed Data Management and Sharing Plan, explicitly describing how and where data will be shared. This turns data sharing from an optional best practice into a contractual obligation for receiving federal funds. In Europe, major funding and universities bodies likewise require data-sharing plans, although approaches vary across countries (Swiss National Science Foundation 2025). Many of these policies currently lack technical specificity, which means researchers can fulfill the letter of the requirement without making data truly reusable. This gap highlights the need for domain-specific guidelines tailored to HCM and behavioural data.

Scientific journals have also established data availability policies as per some established data types that demonstrably influence researcher behaviour (Springer Nature 2025). Once the HCM field coalesces around suitable repositories and standards, we should request high-impact journals to extend such requirements to HCM datasets as well. Studies show that journal data policies do increase data-sharing compliance in practice (Thelwall and Kousha 2017). For the HCM community, these policy developments create both urgency and opportunity. As external mandates increasingly compel data sharing, the community must define its own standards, repositories, and best practices to guide researchers. In this way, mandatory sharing can be transformed from an administrative burden into an opportunity that advances the field, ensuring that compliance leads to genuinely useful data resources (Fraga-González et al. 2025).

3.2.2 Community Governance

Community governance underpins scientific data-sharing initiatives by establishing clear rules, procedures, and decision-making structures that protect contributors while maximizing scientific value. Good governance builds long-term trust by ensuring that issues like attribution, representation, and misuse are properly addressed. With strong policy frameworks, researchers' concerns can be tackled head-on turning potential barriers into drivers of data sharing (Woods and Pinfield 2022).

Well-governed communities implement data protection measures that encourage sharing. These policies directly address researchers' fears about being preempted, which surveys have identified as a primary factor delaying data sharing (Tenopir et al. 2020). The European Bioinformatics Institute employs tiered embargo periods that protect data generators prior to publication while ensuring eventual public access (Cerezo et al. 2025). Well-governed communities establish guardrails against data misuse and protect contributors legally, building essential trust (Kwon and Motohashi 2021).

Communities must define clear parameters for data access and reuse through trust models and permission frameworks. Most sponsors will not release raw HCM video or cage-level datasets openly because of intellectual property and data rights concerns. The governance solution is a tiered model that protects what must be closed while enabling reuse of other research outputs.

This model is tiered at different levels. Metadata, schemas, and ontologies are open by default to facilitate interoperability. Raw datasets are housed in controlled-access environments such as Trusted Research Environments (TRE) used in federated "model-to-data" architectures. In these environments, raw data do not leave; only aggregated or otherwise derived outputs may be exported after output checking and disclosure control. Released models should be accompanied by documented provenance (model cards) which describe intent, performance, training data lineage, and limitations. Leading enclaves like OpenSAFELY (Williamson et al. 2020) illustrate this practice by restricting downloads to aggregate results following review. As discussed previously, this model could use embargo periods and contributor-first access to protect background intellectual property and patents. Foreground contributions would receive licenses under standard Data Use Agreements that require attribution, ban re-identification and competitive deconvolution, and define audit procedures and proportionate sanctions. A neutral rights registry enforces a give-to-get rule that trades reciprocal access for contribution, balancing data use with data sharing. This balanced governance approach keeps industry engaged while delivering interoperability and measurable scientific value.

Tiered governance requires granular permission systems that allow contributors to specify how researchers can use their data. Established intervention mechanisms for addressing violations build contributor confidence by ensuring recourse when problems arise (Chan et al. 2021). As data management and data sharing challenges grow across communities, the HCM field can borrow proven solutions that academics and data generators have designed from the ground-up (Eke et al. 2022).

The International Brain Laboratory (IBL) offers a real-world example of a comprehensive governance approach. The IBL maintains a transparent mission, phased data-release policies, and consensus-based adoption of data standards (e.g. Neurodata Without Borders, NWB (Rübel et al. 2022)), demonstrating that coordinated governance can empower contributors while promoting broad access (Wool 2020). Similar principles including clear publication rights, attribution policies, and decision transparency can be adapted to HCM consortia to ensure fair and sustainable collaboration.

3.3 Technical and Interoperability Challenges

The growing diversity of HCM systems for laboratory rodents increases the risk of inconsistencies in behavioural data annotation, which hinders cross-study comparisons, large-scale data integration, and the effective use of machine learning models on pooled datasets. This impacts both the HCM field's flexibility to align with emerging technologies and community buy-in due to vulnerability to scientific misinterpretation. Without harmonised processes for collecting, annotating, and sharing behavioural data, results across different labs and systems often remain incompatible, leading to data silos. This lack of standardisation in behavioural definitions, data formats, and annotation methodologies poses significant ethical concerns (unnecessary duplicative experiments) and creates friction in scientific progress. Modern technology can significantly lower the barriers to data sharing by making it easy to store, annotate, and access large datasets. Successful platforms often provide semi-automated pipelines, ontology support, and real-time error checking to assist researchers with submission (Bains et al. 2025).

Researchers often cite technical skills for manag repositories and attribution systems ing big data as obstacles to sharing (Hendriks et al. 2022). In the HCM context, deploying user-friendly tools (such as LLM-enriched plugins translating natural language to database queries) that streamline metadata annotation, automate uploads, and support standardised formats is crucial for easing technical burdens on researchers. The Swiss Personalised Health Network's Schema Forge follows this approach in automating translation from spreadsheet to an enriched contextual data type ready for complex interoperability (Touré et al. 2025). In neuroscience, the Neuromorph has addressed this challenge in building a metadata portal to structure and manage contextual information and terminology, plus the framework can be developed iteratively as an ongoing resource (Bijari et al. 2020).

Beyond metadata standardisation, HCM data present unique technical challenges for storage and sharing. Longitudinal monitoring generates extremely large files, particularly when video recording is involved. A single cage video-monitored for several weeks can produce terabytes of data, creating significant storage demands that exceed typical laboratory infrastructure. The volume challenge is compounded by heterogeneous HCM data, which span multiple modalities including video recordings, sensor outputs, environmental parameters, and derived behavioural metrics, each requiring different handling approaches.

Processing requirements present another barrier to effective data sharing. Complex behavioural analysis often requires specialised computational resources and expertise, particularly for video data or machine learning applications. Smaller labs may lack the infrastructure to both store and process these rich datasets, limiting their ability to contribute to or benefit from shared resources. Federated approaches that distribute processing could help address this imbalance, but implementing such systems requires coordination and investment.

Storing, processing, and maintaining HCM datasets cost substantial resources requiring immediate attention. Without sustainable funding, HCM data sharing cannot develop as needed. Table 1 shows how other scientific fields secured funding for repositories through diverse strategies. The HCM community lags behind: it has no community or mandated standard for data deposition (Springer 2025). Unless communities establish robust economic models (repositories and attribution systems), they risk failure.

Most industry data owners will not release HCM data openly. However, successful models in Table 1 show that communities still create value by combining open metadata with governed access to raw datasets. These successful models share a pattern: neutral portals, common schemas, automated quality control at ingestion, and analytical tools within secure environments. The HCM community should follow this approach and build trusted data and environments to protect intellectual property and enable collaboration.

Storage, processing, and funding barriers prevent realisation of all three motivations: they limit ethical benefits by making data reuse difficult, hinder scientific advantages through poor interoperability, and block computational innovations that require well-structured, accessible datasets.

3.4 Conclusion on Data and Metadata Sharing Challenges

Three interconnected barriers prevent the HCM field from realising benefits. First, researchers resist sharing data because current incentive structures emphasise novel findings over replication, undermining animal welfare. Second, inadequate governance frameworks leave questions about attribution, control, and misuse unresolved. Third, technical hurdles in storage, processing, and standardisation create practical barriers even for motivated researchers. These barriers hinder the development and sharing of AI-ready datasets to develop innovative computational analyses. While we have shown clear value-added for communities when sharing data, to nurture this in the HCM community it will be essential to continuously demonstrate value transfer back to data sharers.

Table 1 Examples of funded repositories and standardisation initiatives

Initiative	Funding model	Repository focus	Outcome	Lessons for HCM community
AMP-AD / AD Knowledge Portal (Greenwood et al. 2020)	Public-private (NIH + pharma + sage)	Alzheimer's genomics, imaging, and clinical trial metadata	Open multi-omic repository with reproducible workflows and managed access that seeded extensive secondary analyses	Pair open metadata and governed data access with analysis recipes and contributor-first access to sustain incentives
eTOX / eTOXsys (Cases et al. 2013)	EU funded; public and private funding, innovative health initiative (IHI)	Preclinical toxicology database aggregating legacy GLP reports from EFPIA companies, curated with ontologies for cross-study analysis	Built a large database covering >8000 studies on ~2000 compounds and ~9 million data points; made available via the eTOXsys platform under governed access	Use an honest-broker model to pool sensitive preclinical data under strict DUAs, harmonise terms up front, and ship a queryable interface so that secondary use happens at scale
IMPC (Groza et al. 2023)	International funders (NIH, EU, RIKEN)	Nonclinical mouse genetics and behaviour phenotyping	A durable, standardised pipeline and portal that link phenotypes to human disease across thousands of alleles	Treat "standard pipeline + portal + ontology" as a single product. Predefine minimal required metadata and make the portal do the heavy lifting
MouseBytes (Beraldo et al. 2019)	Public (CIHR, NSERC) + philanthropy	Touchscreen cognitive task data for rodents	Deployed across labs for multi-site touchscreen datasets with built-in QC and visual analytics	Build domain-specific pipelines with automated QC, a minimal schema, and an analysis front end so that data are useful the moment they land
NC3Rs Data Sharing Initiatives (Percie du Sert et al. 2020)	UK public grants	Reporting standards (ARRIVE) for animal research	ARRIVE 2.0 is widely adopted by journals and funders, and EDA operationalises better design and reporting	Do not publish a checklist alone. Pair the checklist with a usable design tool and reviewer-facing aids
OpenSAFELY (Williamson et al. 2020)	UK public funding (NHS, Wellcome, MRC)	Electronic health records for COVID-19 research via TRE	Operational TRE with 60+ publications; processes 58 M patient records; only aggregate outputs leave secure environment	Implement "model-to-data" architecture where analysis code goes to data, not vice versa. Raw data stay in place; export only aggregate results after automated and manual disclosure review
Virtual Fly Brain (Osumi-Sutherland et al. 2012, 2014; Court et al. 2023)	Wellcome Trust and UK research councils, with additional university-level support	Multi-modal drosophila neuroanatomy database and knowledgebase integrating 3D images, neuron connectivity, and gene expression; curated from hundreds of papers; accessible via web app and API	Operational, continually updated repository with versioned dataset releases (e.g. v4, 2025-07-30) and browsable dataset pages; integrates knowledge and images from multiple bulk datasets with cross-search and programmatic access	Pair an image-rich atlas with a knowledge graph and API. Ship regular, named releases and dataset landing pages so that derived features are reproducible and citable. Keep curation close to the literature to align labels and anatomy across labs

Addressing these challenges requires three coordinated efforts: shifting cultural incentives, developing governance structures, and building technical solutions. The following sections detail practical strategies for building effective and robust data-sharing infrastructure, prioritizing both data management and standardised metadata frameworks.

4 Building FAIR Infrastructure for HCM Data Sharing

The FAIR principles provide a unified framework for data infrastructure. This section describes the semantic infrastructure for interoperability and reusability, and finally physical systems for findability and accessibility. Figures 2 and 3 illustrate how these technical layers work together to enable data sharing, which can then support the cultural and governance solutions discussed elsewhere.

The FAIR principles maximise data reuse in nonclinical research (Wilkinson et al. 2016). A community working towards the FAIR principles follows a "FAIRification" progression from raw data to integrated systems, as Fig. 2 illustrates. When researchers

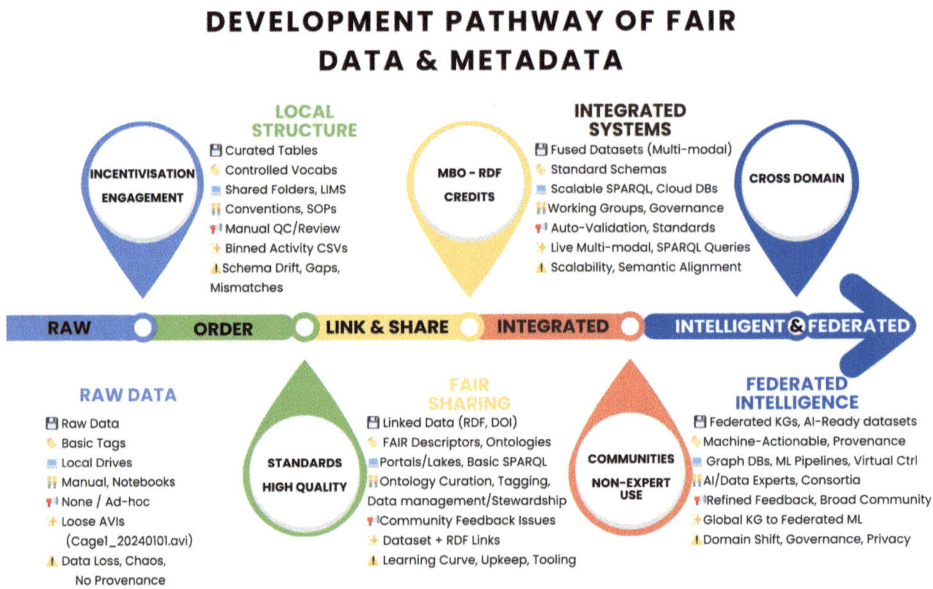

Fig. 2 Development pathway of FAIR data and metadata. This figure illustrates the evolutionary progression of data and metadata management practices in HCM research, organised into five developmental stages of increasing impact and interoperability. The horizontal arrow represents the development pathway from raw data collection to federated intelligence. Each stage shows characteristic features across elements such as infrastructure and tools, practices and people and challenges. This pathway indicates how progression enables the collaborative, AI-ready research ecosystem envisioned for HCM data sharing while delivering value continuously. SPARQL: **SPARQL** **P**rotocol **a**nd **R**DF **Q**uery **L**anguage

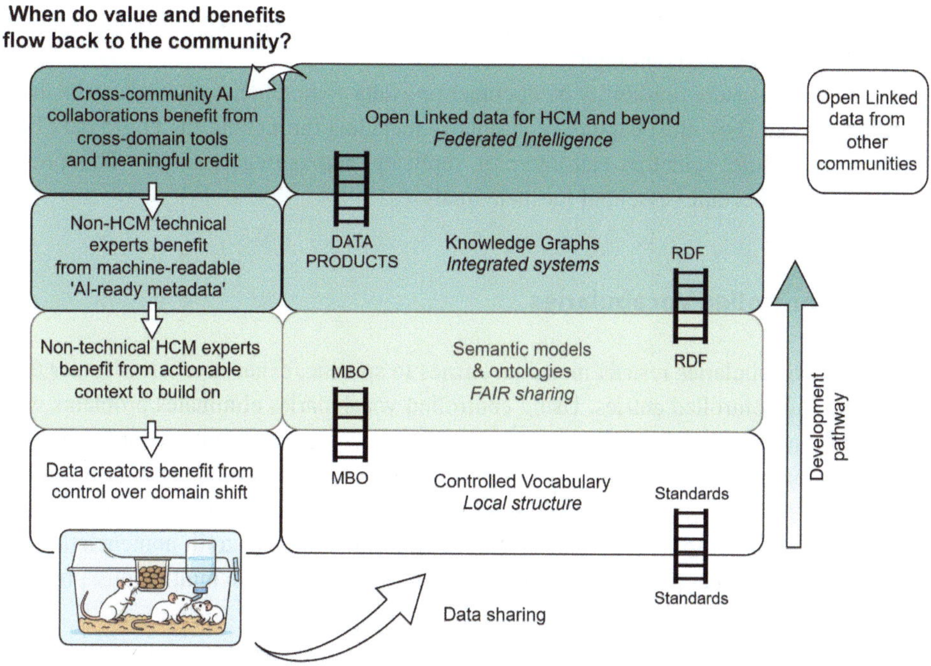

Fig. 3 Technical architecture built with strong foundations delivers value to HCM data creators. This figure illustrates the developmental pathway required to achieve semantic interoperability in HCM, emphasising the critical dependencies between technical stages. The pathway begins with an incentivised and engaged HCM community including data creators using existing standards to develop a controlled vocabulary. Stakeholders with relevant skills then formalise controlled vocabulary into ontologies and semantic models (using resources like MBO). Provided languages like RDF are available to produce machine-readable resources, then the HCM community will build knowledge graphs for large-scale AI applications. finally, a mature HCM community can produce open-linked interoperable data to collaborate with tools and infrastructure in other domains

standardise and share datasets, they enable data integration and analysis. The HCM community must build two complementary systems for FAIR architecture: semantic systems (for interoperability) and physical systems (for discovery and access). This hybrid infrastructure enables AI to extract new patterns, predict behavioural outcomes, and accelerate discovery.

4.1 Semantic Infrastructure: Enabling Interoperability and Reusability of HCM Data

The HCM community achieves interoperability and reusability by adopting machine-readable formats. These formats link HCM datasets with nonclinical data from other fields, enabling cross-study analyses and machine learning applications. To make this integration possible, the HCM community must standardise metadata through common vocabularies and shared ontologies.

Data sharers ensure reusability by documenting data comprehensively and establishing clear licensing. They must capture high-quality metadata throughout the entire data lifecycle so that future scientists can interpret, replicate, and aggregate results. This provenance tracking becomes essential for meta-analyses.

4.2 Controlled Vocabularies

Controlled vocabularies restrict metadata entries to specific, exhaustive terms rather than free text or uncontrolled entries. Using controlled vocabularies eliminates problems with synonyms and spelling variations and standardises how the community records information. For example, specifying the "sex of the animal" using a controlled term (e.g. "male" or "female" linked to an ontology ID) ensures consistent querying of sex across datasets. Domain-specific vocabularies (such as the Jackson Laboratory's strain nomenclature for mouse models) further promote harmonisation of key descriptors in multi-centre projects.

4.3 Enhancing Interoperability Using Ontologies

Ontologies extend controlled vocabularies by defining formal relationships between groups of terms. They create a descriptive 'semantic' layer to enable automated reasoning and complex data integration. In HCM research, ontologies can link observed behaviours, physiological metrics, and environmental conditions, allowing more advanced cross-study analyses. For instance, the Ontology for Biomedical Investigations (OBI) provides a general framework that could be extended to cover HCM-specific parameters, while the Mammalian Phenotypic Ontology (Smith and Eppig 2012) defines and describes gross phenotypic characteristics. These semantic layers could be integrated to describe one interoperable HCM dataset. Packaging datasets with rich semantic metadata using approaches like RO-Crate—aligned with Linked Data principles—facilitates transparent sharing and integration of HCM data across platforms.

HCM community members with technical skills can enhance interoperability by using machine-readable data formats and standardised Application Programming Interfaces (APIs), which enable automated queries across datasets. Using formats like JSON-LD or RDF together with query languages such as SPARQL (SPARQL Protocol and RDF Query Language) allows different databases to be searched and linked. These tools are the components of knowledge graphs and have been essential in formalising the semantic model within Virtual Fly Brain (Court et al. 2023).

Researchers assign each animal a privacy-preserving GUID at acquisition, mapping this identifier to cage ID and study ID. A separate, access-restricted key file stores ear-tag or microchip numbers to maintain privacy. Strain identification uses RRIDs in this format:

RRID:IMSR_JAX:000664 for C57BL/6 J. Behavioural labels reference MBO terms, protocols map to the Ontology for Biomedical Investigations (OBI), measurement units use the Units Ontology (UO), and chemicals reference the Chemical Entities of Biological Interest ontology (ChEBI). Storing each term as a Compact URI (CURIE) in the metadata allows downstream tools to resolve definitions automatically, enabling the cross-study queries described next.

Consider how researchers would use these tools in practice. An ontology-based HCM data system allows users to integrate behavioural measures such as grooming and rearing by mapping each to a standardised ontology term. For a researcher querying a community database with "locomotion speed in 12–16 week-old male mice with an ASD-related mutation", standardised metadata would enable them to retrieve all relevant datasets. This is because every study used the same controlled terms for metrics, species, age, and genotype. Without standardisation, one researcher labels a mutation as "Mybpc3^{tm1Rmos} heterozygous", while another calls it "HCM mutant", fragmenting results and missing data. By using an ontology to standardise and semantically link these descriptors, researchers can aggregate and compare data accurately, enabling robust meta-analyses and improving reproducibility across studies.

4.4 Exploiting Interoperability with AI

Interoperable HCM datasets unlock advanced AI applications. When researchers structure metadata using controlled vocabularies and ontologies, they create machine-readable datasets that AI systems can analyse independently.

Ontology-enriched systems create opportunities for AI and machine learning applications: AI models can exploit structured, machine-readable semantics to detect behavioural patterns and infer latent variables. Conversely, machine learning can assist in ontology development by discovering new relationships among entities, suggesting missing links, or dynamically refining behavioural taxonomies. Together, these AI-driven and ontology-driven processes form a virtuous cycle that continually improves interpretability and scientific insight. Integrating Large Language Models (LLMs) with domain-specific knowledge graphs grounded in formal ontologies will enhance interpretability and enable AI systems to reason over HCM data.

LLMs can act as explainable interfaces to knowledge graphs, translating complex semantic relationships into human-readable summaries that clarify why models reach certain conclusions. For example, an LLM grounded in an HCM ontology could explain that a classifier identified increased "social withdrawal" because it detected a decrease in interaction events and a rise in solitary grooming—both linked through defined ontology terms. This ability to contextualise model outputs within established behavioural frameworks enhances transparency and trust in automated analyses.

This semantic infrastructure improves data discovery and sharing, directly supporting FAIR principles. Researchers can then confidently merge, query, and reanalyse HCM data across studies and platforms. However, semantic structure alone is insufficient; researchers also need physical infrastructure to store, access, and discover these well-described datasets.

At each technical stage, the community will benefit from deliverables such as control over domain shift and AI-ready metadata. Added value flows back to the data creators who began the data ecosystem. Bypassing any foundational stage will lead to technical debt and reduced interoperability of the subsequent stage

4.5 From Metadata Standards to Implementation

Effective metadata standards require integration into existing workflows. HCM software and laboratory information management systems like *Metadatapp* that embed standardised metadata frameworks automatically capture consistent metadata during experiments.

Automated integration transforms abstract guidelines into practical tools. These tools enhance research reproducibility and minimise additional workload. By adopting semantic formats like JSON-LD or RDF to build knowledge graphs and semantic models, and exposing metadata through standardised APIs, HCM metadata can be structured for automatic validation, aggregation, and interoperability across systems. With a unified HCM metadata schema, researchers can establish automated analysis pipelines—similar to how the BIDS standard allows neuroimaging labs to run analyses without manual reconfiguration (Bouchard et al. 2025). In the HCM context, this could mean that datasets from different labs can be retrieved and re-analysed in a common pipeline with no need for custom formatting.

To implement standards effectively, the community needs a robust support framework. Clear documentation and training resources are necessary to help laboratories adopt the standard correctly. User guides, examples, and templates help researchers annotate their experiments correctly. Periodic updates (with thorough release notes) and pilot testing ensure the standard keeps pace with technological and experimental advances.

As HCM technologies advance, metadata standards will broaden to accommodate new data types and analyses. Standards will include details about explainable machine learning, key for translating information across stakeholders and expertise (Chen et al. 2022, 2023). Standards must integrate across different biological data domains (genomic, transcriptomic, proteomic data, etc.), requiring cross-domain metadata frameworks to support meaningful data fusion. The HCM community must balance depth with usability when expanding standards. Overly complex requirements risk overwhelming researchers and disengaging potential data generators. Ongoing dialogue between metadata experts and frontline scientists will be critical to ensure that standards evolve in tandem with technology, creating an interconnected ecosystem that continues to foster reproducible and collaborative science. Standards will evolve as technology advances, requiring clear version control for datasets and metadata. Version control systems allow researchers to track changes transparently, reference specific dataset versions when reproducing analyses, and preserve data provenance over time. This continual refinement process ensures the standard stays current and robust, seamlessly integrating expert feedback over time.

4.6 Follow Examples of Consensus-Built Metadata Standards

Community consensus on data and metadata standards addresses HCM research challenges as comparable communities have demonstrated. Existing guidelines like ARRIVE have established important groundwork by specifying key experimental details critical for reproducibility (on behalf of the IICARus Collaboration et al. 2019). However, studies show that checklists alone cannot improve reporting standards; journals need stringent editorial policies focusing on key quality items (Van Den Dolder et al. 2025; Rasmussen et al. 2025).

Beyond general reporting guidelines, several community initiatives have proposed formal metadata standards under the "Minimum Information" umbrella. For instance, the Minimal Metadata set for nonclinical studies initiative united academic and industry experts to define core in vivo metadata fields relevant across multiple sectors (Moresis et al. 2024). The Kavli Foundation initiated Neurodata Without Borders (NWB), a consortium of researchers and foundations with a shared interest in breaking down the obstacles to data sharing. By uniting multiple groups including the Allen Institute and Janelia Research Campus to agree on a common schema for electrophysiology data, NWB enabled aggregation and comparison of previously incompatible datasets. NWB's success is underscored by free access to the DANDI Archive and robust API support, ensuring shared data remain FAIR and readily reusable.

In nonclinical imaging, the National Cancer Institute's Co-Clinical Imaging Metadata Information standard defines critical metadata elements, such as instrument settings and animal strain, to improve reproducibility in multi-centre studies (Moore et al. 2023). These examples show that researchers, data curators, and publishers must all participate in establishing widely accepted metadata conventions. As shown, journals and funding bodies can drive adoption of standards in their requirements. When the HCM community adopts consensus standards, data become more comparable and reproducible research is driven forwards.

4.7 Physical Infrastructure: Ensuring Findability and Accessibility of HCM Data

Semantic infrastructure creates machine-readable, interoperable datasets. However, users also need physical infrastructure to discover and access datasets. In immature infrastructures, data often exist in local, unstructured formats as seen in Fig. 2.

Accessibility is achieved through open, non-proprietary formats and documented APIs that support programmatic access. An HCM dataset may be deposited in a public repository where metadata describe experimental details, ensuring anyone can access and interpret the data. Secured authentication mechanisms can balance openness with governance, allowing for tiered access that protects sensitive data while ensuring eventual public availability, a model exemplified by the European Bioinformatics Institute.

The choice of where and how researchers share data and metadata significantly impacts its visibility, reuse, and the burden on the researcher or contributor (Dorta-González and Dorta-González 2023). Studies demonstrate that data shared in open access repositories receive substantially more citations than data shared through other means, and publications that include data availability statements linking directly to established repositories show measurably higher citation rates (Colavizza et al. 2020). These benefits stem from the enhanced visibility and searchability that well-designed repositories provide, making data more discoverable for potential users.

For the HCM community specifically, several storage models offer distinct advantages and limitations:

1. *Local repositories* hosted at individual institutions provide direct control over data access and governance. They offer clarity in ownership delineation and more predictable long-term costs, as demonstrated by initiatives like the International Mouse Phenotyping Consortium (IMPC). However, these systems face significant scalability challenges as datasets grow in volume and complexity. Hardware costs, specialised IT expertise requirements, and vulnerability to cyberattacks limit their practicality for extensive collaborative networks. For smaller labs or those with modest data volumes, this approach may still be appropriate, particularly when sharing specialised datasets with niche user communities.
2. *Federated repository networks* distribute data across multiple institutional sites while sharing both costs and management responsibilities. This model has gained popularity in large academic projects, balancing local control with broader accessibility. The Canadian Open Neuroscience Platform exemplifies this approach, utilising a federated structure with specialised crawlers to extract metadata from datasets stored globally across institutions (Poline et al. 2023). Federated systems can provide good geographical distribution of resources, reducing latency for users in different regions while maintaining institutional autonomy. However, they still require substantial coordination and technical expertise to maintain interoperability across distributed nodes.
3. *Cloud-based infrastructure* offers virtually unlimited scalability and integration with computational resources for on-demand processing. These approaches deploy "Software as a Service" models that minimise local IT expertise requirements for patching, security, and server management. Commercial cloud platforms provide reliable access and robust security frameworks but their cost structures often align poorly with academic project budgets and funding cycles, requiring careful prediction and monitoring of expenses. Concerns regarding data sovereignty, such as the physical location of cloud servers, must also be addressed when storing sensitive information. Community or academic cloud initiatives like the European Open Science Cloud

demonstrate how research communities can develop shared infrastructure with appropriate governance.

To address the challenge of managing data collected from different HCM systems, researchers from COST TEATIME launched the Cooperative Home Cage Analysis Infrastructure (Bains et al. 2025). This initiative developed concrete solutions dedicated to the annotation, collection, and storage of HCM data. Adopting a 'FAIR-by-design' approach ensures long-term utility throughout the data lifecycle. The technical solutions developed in this initiative are aimed at the data representation level, the metadata annotation schema, and the technology for sharing data. The infrastructure emphasises interoperable standards that work across diverse storage systems, prioritising accessibility and reuse potential over specific technological implementations. This approach recognises that effective data sharing depends not just on where data are stored, but on how they are organised, described, and made accessible across systems.

4.8 Complex Infrastructure Requires Technical Support

While appropriate storage infrastructure forms the foundation for data sharing, technical support systems determine whether researchers can effectively utilise these resources. Surveys of neuroscientists identify cost and time investment as the most significant obstacles to data sharing (Hendriks et al. 2022). However, research demonstrates that well-curated datasets receive substantially more use, suggesting that these investments ultimately enhance scientific impact (Hemphill et al. 2022).

Several organisations provide models for comprehensive technical support. The Swiss Personalised Health Network (Touré et al. 2023) and EBRAINS (Appukuttan et al. 2023) offer specialised training programs for researchers working with complex datasets. The Jackson Laboratory has established data submission guidelines for mouse genetic data that balance accessibility with quality control, implementing peer review processes for submitted data to maintain high standards while continuously expanding their repository.

Emerging initiatives like FAIR3R in France and BioFAIR (Soranzo et al. 2023) funded by UK Research & Innovation are leveraging modern software tools to "FAIRify" datasets into collaboration-ready data products with minimal technical input required from data providers. Complementary experiment-level solutions such as Metadatapp operationalise the same principles directly within preclinical research workflows, automatically capturing standardised, ontology-linked metadata during data acquisition to reduce user burden and ensure datasets are FAIR-by-design. These platforms can also incorporate automated "FAIRness" checkers that score each dataset's compliance with FAIR principles, ensuring adherence to quality and interoperability benchmarks (Gaignard et al. 2023; Poveda-Villalon et al. 2024). Another approach over retroactive data management could be to ensure FAIRness of data and metadata throughout the data lifecycle (FAIR-IMPACT 2022). By systematically applying the FAIR principles, the HCM community can build a collaborative data ecosystem that enhances reproducibility and accelerates discoverability. This evolution is supported by new models like the FAIR Digital Objects (FDOs) framework, which packages data and metadata into self-contained, machine-actionable objects (Bonino Da Silva Santos et al. 2023).

These approaches recognise that reducing technical barriers is essential for widespread adoption of data sharing practices. The European Union has proposed a €200 billion AI-continent action plan aiming to fund infrastructure, skills, and development towards AI innovation, with importance put on the curation of high-quality datasets. Powerful and coordinated initiatives like this indicate that regulators understand the scale required to solve cutting-edge data problems and offer opportunities for cross-field engagement to drive forward computational innovation in HCM. Together, semantic and physical infrastructures anchored in FAIR principles create a robust ecosystem for HCM data sharing.

5 FAIR Implementation Review for HCM

The preceding sections established why semantic and physical infrastructures matter for HCM data sharing. This section reviews brief, actionable guidelines for implementing each FAIR principle. Research institutions, data generators, and repository managers can adopt these practices to ensure their HCM datasets achieve maximum discoverability, accessibility, interoperability, and reusability.

Findable Assign persistent identifiers at every level that matters for discovery and attribution: a DataCite DOI for each dataset and version; ORCID for contributors; ROR for the research institute; and a privacy-preserving per-animal GUID that never leaves the enclave in identifiable form. Publish a searchable landing page with minimal, indexed metadata and a clear license or DUA reference.

Accessible Host landing pages on stable HTTPS endpoints with short-lived, tokenised links, audit logs, and documented access paths. For controlled data, use a trusted research environment or federated "model-to-data" workflow so that analytics go to the data. Expose only derived features and quality summaries outside the secure boundary.

Interoperable Use shared vocabularies and IDs so that files and features line up across studies: link species and strains to RRIDs and NCBI Taxonomy, behaviours to the Mouse Behaviour Ontology, protocols and instruments to OBI terms, measurements to Units of Measurement (UO), and chemicals to ChEBI. Package metadata as JSON-LD or RO-Crate so that machines can follow the links.

Reusable Provide a machine-readable license or DUA, version histories, data quality flags, and model cards that record training data, validation, and known limits. Include enough contextual metadata to reproduce how a feature was derived from raw signals.

6 Case Study—Standardising HCM Behavioural Data and Metadata for Interoperability

The multitude of HCM platforms currently available introduces divergent annotation practice (De Chaumont et al. 2019; Sturman et al. 2020; Burand Jr. et al. 2023; Lapp et al. 2023). Recognizing this challenge, the TEATIME consortium has taken initial steps toward harmonisation by defining a HCM system in formal terms and categorizing core HCM components (arena, sensors, environment, etc.) across systems to enable meaningful comparisons [see Fig. 1 in (Bains et al. 2025)]. Building on this foundation, we propose a standardised framework that integrates a consensus-based ethogram with a formal ontology, the MBO (Huzard et al. 2025), to harmonise behavioural descriptions across platforms.

6.1 Standardised Ethogram

An ethogram is a list of species-specific behaviours describing the elements and functions of each behaviour, intended to objectively describe and record animal activities using a common behavioural lexicon. Although numerous rodent ethograms exist for particular experiments or strains (Bardi et al. 2011; Lapp et al. 2023), few comprehensive ethograms for spontaneous, naturalistic behaviour in laboratory mice have been published to date. By devising a shared, standardised description of behaviours and annotations, researchers can directly compare and integrate data from different experiments and even pool datasets across institutions and HCM systems.

However, traditional ethograms are not machine-readable. Different HCM systems define and label behaviours inconsistently, making dataset integration difficult, reducing the power of these models and impeding progress in behaviour prediction.

6.2 Formal Ontology for the Ethogram—Mouse Behaviour Ontology

Formal ontologies overcome ethogram limitations by providing a rigorously structured framework for describing behaviours and the relationships between behaviours, states, and events in a machine-readable format. Machine-readable formats address concerns about misinterpreting complex data (Hendriks et al. 2022). Mapping mouse ethograms of spontaneous behaviours to a formal ontology allows machine readability of behavioural definitions, paving the way to cutting-edge analytical innovation. Another advantage of this approach lies in exposing the semantic relationships among behaviours. Ontologies encode behaviours as well-defined classes (and subclasses) with properties that describe their features and connections, enabling representation of hierarchical relationships ("is-a" types), temporal sequences (e.g. precedes or overlaps), causal links (e.g. results-from), and functional roles (e.g. serves-function-of). For example, a high-level class like self-maintenance behaviour may include sub-behaviours such as grooming, eating, and drinking, each linked by an *is-a* relationship to the parent class. Likewise, a behaviour sequence like *exploration* → *rearing* → *sniffing* can be formally represented with temporal relationships, allowing the ontology to capture typical behaviour orderings or detect unusual transitions.

Formalising behavioural knowledge enables automated reasoning. Description logic reasoners (using Web Ontology Language—OWL—with reasoning tools like HermiT or SPARQL) derive implicit information from explicit facts. For example, if the ontology states that *grooming* is a subtype of *self-maintenance behaviour*, any dataset that records grooming events automatically gains the broader *self-maintenance* label—even if it never appeared in the raw annotations. A reasoner can push the inference further: knowing that a *grooming* bout took place in *Cage A*, and that *Cage A* sits on *Rack 3* inside *Room 12*, it materialises the full location so that you can later ask, within a SPARQL query, corresponding to the request: "Show me every act of self-maintenance that happened in Room 12 but wasn't originally tagged as grooming." In this way, logical inference fills in for higher-level behavioural categories and contextual details from low-level observations, enriching the dataset and simplifying downstream analyses.

Ethogram-ontology links enable two types of scalability: horizontal and vertical. *Horizontal scalability* refers to the ontology's ability to integrate behavioural data with other domains by establishing formal links to external ontologies (Hoehndorf et al. 2014). For example, behaviours annotated in MBO could be connected to entries in the Gene Ontology (for genetic annotations), then to a mental health ontology (e.g. the Mental Disease Ontology) to provide rich context about genetic or pathological factors associated with certain behaviours. These cross-domain links allow researchers to ask complex questions—such as correlating spontaneous behaviours with underlying genetic mutations or disease models—by merging data across traditionally separate knowledge domains. *Vertical scalability*, on the other hand, describes the ontology's utility across different scales of research operations. An individual laboratory could adopt MBO to ensure consistent annotation within its own experiments, improving reproducibility and easing collaboration with other labs by capturing datasets with sharing in mind. Meanwhile, large-scale endeavours (pharmaceutical companies, multi-centre consortia engaged in high-throughput phenotyping) could leverage MBO as a common reference to harmonise vast amounts of behavioural data generated at different sites. The ontology serves both as a reference knowledge base for organizing behavioural concepts and as infrastructure for collaborative, multi-scale research in academia and industry alike.

7 Roadmap to Open Data and Metadata Sharing in the HCM Community

This roadmap outlines a phased strategy to build a sustainable, community-driven open data ecosystem for HCM. Figure 4 illustrates this strategy, showing how progression through foundation building, incentive development, scaling efforts, and innovation initiatives can transform the current fragmented landscape into a collaborative, interoperable research ecosystem.

Phase 1: Foundation Building—The community establishes the governance and technical groundwork for sharing.

- A representative steering committee (with data generators, analysts, and infrastructure experts) will establish a governance framework. Committee members will define policies on data embargo periods, attribution requirements, and decision-making procedures, following models like the International Brain Laboratory (which balances contributor protection with open science goals).
- Define technical standards by using minimal required metadata fields for HCM experiments (Moresis et al. 2024). Organisations like the Pistoia Alliance are actively building ARRIVE and FAIR compliant metadata standards for in vivo data; emerging standards should be reviewed. New standards should only be defined if existing standards are not fit for purpose.
- Incorporate provenance tracking so that each dataset preserves its context. Share and version Standard Operating Procedures (following the International Mouse Phenotyping Consortium (Koscielny et al. 2014)) to capture further context in datasets.
- Develop recommendations for standard formats for common data types (video recordings, activity sensor data, physiological signals, etc.) and behaviour classes (Huzard et al. 2025).
- Select an initial repository infrastructure suited to community requirements and existing resources. Depending on scale and funding, this could be a centralised cloud repository, a federated system as presented by the HCM community (Bains et al. 2025), or an on-premises server network.
- Implement basic persistent identifiers (DOIs) and unique resource identifiers (RRIDs) for datasets from the outset to ensure proper credit, tracking, and findability through data linking. Follow the strategic roadmap produced by members of the TEATIME community (Petit-Demouliere et al. 2025). Record a DataCite DOI for each dataset and version, ORCID for contributors, ROR for the research institute, and the funder's Crossref Funder ID. Expose these on the dataset landing page and in JSON-LD so that the record is indexable across catalogues.
- Publish a tiered IP and data-rights policy. Codify open by default for metadata and schemas, controlled access for raw datasets, and public release of derived features and model cards. Include a template Data Use Agreement (DUA), standard license options,

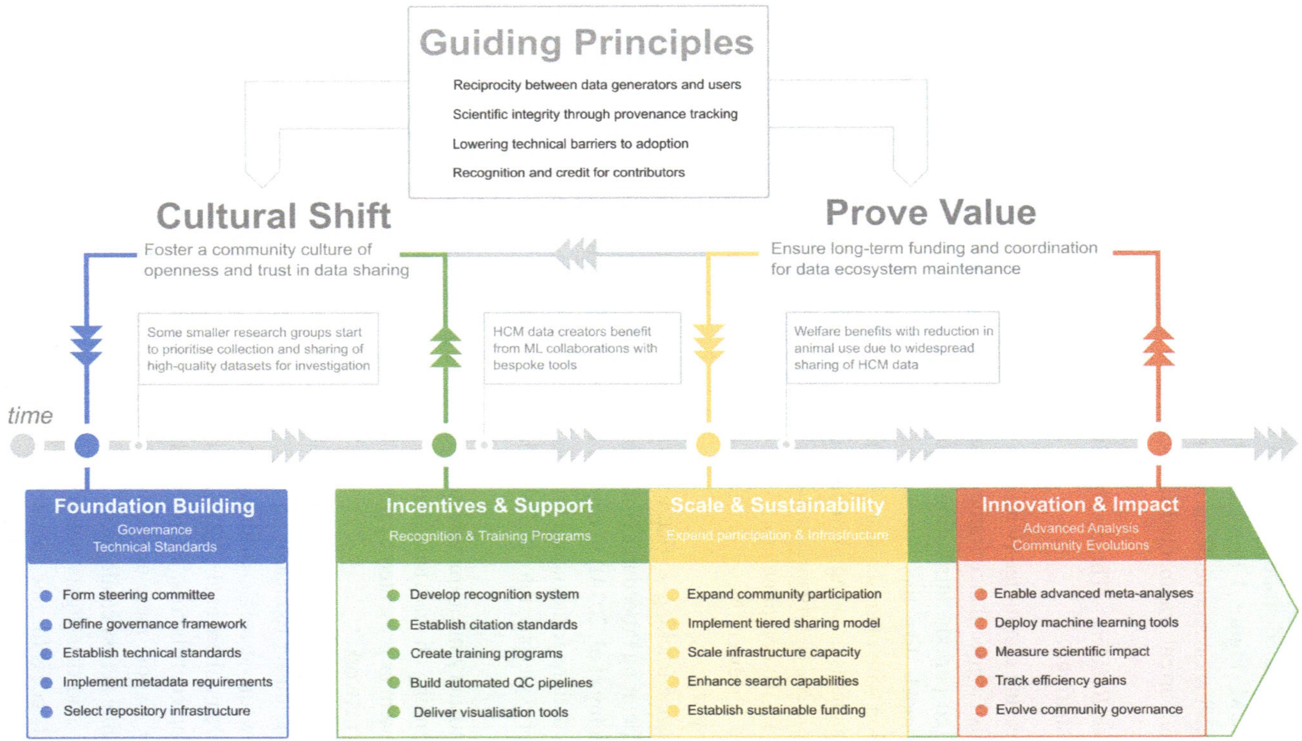

Fig. 4 Community roadmap to enable open data practices in HCM research. The roadmap progresses chronologically from left to right, with each phase building upon the achievements of previous stages to ensure systematic adoption and long-term impact, provided listed actions are fulfilled. The process begins with a necessary cultural shift to foster openness, trust, and shared responsibility within the research community through building governance and technical foundations while incentivising progress and providing support. These steps are not necessarily linear; as incentives are shaped they will feed back into foundation building. Once foundations are in place, the focus will shift to scaling technology and processes and providing sustainable innovation and impact. Again, this pathway is not always linear, and we have indicated that impact will guide how we scale and where the field prioritises sustainability, and these factors may shape how we govern, support, and incentivise further progress. Together, these steps provide a pathway for transforming HCM data into a reusable, ethical, and impactful scientific resource

embargo windows, a neutral rights registry, give-to-get reciprocity, and an audit and sanctions path.

Phase 2: Incentives and Support—Once governance is in place, focus shifts to encouraging participation and making data sharing rewarding and user-friendly.

- Implement and prove recognition and reward systems for data contributors. For example, create public contributor profiles highlighting each lab's shared datasets and their reuse impact. Work with academic journals to establish formal citation practices for HCM datasets. Provide dashboards that track dataset downloads and derived publications, demonstrating the value of sharing.
- Develop technical support and training programs. Use successful models such as the Swiss Personalised Health Network and the EBRAINS platform in neuroscience to provide workshops or online training to help researchers prepare and upload data in the standard formats. Set up automated quality control pipelines (Gaignard et al. 2023; Poveda-Villalon et al. 2024) that validate incoming datasets against metadata standards, see Table 1. These pipelines reduce contributor burden by catching errors automatically.
- Deliver early tangible benefits to data users. Build analysis and visualisation tools optimised for the shared HCM data formats (similar to what the Mouse Phenome Database offers for integrated data). Easy-to-use visualisation interfaces help researchers identify patterns across datasets. This shows immediate scientific advantages and incentivises further contributions.
- Stand up secure analytics without moving data. Pilot a trusted research environment or federated "model-to-data" workflow with at least two pharma sites. Pre-specify what can leave the enclave (derived features, QC summaries, model cards) and what cannot (raw video, identifiers).

Phase 3: Scale and Sustainability—With initial adoption underway, the focus turns to scaling up the network and ensuring long-term sustainability.

- Expand community participation by leveraging early successes. Use case studies showing how shared data enabled discoveries to recruit additional labs. Introduce a tiered data sharing model that addresses concerns about competition—for instance, allowing researchers to set an embargo period during which only consortium members can access their new data, before full public release.
- Strengthen and scale the infrastructure, both horizontally and vertically. Increase repository capacity as usage grows and functionality according to clear requirements. Implement advanced search and query capabilities to improve data discoverability. Introduce automated data cleaning and standardisation tools that enhance data quality as they are uploaded, minimizing the effort required from contributors.
- Establish a sustainable funding and management model. Transition from reliance on initial grants to a consortium-based funding structure with multiple stakeholders (research institutions, funding agencies, possibly industry partners) to share costs. The

examples in Table 1 demonstrate diverse funding models that have sustained other non-clinical data initiatives. The HCM community should evaluate which model best fits its needs and governance structure. Develop a long-term business plan that keeps the repository open and free to use, while ensuring resources for maintenance and future upgrades are secured.

Phase 4: Innovation and Impact—In the long term, the emphasis is on maximizing scientific innovation and community governance as data sharing becomes the norm.

- Enable advanced meta-analyses and machine learning on the aggregated data. Deploy tools that can analyse combined datasets for patterns or biomarkers that wouldn't be detectable in smaller samples. Facilitate cross-modal studies that link HCM data with other data types (e.g. genomics, phenotypics, or imaging data), providing an integrated view of animal biology.
- Measure and communicate the scientific impact of the open-data initiative. Track metrics such as the number of secondary publications, new hypotheses generated, or cross-institution collaborations that arose thanks to shared HCM data. Publicise success stories where integrated datasets led to breakthroughs and quantify efficiency gains (e.g. reduction in duplicate experiments) resulting from data reuse.
- Evolve governance as the community grows. Introduce more nuanced permission and data-use agreements that let data contributors specify how their data can be used (for example, distinguishing between exploratory analysis vs. inclusion in nonclinical meta-studies). Establish regular community feedback mechanisms and update policies accordingly, so that the data sharing platform continues to meet researchers' needs and ethical standards as technology and priorities change.

Across all phases of this roadmap, reciprocity between data generators and data users remains a guiding principle. By addressing concerns about scientific integrity through rigorous provenance tracking, providing recognition and credit for contributors, lowering technical barriers with strong support, and delivering concrete scientific benefits from shared data, the community can turn the challenges identified in this chapter into stepping stones toward a thriving open data ecosystem in HCM research.

7.1 Leadership Challenges for the HCM Community

The vision of a federated network for HCM data promises to revolutionise nonclinical research, enhancing animal welfare, accelerating scientific discovery, and encouraging cutting edge computational analysis. This chapter has explored how the HCM community can achieve comprehensive data sharing and identified the obstacles hindering progress. The community roadmap (Fig. 4) integrates these insights into actionable phases. We reiterate the obstacles to federated data sharing below in a series of leadership challenges for the HCM community.

For Animal Welfare Advocates and Ethical Review Boards How can we ensure that shared data genuinely advance the 3Rs? Will historical control data truly reduce the number of animals needed, and can automated monitoring refine care without becoming a substitute for human oversight?

For Researchers and Scientific Leaders Does standardising complex behavioural data risk losing essential experimental nuance? Will the digital biomarkers generated by continuous monitoring truly improve the translatability of animal findings to human medicine, or will they create a new set of data that is difficult to interpret? How do we ensure that data sharing delivers tangible, visible benefits back to the researchers who contribute data, beyond abstract promises of future scientific progress? How do we make data FAIRification and AI tools accessible to researchers without deep technical expertise?

For Data Scientists and Technologists Are we prepared for the technical and financial investment required to make massive HCM datasets truly "AI-ready"? Is simply having ontology-annotated data enough to bridge the gap between biological knowledge and scalable machine learning applications? What metadata quality standards are needed to ensure historical data can be confidently repurposed? Do we have mechanisms to facilitate effective collaboration between domain scientists, data engineers, and AI specialists?

For Funders, Institutions, and Industry Partners Who will pay? What sustainable funding models can support the creation, governance, and long-term maintenance of the repositories and tools that form the backbone of this infrastructure?

For the Entire Scientific Community How do we overcome the significant cultural, financial, and practical barriers to ensure widespread adoption? What incentives will convince individual labs that sharing their data will empower their science, not just burden them with new requirements? More critically: how do we demonstrate and deliver tangible value back to data creators who invest time in high-quality annotation and sharing? Finally, how do we govern and transition this diverse and federated community through the necessary cultural change?

8 Conclusion

The HCM community must share data and metadata for three reasons: ethical imperatives, scientific advantages, and computational opportunities. Common ontologies like the MBO and comprehensive metadata frameworks provide shared language for data interoperability and machine-readability. These consensus standards enhance data comparability, enable robust meta-analyses, and drive more reproducible research. Without this technical foundation, even willing collaborators cannot effectively share or reuse datasets across laboratories and platforms.

Data sharing must deliver tangible benefits to contributors: improved welfare monitoring, novel detection of subtle phenotypes, and integrated simulations. Early successes in federated learning, virtual control groups, and cross-platform behavioural analysis provide proof-of-concept, but broader adoption will require visible returns on the substantial effort required for high-quality data annotation and sharing, while moving in tandem with a cultural shift towards sharing.

Building an open data and metadata ecosystem for HCM demands long-term funding, training programs, and governance structures to maintain repositories and evolve standards with technology. The roadmap we have outlined is a step towards this goal, but success ultimately depends on continued collaboration across institutions, disciplines, and stakeholder communities. While achieving comprehensive data and metadata sharing presents significant challenges, the demonstrated success in other scientific domains shows this transformation is both feasible and valuable.

References

Al Khatib HS, Neupane S, Kumar Manchukonda H et al (2024) Patient-centric knowledge graphs: a survey of current methods, challenges, and applications. Front Artif Intell 7:1388479. https://doi.org/10.3389/frai.2024.1388479

Aldarondo D, Merel J, Marshall JD et al (2024) A virtual rodent predicts the structure of neural activity across behaviours. Nature 632:594–602. https://doi.org/10.1038/s41586-024-07633-4

Appukuttan S et al (2023) EBRAINS live papers - interactive resource sheets for computational studies in neuroscience. Neuroinformatics 1:101–113. https://doi.org/10.1007/s12021-022-09598-z

Bains R, Huzard D, McCutcheon J et al (2025) Too big to lose – a FAIR repository for biomedical data derived from home-cage monitoring. https://doi.org/10.31219/osf.io/fsg83_v1

Baran SW, Lim MA, Do JP et al (2021) Digital biomarkers enable automated, longitudinal monitoring in a mouse model of aging. J Gerontol A Biol Sci Med Sci 76:1206–1213. https://doi.org/10.1093/gerona/glab024

Baran SW, Bratcher N, Dennis J et al (2022) Emerging role of translational digital biomarkers within home cage monitoring technologies in preclinical drug discovery and development. Front Behav Neurosci 15:758274. https://doi.org/10.3389/fnbeh.2021.758274

Bardi M, Franssen CL, Hampton JE et al (2011) Paternal experience and stress responses in California mice (Peromyscus californicus). Comp Med 61:20–30

Beck T, Hancock J, Mallon A-M (2009) Developing a mammalian behaviour ontology. Nat Preced. https://doi.org/10.1038/npre.2009.3565.1

Beraldo FH, Palmer D, Memar S et al (2019) MouseBytes, an open-access high-throughput pipeline and database for rodent touchscreen-based cognitive assessment. eLife 8:e49630. https://doi.org/10.7554/eLife.49630

Bijari K, Akram MA, Ascoli GA (2020) An open-source framework for neuroscience metadata management applied to digital reconstructions of neuronal morphology. Brain Inform 7:2. https://doi.org/10.1186/s40708-020-00103-3

Bogue MA, Philip VM, Walton DO et al (2019) Mouse phenome database: a data repository and analysis suite for curated primary mouse phenotype data. Nucleic Acids Res:gkz1032. https://doi.org/10.1093/nar/gkz1032

Bonino Da Silva Santos LO, Sales TP, Fonseca CM, Guizzardi G (2023) Towards a conceptual model for the FAIR digital object framework. In: Aussenac-Gilles N, Hahmann T, Galton A, Hedblom MM (eds) Frontiers in artificial intelligence and applications. IOS Press

Bouchard AE, Wong D, Bogner W et al (2025) MRS-BIDS, an extension to the brain imaging data structure for magnetic resonance spectroscopy. Sci Data 12:1384. https://doi.org/10.1038/s41597-025-05543-2

Bult CJ, Blake JA, Smith CL et al (2019) Mouse Genome Database (MGD) 2019. Nucleic Acids Res 47:D801–D806. https://doi.org/10.1093/nar/gky1056

Burand AJ Jr, Waltz TB, Manis AD et al (2023) HomeCageScan analysis reveals ongoing pain in Fabry rats. Neurobiol Pain 13:100113. https://doi.org/10.1016/j.ynpai.2022.100113

Campbell HA, Micheli-Campbell MA, Udyawer V (2019) Early career researchers embrace data sharing. Trends Ecol Evol 34:95–98. https://doi.org/10.1016/j.tree.2018.11.010

Cases M, Pastor M, Sanz F (2013) The eTOX library of public resources for in Silico toxicity prediction. Mol Inform 32:24–35. https://doi.org/10.1002/minf.201200099

Cerezo M, Sollis E, Ji Y et al (2025) The NHGRI-EBI GWAS catalog: standards for reusability, sustainability and diversity. Nucleic Acids Res 53:D998–D1005. https://doi.org/10.1093/nar/gkae1070

Challenge.gov (2025) NIH data sharing index (S-index) challenge. In: NIH Data Shar. Index -Index Chall. https://www.challenge.gov/?challenge=nih-data-sharing-index-s-index-challenge. Accessed 21 May 2025

Chan V, Gherardini PF, Krummel MF, Fragiadakis GK (2021) A "data sharing trust" model for rapid, collaborative science. Cell 184:566–570. https://doi.org/10.1016/j.cell.2021.01.006

Chen H, Lundberg SM, Lee S-I (2022) Explaining a series of models by propagating Shapley values. Nat Commun 13:4512. https://doi.org/10.1038/s41467-022-31384-3

Chen H, Covert IC, Lundberg SM, Lee S-I (2023) Algorithms to estimate Shapley value feature attributions. Nat Mach Intell 5:590–601. https://doi.org/10.1038/s42256-023-00657-x

Christensen G, Dafoe A, Miguel E et al (2019) A study of the impact of data sharing on article citations using journal policies as a natural experiment. PLoS One 14:e0225883. https://doi.org/10.1371/journal.pone.0225883

Colavizza G, Hrynaszkiewicz I, Staden I et al (2020) The citation advantage of linking publications to research data. PLoS One 15:e0230416. https://doi.org/10.1371/journal.pone.0230416

Court R, Costa M, Pilgrim C et al (2023) Virtual Fly brain—an interactive atlas of the drosophila nervous system. Front Physiol 14:1076533. https://doi.org/10.3389/fphys.2023.1076533

De Chaumont F, Ey E, Torquet N et al (2019) Real-time analysis of the behaviour of groups of mice via a depth-sensing camera and machine learning. Nat Biomed Eng 3:930–942. https://doi.org/10.1038/s41551-019-0396-1

De Vries SE, Siegle JH, Koch C (2023) Sharing neurophysiology data from the Allen Brain Observatory. eLife 12:e85550. https://doi.org/10.7554/eLife.85550

Dorta-González P, Dorta-González MI (2023) The influence of funding on the open access citation advantage. J Scientometr Res 12:68–78. https://doi.org/10.5530/jscires.12.1.010

Eke DO, Bernard A, Bjaalie JG et al (2022) International data governance for neuroscience. Neuron 110:600–612. https://doi.org/10.1016/j.neuron.2021.11.017

FAIR-IMPACT (2022) Metadata and Ontologies (WP4). https://fair-impact.eu/wp4-metadata-and-ontologies. Accessed 29 May 2025

Fraga-González G, Van De Wiel H, Garassino F et al (2025) Affording reusable data: recommendations for researchers from a data-intensive project. Sci Data 12:258. https://doi.org/10.1038/s41597-025-04565-0

Gaignard A, Rosnet T, De Lamotte F et al (2023) FAIR-checker: supporting digital resource findability and reuse with knowledge graphs and semantic web standards. J Biomed Semant 14:7. https://doi.org/10.1186/s13326-023-00289-5

Greenwood AK, Montgomery KS, Kauer N et al (2020) The AD knowledge portal: a repository for multi-omic data on Alzheimer's disease and aging. Curr Protoc Hum Genet 108:e105. https://doi.org/10.1002/cphg.105

Groza T, Gomez FL, Mashhadi HH et al (2023) The international mouse phenotyping consortium: comprehensive knockout phenotyping underpinning the study of human disease. Nucleic Acids Res 51:D1038–D1045. https://doi.org/10.1093/nar/gkac972

Guinney J, Wang T, Laajala TD et al (2017) Prediction of overall survival for patients with metastatic castration-resistant prostate cancer: development of a prognostic model through a crowdsourced challenge with open clinical trial data. Lancet Oncol 18:132–142. https://doi.org/10.1016/S1470-2045(16)30560-5

Hemphill L, Pienta A, Lafia S et al (2022) How do properties of data, their curation, and their funding relate to reuse? J Assoc Inf Sci Technol 73:1432–1444. https://doi.org/10.1002/asi.24646

Hendriks S, Ramos KM, Grady C (2022) Survey of investigators about sharing human research data in the neurosciences. Neurology 99. https://doi.org/10.1212/WNL.0000000000200886

Hoehndorf R, Hancock JM, Hardy NW et al (2014) Analyzing gene expression data in mice with the neuro behavior ontology. Mamm Genome Off J Int Mamm Genome Soc 25:32–40. https://doi.org/10.1007/s00335-013-9481-z

Hood ASC, Sutherland WJ (2021) The data-index: an author-level metric that values impactful data and incentivizes data sharing. Ecol Evol 11:14344–14350. https://doi.org/10.1002/ece3.8126

Huzard D, Restivo L, Rivalan M (2025) MBO. https://doi.org/10.17605/OSF.IO/S8KR9

Kavianpour S, Sutherland J, Mansouri-Benssassi E et al (2022) Next-generation capabilities in trusted research environments: interview study. J Med Internet Res 24:e33720. https://doi.org/10.2196/33720

Koscielny G, Yaikhom G, Iyer V et al (2014) The international mouse phenotyping consortium web portal, a unified point of access for knockout mice and related phenotyping data. Nucleic Acids Res 42:D802–D809. https://doi.org/10.1093/nar/gkt977

Kwon S, Motohashi K (2021) Incentive or disincentive for research data disclosure? A large-scale empirical analysis and implications for open science policy. Int J Inf Manag 60:102371. https://doi.org/10.1016/j.ijinfomgt.2021.102371

Lapp HE, Salazar MG, Champagne FA (2023) Automated maternal behavior during early life in rodents (AMBER) pipeline. Sci Rep 13:18277. https://doi.org/10.1038/s41598-023-45495-4

Li R, Hill N, D'Arcy C et al (2022) Health data sharing platforms: serving researchers through provision of access to high-quality data for reuse. Health Data Sci 2022:9768384. https://doi.org/10.34133/2022/9768384

Mao A, Huang E, Gan H, Liu K (2022) FedAAR: a novel federated learning framework for animal activity recognition with wearable sensors. Animals 12:2142. https://doi.org/10.3390/ani12162142

Miller J, Ross JS, Wilenzick M, Mello MM (2019) Sharing of clinical trial data and results reporting practices among large pharmaceutical companies: cross sectional descriptive study and pilot of a tool to improve company practices. BMJ:l4217. https://doi.org/10.1136/bmj.l4217

Moore SM, Quirk JD, Lassiter AW et al (2023) Co-Clinical Imaging Metadata Information (CIMI) for cancer research to promote open science, standardization, and reproducibility in preclinical imaging. Tomography 9:995–1009. https://doi.org/10.3390/tomography9030081

Moresis A, Restivo L, Bromilow S et al (2024) A minimal metadata set (MNMS) to repurpose nonclinical in vivo data for biomedical research. Lab Anim 53:67–79. https://doi.org/10.1038/s41684-024-01335-0

Mosleh M, Roshani S, Coccia M (2022) Scientific laws of research funding to support citations and diffusion of knowledge in life science. Scientometrics 127:1931–1951. https://doi.org/10.1007/s11192-022-04300-1

On behalf of the IICARus Collaboration, Hair K, Macleod MR, Sena ES (2019) A randomised controlled trial of an intervention to improve compliance with the ARRIVE guidelines (IICARus). Res Integr Peer Rev 4:12. https://doi.org/10.1186/s41073-019-0069-3

Osumi-Sutherland D, Reeve S, Mungall CJ et al (2012) A strategy for building neuroanatomy ontologies. Bioinformatics 28:1262–1269. https://doi.org/10.1093/bioinformatics/bts113

Osumi-Sutherland D, Costa M, Court R, O'Kane CJ (2014) Virtual Fly brain – using OWL to support the mapping and genetic dissection of the Drosophila brain. CEUR Workshop Proc 1265:85–96
Percie du Sert N, Hurst V, Ahluwalia A, Alam S, Avey MT, Baker M et al (2020) The ARRIVE guidelines 2.0: updated guidelines for reporting animal research. PLoS Biol 18(7):e3000410. https://doi.org/10.1371/journal.pbio.3000410
Petit-Demouliere B, Huzard D, Forrest H et al (2025) Federated FAIR repository for home-cage monitoring and behaviour: strategic roadmap. https://doi.org/10.5281/ZENODO.17265237
Poline J-B, Das S, Glatard T et al (2023) Data and tools integration in the Canadian open neuroscience platform. Sci Data 10:189. https://doi.org/10.1038/s41597-023-01946-1
Poveda-Villalon M, Garijo D, Gonzalez-Beltran A et al (2024) Ontology engineering and the FAIR principles: a gap analysis toward a FAIR-by-design methodology. In: Trojahn C, Garijo D, Villalón MP, Bernabé CH, Lin AY (eds) FOAM 2024 – FAIR principles for ontologies and metadata in knowledge management, Enschede, Netherlands, p 15p
Rasmussen CLM, Burkhart A, Moos T, Thomsen LB (2025) Reporting preclinical gene therapy studies in the field of Niemann-Pick type C disease according to the ARRIVE guidelines. Orphanet J Rare Dis 20:214. https://doi.org/10.1186/s13023-024-03479-1
RELACS Consortium, Bonapersona V, Hoijtink H et al (2021) Increasing the statistical power of animal experiments with historical control data. Nat Neurosci 24:470–477. https://doi.org/10.1038/s41593-020-00792-3
Rübel O, Tritt A, Ly R et al (2022) The Neurodata without borders ecosystem for neurophysiological data science. eLife 11:e78362. https://doi.org/10.7554/eLife.78362
Sabnis GS, Churchill GA, Kumar V (2025) Machine vision-based frailty assessment for genetically diverse mice. GeroScience. https://doi.org/10.1007/s11357-025-01583-z
Smith CL, Eppig JT (2012) The mammalian phenotype ontology as a unifying standard for experimental and high-throughput phenotyping data. Mamm Genome 23:653–668. https://doi.org/10.1007/s00335-012-9421-3
Soranzo N, Andrews R, Beck T, et al (2023) BioFAIR: a new BioCommons infrastructure for the UK life science
Springer Nature (2025) Mandated data types
Steger-Hartmann T, Sanz F, Bringezu F, Soininen I (2025) IHI VICT3R: developing and implementing virtual control groups to reduce animal use in toxicology research. Toxicol Pathol 53:230–233. https://doi.org/10.1177/01926233241303906
Sturman O, Von Ziegler L, Schläppi C et al (2020) Deep learning-based behavioral analysis reaches human accuracy and is capable of outperforming commercial solutions. Neuropsychopharmacology 45:1942–1952. https://doi.org/10.1038/s41386-020-0776-y
Sudhahar S, Ozer B, Chang J et al (2024) An experimentally validated approach to automated biological evidence generation in drug discovery using knowledge graphs. Nat Commun 15:5703. https://doi.org/10.1038/s41467-024-50024-6
Swiss National Science Foundation (2025) Data Management Plan (DMP) – Guidelines for researchers
Tan SZK, Baksi S, Bjerregaard TG et al (2025) Digital evolution: Novo Nordisk's shift to ontology-based data management. J Biomed Semant 16:6. https://doi.org/10.1186/s13326-025-00327-4
Tenopir C, Rice NM, Allard S et al (2020) Data sharing, management, use, and reuse: practices and perceptions of scientists worldwide. PLoS One 15:e0229003. https://doi.org/10.1371/journal.pone.0229003
Thelwall M, Kousha K (2017) Do journal data sharing mandates work? Life sciences evidence from Dryad. Aslib J Inf Manag 69:36–45. https://doi.org/10.1108/AJIM-09-2016-0159
Touré V, Krauss P, Gnodtke K et al (2023) FAIRification of health-related data using semantic web technologies in the Swiss Personalized Health Network. Sci Data 10:127. https://doi.org/10.1038/s41597-023-02028-y

Touré V, Unni D, Krauss P et al (2025) The SPHN Schema Forge—transform healthcare semantics from human-readable to machine-readable by leveraging semantic web technologies. J Biomed Semant 16:9. https://doi.org/10.1186/s13326-025-00330-9
UK Health Data Research Alliance, NHSX (2021) Building trusted research environments – principles and best practices. Towards TRE Ecosystems, Zenodo. https://zenodo.org/record/5766512
Ulfhake B, Lerat H, Honetschlager J et al (2022) A multicentre study on spontaneous in-cage activity and micro-environmental conditions of IVC housed C57BL/6J mice during consecutive cycles of bi-weekly cage-change. PLoS One 17:e0267281. https://doi.org/10.1371/journal.pone.0267281
Van Den Dolder FW, Dinani R, Warnaar VAJ et al (2025) Experimental models of hypertrophic cardiomyopathy. JACC Basic Transl Sci:S2452302X24003966. https://doi.org/10.1016/j.jacbts.2024.10.017
Vaxenburg R, Siwanowicz I, Merel J et al (2024) Whole-body simulation of realistic fruit fly locomotion with deep reinforcement learning
Von Kortzfleisch VT, Karp NA, Palme R et al (2020) Improving reproducibility in animal research by splitting the study population into several 'mini-experiments.'. Sci Rep 10:16579. https://doi.org/10.1038/s41598-020-73503-4
Wilkinson MD, Dumontier M, Aalbersberg IJJ et al (2016) The FAIR guiding principles for scientific data management and stewardship. Sci Data 3:160018. https://doi.org/10.1038/sdata.2016.18
Williamson EJ, Walker AJ, Bhaskaran K et al (2020) Factors associated with COVID-19-related death using OpenSAFELY. Nature 584:430–436. https://doi.org/10.1038/s41586-020-2521-4
Wilson SL, Way GP, Bittremieux W et al (2021) Sharing biological data: why, when, and how. FEBS Lett 595:847–863. https://doi.org/10.1002/1873-3468.14067
Woods HB, Pinfield S (2022) Incentivising research data sharing: a scoping review. Wellcome Open Res 6:355. https://doi.org/10.12688/wellcomeopenres.17286.2
Wool LE (2020) Knowledge across networks: how to build a global neuroscience collaboration. Curr Opin Neurobiol 65:100–107. https://doi.org/10.1016/j.conb.2020.10.020
Ye S, Filippova A, Lauer J et al (2024) SuperAnimal pretrained pose estimation models for behavioral analysis. Nat Commun 15:5165. https://doi.org/10.1038/s41467-024-48792-2
Zentrich E, Talbot SR, Bleich A, Häger C (2021) Automated home-cage monitoring during acute experimental colitis in mice. Front Neurosci 15:760606. https://doi.org/10.3389/fnins.2021.760606

Education and Training School in Home Cage Monitoring: The 'Whys' and 'Hows'

Nuno Henrique Franco, Silvia Mandillo, and Lior Bikovski

Abstract

The adoption of Home Cage Monitoring (HCM) systems, as well as its effective and ethical use, requires proper education and training in this technology. This chapter explores the critical role of training in preparing researchers to handle the complexities associated with HCM. Effective education should focus on knowledge on the capabilities of HCM systems, their possible applications, technological hurdles, experimental design issues, and animal welfare implications. Hands-on training promotes proficiency, enabling users to set up, calibrate, and troubleshoot HCM systems effectively and tailor them to their own research models and scientific objectives, ensuring consistent data quality and reliable analysis. Training, moreover, aims at standardization, enabling researchers to adopt shared protocols and practices that facilitate comparability across studies and strengthen the credibility of HCM research.

The COST Action TEATIME (Action CA20135 'Improving biomedical research by automated behaviour monitoring in the animal home cage') held four editions of yearly

N. H. Franco
Universidade do Porto, Porto, Portugal

S. Mandillo
Institute of Biochemistry and Cell Biology (IBBC), National Research Council (CNR), Monterotondo (Rome), Italy

L. Bikovski (✉)
Myers Neuro-Behavioral Core Facility, Gray Faculty of Medical & Health, Tel Aviv University, Tel Aviv, Israel

Department of Human Molecular Genetics & Biochemistry, Gray Faculty of Medical & Health, Tel Aviv University, Tel Aviv, Israel
e-mail: liorbiko@tauex.tau.ac.il

S. Gaburro, S. Mandillo (eds.), *Home Cage Monitoring in Rodents: A Global Effort*,
https://doi.org/10.1007/978-3-032-19781-8_11

1-week training schools, two for novice and two for advanced users. It was decided early on that representatives of industry partners should join the roster of trainers to bring their expertise in specific HCM systems. It was also agreed that their contributions should be free of advertising or promotion of the companies and systems presented, and of course, of any negative comparisons between competing systems. A training school manual was drafted for future reference.

These structured educational programs helped reduce the learning curve for HCM use, facilitating adoption and use of this technology and saving time and resources for research institutions. Moreover, they fostered a collaborative community of both early career and established HCM users, along with an open collaboration between academia and industry, promoting knowledge exchange and continuing skill development.

The collection of trainees' feedback and prompt integration of necessary changes, along with a reflection on course contents and teaching approaches, allowed by a stable course faculty well-coordinated with the core project management team, were key to the courses' success. While there are several specificities of the courses relating to their subject—i.e. HCM systems—we believe that several conclusions laid out in this chapter are of general applicability and provide a template to guide future organizers of similar training events, either under the auspices of COST actions or another funding framework.

Keywords

Education and training · Knowledge transfer · Home cage monitoring · Standardization and reproducibility through training · 3Rs

1 Why Have Structured Education and Training in HCM?

Contemporary biomedical education and training programs shape the outcomes and capabilities of researchers and scientists, ultimately impacting scientific progress. Modern training could be divided into Broad vs. Specialized Graduate Biomedical Education and Training (Costello 2009). Both are needed when discussing training on unique systems such as those providing home cage monitoring (HCM). Broad teaching should provide the theoretical context for understanding the research needs and the collected data, while specialized training would provide the "know-how" to use the system and provide troubleshooting when needed.

HCM technologies represent a transformative advancement in behavioural research, enabling non-invasive, automated, and high-resolution data collection from laboratory animals, showing spontaneous behaviour without human interference, and allowing animals to perform the needed tasks voluntarily, under specific circumstances. However, the sophisticated equipment and software used in these systems impose a steep learning curve. Moreover, learning to use HCM systems through trial and error is not only time-consuming and resource-intensive, but can also potentially lead to unnecessary use of animals. Structured training programs can significantly ease this learning curve by providing clear, step-by-step instructions and opportunities for guided practice. Efficient training enables trainees to rapidly acquire operational independence, minimizing errors that could necessitate costly troubleshooting or equipment replacement or deter untrained researchers from adopting this technology. In research settings where time and resources are often constrained, this efficiency will translate into more streamlined workflows and higher productivity through the effective, ethical, and consistent use of HCM technology.

As with every scientific tool producing large datasets, there is a need to understand such data and to standardize its processing, analysis, and reporting, so protocols can be reproduced and results replicated (Lapchak and Zhang 2018; Gonzalez Soltero et al. 2024). Without adequate education and training, users may struggle with implementing and using HCM, risking suboptimal data acquisition, compromised animal welfare, and inefficient use of resources. These challenges might also deter untrained researchers from adopting this technology. Therefore, education and training in HCM systems are indispensable for equipping researchers with the knowledge and skills necessary to use these technologies effectively, ethically, and consistently.

While the theoretical concepts around home cage systems are applicable across different systems (e.g. PhenoTyper, Intellicage, or DVC), researchers must gain scientific and technical expertise in the specific HCM system they intend to use, as well as understand its potential and limitations. Each HCM system has various complex components, including sensors, video cameras, RFID tags, telemetry devices, and analysis software, each with distinct operational principles and limitations that are unique to that system. For example, the PhenoTyper cage system (Noldus systems) uses camera-based tracking technology, Intellicage (TSE systems) uses RFID tracking technology, and the DVC uses EMF capacitance sensors, making the technological training for each system completely different. Such systems, moreover, yield different datasets. Mastery of these technologies, moreover, requires theoretical knowledge of specific behaviours expected for each HCM environment and hands-on experience in assembling, upgrading, and troubleshooting such systems. Structured training programs ensure users are equipped to set up, calibrate, and maintain the equipment, optimizing its performance and reliability. Studies demonstrate that operator proficiency directly correlates with data accuracy, emphasizing the value of proper training in reducing errors during data collection and analysis (Srinivasan et al. 2021; Bau-Gaudreault et al. 2021). By understanding the nuances of each HCM component, users can avoid common pitfalls, such as miscalibration or improper maintenance, which could compromise research outcomes.[1] While invaluable, the continuous data streams generated by HCM systems are challenging to manage and interpret without specialized training. Education in experimental design, along with data handling and analysis,

[1] In this book, Chapter "From Sensors to Insights: Technologies for Home Cage Monitoring in Preclinical Research" presents details, pros/cons, and specific considerations on all the different HCM technologies that are available.

equips users with the skills to avoid commons sources of bias, apply appropriate filters, focus on relevant behaviours, and interpret patterns in ways aligned with their research objectives. This improves data validity and reliability, which is critical for drawing meaningful scientific conclusions. Training also reduces the likelihood of errors during data processing, which can skew results and lead to flawed interpretations. By fostering a thorough understanding of data workflows, training supports the production of scientifically robust outcomes that advance the field. An overview on HCM data management and analysis is presented in Chapter "Study Design and Data Analysis in Home Cage Monitoring Experiments" of this book.

Given how central ethical considerations are in animal research, as well as the direct impact of housing conditions on animal welfare, proper training should emphasize on the importance of minimizing stress and discomfort for the animals being studied. Users must hence learn to recognize how factors such as system placement, environmental noise, device calibration, and husbandry choices can affect animal well-being and, consequently, how they perform in behavioural tests. Training should also provide guidelines on how to maintain low-stress environments and mitigate potential stressors, ensuring compliance with ethical standards and welfare regulations. Such awareness is critical, as improper use of HCM technologies may unintentionally compromise animal welfare, undermining the primary goal of non-invasive monitoring.

Education and training also promote consistency in the use of HCM systems, as researchers trained in a harmonized way are more likely to adhere to established protocols, ensuring the comparability of their results and promoting reproducibility of research findings. Achieving such consistency enhances the credibility of HCM as a research tool, fostering collaborations among researchers and encouraging broader adoption of these technologies.

The successful adoption and use of HCM systems depend on comprehensive education and training that combine theoretical knowledge with practical expertise. By addressing the complexities of these advanced technologies, structured training programs equip researchers with the tools to navigate challenges, optimize data reliability, and maintain high ethical standards. These programs thus enhance individual proficiency, while promoting consistency and reproducibility across studies and fostering collaboration and broader acceptance of HCM technologies. With these foundational elements in place, the next step is to focus on the strategic selection of faculty and trainees, ensuring the effective delivery and dissemination of this critical knowledge.

2 Faculty and Target Audience

The selection of faculty members and trainees for a scientific training event is crucial to ensure meaningful learning and foster professional and personal interactions. Over years of designing training events, we identified key factors in faculty and trainee composition that optimize knowledge exchange and professional networking. When considering *faculty members* for a training event, it is best to start by discussing the several aspects of the event. First and most important is to define which are the goals of the training event, and based on this, determine what expertise is needed. For example, regarding home cage research methods, one should consider both commercial and do-it-yourself (DIY) systems. Hence, when planning the training events in the TEATIME COST Action initiative, we selected experts in three different commercial systems and added another scientist with a system he had designed and built. This combination of expertise allowed fostering discussion on the connection between the scientific question at hand and the right HCM system to answer it.

Another essential aspect to consider when selecting faculty is the *professional and social context of the experts*, as these will shape how trainees conceive, carry out, and interpret behavioural research. Experienced principal investigators (PIs) working in an academic environment can provide essential theoretical knowledge. Yet, core facility personnel work with varied researchers, animal models, and systems and are therefore exposed to a variety of methods and solutions that PIs are sometimes unaware of. The result is that, on many occasions, core facility personnel may have a higher level of expertise on HCM, animal facility logistics, research design, methodology, and data analysis and interpretation, so their inclusion in course faculty ensures that trainees gain a solid conceptual understanding of home cage systems, their potential applications, and how best to make use of them. However, while both established researchers and core facility personnel are essential to convey knowledge on relevant theoretical concepts and practical aspects of using these systems, it is graduate trainees, postdoctoral researchers, and other early career scientists who actively use them. Thus, incorporating early career scientists into the team of trainers can bring valuable practical first-hand experience, i.e. "real-life know-how", offering insight into real-world applications, troubleshooting, and workflow optimization, as well as greater proximity to trainees' own personal research experiences, questions, and frustrations, making them critical contributors to hands-on training sessions. With subsequent editions of training events, this subset of faculty can be made up of alumni of previous training events. *Alumni* can provide unique insights from the trainees' perspective, bridging the gap between faculty and trainees and improve the training events themselves through their constructive feedback. They also play a key role in promoting networking behaviour, facilitating professional connections, and supporting knowledge dissemination beyond the training event. Another potentially important group to include comprises *industry representatives*. These are the professionals from companies developing HCM technology, who can provide an understanding of the rationale behind system development, discuss technological advancements, the full body of applications of their systems, and highlight potential future directions. Their involvement also facilitates industry-academia interactions, fostering potential collaborations and ensuring academic users stay up to date with cutting-edge tools.

While the selection of faculty is key, it is equally important to identify and segment the *target audience* (see Table 1) for HCM training clearly. Distinguishing among different professional profiles allows tailoring the educational content, depth, and learning methods

Table 1 Target audiences for Home Cage Monitoring (HCM) training, their main challenges, and recommended focus areas

Audience group	Main needs and challenges	Recommended training focus
Animal technicians	Daily operation of HCM systems, animal handling, welfare assessment, and technical maintenance	Hands-on sessions on calibration, welfare monitoring, troubleshooting, and recognition of stress behaviours
Early career scientists (PhD students, postdocs)	Understanding system capabilities, data interpretation, and experimental design	Theoretical background, data analysis workshops, study design exercises, and networking with peers
Senior scientists / principal investigators	Strategic implementation of HCM in research programs, supervision of projects	Modules on experimental design, reproducibility, and integration of HCM data into larger research frameworks
Facility managers and core staff	System logistics, scheduling, equipment upkeep, training others	Operational planning, protocol standardization, and managing multi-user environments

to meet their specific needs. The following segmentation provides a framework for designing targeted training programs:

The table outlines distinct participant groups and highlights their specific educational needs and practical training priorities, providing a framework for designing role-appropriate HCM training programs. Recognizing these distinct roles enhances the overall impact of training by ensuring trainees receive content directly applicable to their daily responsibilities.

The next key aspect to consider when selecting participants is *heterogeneity* versus homogeneity, referring to the composition within the group of trainees. We would argue that an effective training event requires a well-balanced and strategically selected group of trainees to ensure engagement, knowledge retention, and post-training impact. In fact, choosing the right mixture of trainees might indeed contribute more to the success of a course than the selection of faculty members. Something worth considering is having at least two trainees from the same institution, to encourage collaboration and knowledge-sharing upon returning to their home institutions. Another suggestion is that, when courses are delivered at introductory and advanced levels, alumni from the introductory course could be integrated into the advanced course to facilitate newcomers' active participation, lead group activities, and improve networking.

It is also important to consider giving preference to *trainees with higher potential to apply and disseminate* what they have learned. In that sense, including first-year PhD trainees will have more impact than last-year PhD trainees, with the same applying to researchers in leadership roles, core facilities' staff, and individuals responsible for implementing home cage monitoring within their organizations. In addition, the audience should include researchers from various fields, such as behavioural neuroscience, pharmacology, toxicology, physiology, or computational biology. A multidisciplinary group allows discussions on the added value of home cage systems across different scientific contexts, experimental setups, and technical demands, enhancing the audience's understanding of their broad applicability and potential. For both types of courses, priority was given to course applicants who were already working—or soon to be working—with HCM technologies.

Another vital point to consider is that training events are important for *networking* and creating sustainable connections that can benefit both faculty and audience. Breakout sessions, hand-on demonstrations, Q&A sessions, as well as coffee breaks and dinner events are all great opportunities for networking. At the TEATIME training events, the addition of deliberately long coffee-breaks, social dinners, and a recommended hotel for all to stay at were strategies designed to spark social interaction. Such structured interactions between faculty, alumni, and trainees facilitate the development of professional networks, leading to future research partnerships and technological advancements. These include deliberate actions by faculty members to actively engage with trainees during breaks, asking about their work, connecting them with other trainees and faculty members working on similar problems, and breaking up clusters of people from the same country and institutions. From faculty to industry and trainees, all should understand the value given to the social and professional networking aspects of the training event. And, selecting faculty members with the skills to encourage social communication between and with trainees will contribute to foster social interaction from the first moment and establish the success of the training event years onwards.

Beyond trainees and faculty selection, careful attention to *logistical arrangements* is crucial for a seamless and productive training event. A central venue, ideally within an academic setting, fosters an engaging learning environment while ensuring access to necessary facilities. Nearby accommodations, preferably in a single hotel, encourage informal interactions between faculty and trainees, enhancing networking and collaboration. Thoughtful catering, provided in the vicinity (to avoid wandering about and delays after breaks, to maximize the time allowed for networking), should accommodate dietary restrictions, including allergies, religious preferences, and budget-friendly options for trainees, ensuring inclusivity. Training rooms must be well-equipped and suited for both theoretical and practical sessions, while strategically located coffee breaks provide essential opportunities for discussion. Faculty availability should be maximized, with incentives, where possible, to ensure their full participation. Additionally, having a dedicated person on call for technical issues can prevent disruptions and optimize learning time.

The success of scientific training events, such as those held by TEATIME on HCM systems, depends heavily on the *thoughtful selection* of location, faculty, and trainees, with special attention to diversity (e.g. gender balance, geographic diversity, early career vs. senior scientists). By balancing theoretical expertise, practical experience, and diverse perspectives, training programs can optimize knowledge transfer, foster professional networks, and ensure long-term impact. While a diverse faculty integrating experienced researchers, early career scientists, and industry representatives provides a holistic learning experience, a strategically selected, multidisciplinary audience maximizes engagement and knowledge dissemination. With a strong foundation in faculty and trainee selection, the next critical step is to define clear learning outcomes that are based on faculty abilities and audience needs and abilities, while adopting effective educational approaches to ensure the training achieves its goals.

When considering training initiatives in HCM, the planning programme should be *adaptable* to diverse institutional, cultural, and economic settings. The following principles ensure transferability and sustainability:

1. *Scalability*: Depending on available resources and support from the host organization, design modular content that can be implemented as 1-day workshops or extended training schools.
2. *Accessibility:* Use blended learning formats (onsite + online) to widen participation across geographic regions. On-site training has its advantages, but if your potential audience is spread across different locations or even organizations, bringing them all to one location can be challenging.
3. *Cross-disciplinary Collaboration*: Involve professionals from behaviour, physiology, data science, and ethics to ensure integrative training. Proper integration of information from different disciplines is a key feature to effective research, especially in research tools such as HCS.
4. *Industry-Academia Partnerships*: Encourage collaboration while maintaining transparency and neutrality regarding commercial systems. Each one controls vital information for the other. While academia can assist industry in understanding the future of new developments, industry can help academic users better understand how to use the system, including troubleshooting information, the development process, and how different users utilize the system.
5. *Feedback-driven Improvement*: Use structured post-course evaluations and alumni feedback loops to refine future training events. Users are at the forefront of science, testing the limitations of the tools and pointing out the need for developing new ones. Communication with our audience could provide crucial information and fine-tune our programme.

These recommendations are the result of our combined experience from the TEATIME-COST Action initiative, as well as our unique insights gained from our own courses and workshops.

3 Learning Outcomes and Educational Approaches

The learning outcomes (see Table 2) for this training programme reflect a comprehensive approach to equipping trainees with the theoretical knowledge, technical proficiency, and ethical grounding necessary for using home cage monitoring (HCM) systems. By integrating lectures, hands-on training, data analysis workshops, and interactive discussions, the programme ensures trainees can effectively apply HCM methodologies to achieve reliable, ethical, and reproducible research outcomes.

The Table 2 summarizes the main learning outcomes for the TEATIME courses and the educational approaches designed to aid trainees achieve them.

The table summarizes the main theoretical and practical objectives of the training, illustrating how different instructional formats—lectures, workshops, and

Table 2 Core learning outcomes and corresponding educational approaches in the TEATIME Home Cage Monitoring training schools

Learning outcome	Approach
Explain the ethical challenges concerning the use of animals	Lecture on animal ethics and the 3Rs Lecture on the advantages and limitations of current animal models and tests
Apply the 3Rs and ethical principles in the context of HCM research	Lectures and discussions on minimizing stress during monitoring, optimizing housing conditions, and complying with welfare regulations. Discussion on how HCM can further the 3Rs
Explain behaviour by integrating genetic, evolutionary, anatomical, sensory, physiological, developmental, social, and environmental factors	Lectures and discussions on the fundamental principles of behaviour, key research findings, and the various genetic, physiological, environmental, and social factors that influence animal behaviour. (e.g. also adding "meet the experts" interactive sessions)
Describe the theoretical and practical foundations of HCM systems	Lectures on the principles of HCM, including their advantages and challenges, compared to traditional behavioural tests
Design robust and reproducible HCM experiments	Experimental design lecture emphasizing randomization, blinding, sample size calculation, and the avoidance of common pitfalls in research design Scenario-based group work (e.g. for identifying flaws in experiments, selecting an appropriate design, calculate an adequate sample size)
Assemble, calibrate, and troubleshoot HCM systems	Hands-on workshops focusing on real-time monitoring, calibration, and system setup (e.g. "design and print a home cage system" and system-specific demonstrations of HCM systems: PhenoTyper, IntelliCage, and live mouse tracker
Analyse and interpret high-dimensional data generated by HCM systems	Data analysis lectures and workshops exploring statistical approaches, software tools, and advanced techniques for integrating multimodal datasets
Compare strengths and limitations between commercial and home-made HCM systems	Industry-led sessions (e.g. "meet company X") and comparative discussions on home-made and commercial systems
Collaborate effectively within multidisciplinary teams	Interactive sessions, planned networking opportunities, and follow-up training events to strengthen collaborative practices
Implement proper data handling, quality control, and storage practices for HCM	Introductory sessions for all levels on raw data labelling, storage, and metadata management; advanced workshops on data QC, error detection, preprocessing pipelines, and ethical data sharing following FAIR principles

discussions—support skill acquisition and ethical understanding. Ethical principles and the 3Rs (Replacement, Reduction, Refinement) are not separate from HCM training; they are deeply embedded within every stage of it. HCM technologies themselves offer opportunities to enhance animal welfare by minimizing handling, stress, and experimental variability (as described in Chapter "Enhancing Animal Welfare Through Home Cage Monitoring Systems" of this book). Training programs should therefore:

- Integrate ethical reflection into every module, not only as a theoretical lecture but as a practical mindset guiding experiment design and execution. HCM systems should be considered a viable solution that could replace some methods deemed unacceptable by ethics committees today.
- Present case studies demonstrating how HCM data can reveal welfare-related behaviours and guide refinement.
- Encourage trainees to identify ways in which automated systems can reduce animal numbers and improve data quality simultaneously.

Connect explicitly with ethical frameworks presented in other chapters (notably Chapters "Enhancing Animal Welfare Through Home Cage Monitoring Systems" and "The Most Used Rodent Models in Home Cage Monitoring").

Embedding ethics and the 3Rs into HCM training ensures that technological advancement and moral responsibility evolve hand in hand.

Data generated by HCM systems are inherently high-dimensional, continuous, and complex, encompassing behavioural, environmental, and physiological variables that together can reach terabyte-scale volumes. Even apparently simple measures, such as distance travelled, can provide insights not only into motor function but also into motivation, habituation to novel environments, circadian patterns, and welfare-related parameters. This richness, while scientifically valuable, creates significant challenges for data management, storage, and quality control.

For this reason, training programs must explicitly address data stewardship; more specifically, how to organize, label, store, and share datasets in accordance with FAIR data principles (Findable, Accessible, Interoperable, and Reusable; Gonzalez Soltero et al. 2024). Basic instruction should include practical guidance on file naming conventions, metadata annotation, and raw data storage solutions, particularly for large-scale video and sensor data. These topics are essential for novice users, regardless of whether they are technicians, graduate students, or principal investigators, as proper data handling practices ensure reproducibility and prevent information loss. For a detailed dissertation about these principles, see Chapter "Data Sharing and Metadata" of this book.

In addition, data quality control (QC) and integrity assurance must be integrated into advanced training. This includes identifying outliers and missing data, recognizing artifacts caused by system calibration errors, and applying standardized pre-processing workflows. Training at this level should also familiarize participants with current tools and software used for data validation, as well as approaches for secure and ethical data sharing across institutions. As highlighted by Lapchak and Zhang (2018), data quality management is critical to ensure that experimental conclusions are scientifically valid and ethically defensible.

While technicians may not perform detailed analyses, they must understand how their handling and system setup affect data quality. Conversely, postdoctoral researchers and data analysts need hands-on experience in managing, curating, and analysing raw datasets. Incorporating dedicated modules on data QC, storage, and sharing thus enhances the overall scientific rigor and transparency of HCM-based research.

While it is desirable that trainees acquire a strong theoretical basis that will allow them to autonomously plan, execute, and interpret HCM in research, the greatest advantage of face-to-face training courses comprises the practical, *hands-on sessions*, ensuring that trainees can independently set up, calibrate, and troubleshoot HCM systems. These sessions can include real-time monitoring exercises, demonstrations, or system assembling and servicing workshops. Through hands-on practice and guidance from tutors, trainees can develop more confidence to apply HCM in future studies. Building on our combined training experience, we propose a structured curriculum organized into three progressive levels, novice, intermediate, and advanced, designed to support career-long skill development in HCM research (See Table 3).

Such structured progression ensures consistency while allowing flexibility for adaptation across institutions, audience groups (as mentioned above), and contexts. The curriculum can serve as a template for designing both short courses and long-term academic programs (See Table 3).

The table summarizes the core learning objectives, principal activities, and example topics corresponding to each trainee level, illustrating how HCM education evolves from basic operational understanding to advanced experimental design, data analysis, and ethical integration.

Table 3 Learning progression from novice to advanced levels in Home Cage Monitoring (HCM) training

Level	Core learning objectives	Key activities	Example topics
Novice	Understand the theoretical foundations and basic operations of HCM systems	Introductory lectures, demonstrations, guided practical sessions	Principles of HCM, introduction to system components, data types, and animal welfare basics
Intermediate	Apply HCM methods in experimental design and data analysis	Group work, hands-on calibration, troubleshooting, and data processing workshops	Experimental design, data handling, statistical approaches, and identifying artifacts
Advanced	Innovate, optimize, and supervise HCM-based studies	Case-study discussions, multi-system integration, data reproducibility analysis	Advanced analytics, multi-system comparison, data management, and ethical considerations

4 Post-Training Support and Resources

The success of any training programme or school depends not only of the event itself but also on what follows. Training has a lasting impact when learners retain what they have learned, build on it, and stay connected with their peers. This requires post-training support, through knowledgeable people and well-curated educational resources, that will sustain scientific exchange and ongoing learning and professional development.

4.1 Key Individuals: Sustaining Knowledge Through Dialogue

Maintaining communication with key individuals is crucial for reinforcing and expanding on what has been learned. These interactions provide invaluable guidance and support when facing challenges. The main post-training contacts include:

- *Principal Investigators (PIs)*—While not always the most accessible, PIs play a crucial role in post-training education. Ideally, they should be actively involved in knowledge transfer, not just in theory but also in hands-on applications. Former trainees have highlighted the importance of PI engagement, especially in understanding the practical aspects of behavioural tests and home cage monitoring (HCM) systems in daily lab work.
- *Core Personnel and Technicians*—These individuals are instrumental in the practical application of training content. Maintaining an ongoing exchange of knowledge with them is essential for troubleshooting and refining methodologies related to animal handling, experimental tests, and monitoring systems.
- *Industry Representatives*—Establishing an open dialogue with scientific managers and technical support teams from HCM system providers is critical for correctly implementing training insights. These industry experts also help improve tools and protocols by integrating user feedback.
- *Faculty Members from the School*—Instructors and guest lecturers remain a valuable resource even after the training event. They can provide further clarification, answer questions, and act as connectors between different stakeholders, fostering an ongoing exchange of expertise.
- *Fellow Trainees*—Maintaining contact with peers from the training programme is crucial for mutual support and collaboration. These connections often lead to shared problem-solving, technical discussions, and career advice. A notable example from past programs is the spontaneous creation of alumni chat groups, which continue to facilitate discussions and collaborations long after the event.

Collectively, these key individuals contribute to an expanding professional network and build a community dedicated to home cage monitoring and behavioural research. This network, one of the primary goals of the TEATIME COST Action, continues to grow and strengthen over time. Proof is the enthusiastic engagement of former trainees in leading the Action new activities and participating in following training events as faculty members, as well as the Behaviour Forum (https://www.thebehaviourforum.org/) established by TEATIME course faculty and alumni.

4.2 Educational Materials: Enhancing Knowledge Through Reference

In addition to maintaining professional connections, having access to relevant educational materials ensures the longevity and effectiveness of training. Some of the most valuable resources include:

- TEATIME Behaviour Forum—A platform for discussions, knowledge exchange, and updates in the field (TEATIME n.d.)
- Protocols, Manuals, Tutorials, and Online Resources.
- Comprehensive Catalogue and Protocols for widely used HCM systems (available through the TEATIME website and other sources; TEATIME n.d.)
- Instruction manuals and tutorials available on company websites for specific systems (e.g. Spink et al. 2001; Noldus et al. 2002).
- Webinars and online training sessions providing further insights into HCM applications (TEATIME COST Action n.d.)
- Scientific Literature and Bibliography Reviews and research articles discussing the application of HCM systems in various fields such as sleep research, neurodegeneration, animal welfare, developmental studies, and drug screening (e.g. Kahnau et al. 2023; Moore et al. 2024; NC3Rs 2023).
- Additional materials provided during the training programme or recommended by faculty and key individuals afterward.

Dialogue with key individuals and access to educational materials are crucial for sustaining training impact. Ongoing discussions and reference to quality materials help trainees, faculty, and industry professionals to continuously deepen their understanding and use of HCM systems. This also supports broader knowledge dissemination, enabling future trainees and colleagues to benefit from shared expertise.

5 "And What About the Next-Time?"—Improving from One Training Event to the Next

Planning for future events should start with critically assessing the previous one. This involves examining the added value of each session, the quality of networking opportunities, and the effectiveness of each talk from both the speakers' and trainees' perspectives. This feedback from both faculty and trainees—surveys, personal discussions, own notes during the course—will ground a continuous improvement process. Key questions to guide this evaluation include: Which lessons/sections in the training course should be included or excluded in the next iteration? Was the content delivered in the most effective manner? And crucially, what was missing, i.e. what did trainees need, expect, but did not receive?

A notable example of this reflective process comes from the adjustments made between the first and second TEATIME training schools. One of the most frequent comments from trainees was the need to facilitate networking earlier and enable speakers to tailor their talks to the trainees' needs. To address this, we replaced 3 h of the first day with brief 5-min trainee presentations, where attendees introduced themselves, shared their research focus, and outlined their expectations. Although allocating such a significant portion of the first day to introductions might seem excessive, this change had a profound impact. Networking began immediately, evidently as early as the first coffee break, and speakers were able to readily incorporate specific references and ad hoc advice during their lessons, catering to trainees' specific needs.

6 Assessment and Certification

One way to ensure the long-term effectiveness of HCM training is to implement systematic assessment and certification procedures.

Assessment Methods

- *Knowledge Evaluation:* Pre- and post-course questionnaires to measure knowledge gain.
- *Practical Assessment:* Observation during hands-on sessions to evaluate technical proficiency.
- *Project-Based Evaluation:* Short applied projects or data analyses demonstrating integration of theory and practice.
- *Feedback Surveys:* Trainee self-assessment and faculty evaluation to improve course structure.

Certification Pathways

Establishing a recognized certification framework could enhance professional credibility and standardization across Europe and beyond. Certificates could reflect levels of competence (basic, intermediate, advanced) and be endorsed by scientific or ethical bodies (e.g. FELASA, COST, or institutional training centres). This step would help formalize expertise and motivate participation, contributing to standardization in the field, accelerating the development of different systems, and ensuring better replicability between and within different organizations in the future.

7 Conclusion

Education and training in HCM technologies are foundational to their effective application in research settings. By fostering technical proficiency, ensuring data quality, promoting ethical awareness, enhancing efficiency, standardizing practices, and supporting continuing education and training, training programs maximize the potential of HCM systems. These programs not only empower researchers to leverage these advanced technologies, but also contribute to the broader goals of scientific rigor, reproducibility, and ethical responsibility in animal research.

In this chapter, we outlined the key components of designing and delivering an effective training programme (see Fig. 1). We began by addressing the critical question of why training is needed, emphasizing the importance of bridging knowledge gaps or advancing novel methods and technologies for the target audience. From there, we explored the process of selecting faculty and trainees, acknowledging that while options may sometimes be limited—such as when faculty are restricted to a single instructor or the audience consists of internal trainees—understanding the composition and dynamics of the group is essential. This foundation informs the next step: defining learning outcomes and determining the appropriate educational approach, whether hands-on, theoretical, or a combination of both. Finally, we highlighted how the training experience shapes post-training resource

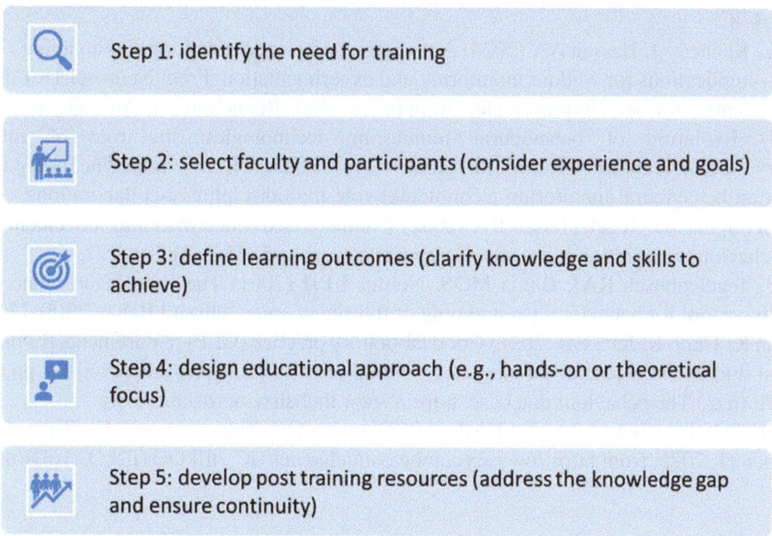

Fig. 1 Flow chart of the different steps to design a new training school

development. By conducting training, educators gain a deeper understanding of the audience's needs and knowledge gaps, allowing them to design follow-up materials and support systems that reinforce learning and encourage continuous skill development. This flow—starting from the purpose of training and ending with long-term resource creation—ensures not only the immediate success of the training but also its sustained impact on advancing expertise and innovation within the field.

Declaration of Interests The authors of this chapter are scientists committed to the well-being of even the smallest living beings. Hence, the suffering of innocent people, including in the Middle East, concerns us deeply. We hope that the principles underpinning good science, reason, cooperation, honesty, and transparency, may also guide efforts towards justice, peace, and the protection of human life.

References

Bau-Gaudreault L, Arndt T, Provencher A, Brayton CF (2021) Relevant clinical pathology resources: emphasis on mice, rats, rabbits, dogs, minipigs, and non-human primates. ILAR J 62(1–2):203–222

Costello LC (2009) Perspective: the effect of contemporary education and training of biomedical scientists on present and future medical research. Acad Med 84(4):459–463

Gonzalez Soltero R, Pino García D, Bellido A, Ryan P, Rodríguez-Learte AI (2024) FAIR data management: a framework for fostering data literacy in biomedical sciences education. BMC Med Res Methodol 24(1):284

Kahnau P, Mieske P, Wilzopolski J, Kalliokoski O, Mandillo S, Hölter SM et al (2023) A systematic review of the development and application of home cage monitoring in laboratory mice and rats. BMC Biol 21(1):256

Lapchak PA, Zhang JH (2018) Data standardization and quality management. Transl Stroke Res 9:4–8

Moore JL, Kennedy J, Hassan AA (2024) Automated home cage monitoring of an aging colony of mice—implications for welfare monitoring and experimentation. Front Neurosci 18:1489308

National Centre for the Replacement, Refinement and Reduction of Animals in Research (2023) Evolution of behavioural monitoring technologies: the role of multidisciplinary collaborations. Retrieved June 11, 2025, from https://nc3rs.org.uk/news/evolution-behavioural-monitoring-technologies-role-multidisciplinary-collaborations

Noldus LP, Spink AJ, Tegelenbosch RA (2002) Computerised video tracking, movement analysis and behaviour recognition in insects. Comput Electron Agric 35(2–3):201–227

Spink AJ, Tegelenbosch RAJ, Buma MOS, Noldus LPJJ (2001) The EthoVision video tracking system—a tool for behavioral phenotyping of transgenic mice. Physiol Behav 73(5):731–744

Srinivasan K, Tikoo K, Jena GB (2021) Good laboratory practice (GLP) requirements for preclinical animal studies. In: Essentials of laboratory animal science: principles and practices, pp 655–677

TEATIME (n.d.) The behaviour database. https://www.thebehaviourdatabase.org

TEATIME COST Action (n.d.) TEATIME COST Action [YouTube channel]. YouTube. Retrieved October 31, 2025, from https://www.youtube.com/channel/UC_4tIkOQsT2kOA1uDRum5SA

Sharing the Knowledge: Communication and Dissemination

Maša Čater and Sabine M. Hölter

Abstract

All the great potential of home cage monitoring (HCM) will remain unrealised if the knowledge about its value is not communicated and disseminated efficiently via appropriate channels to the relevant target audiences. This chapter explains why effective communication and widespread dissemination are so important and describes in detail who are relevant stakeholders, what messages they need to hear, which channels are appropriate for which audience, which tools to use (including AI-driven storytelling), what efforts are involved, and how to evaluate the impact of your communication activities. The necessity of understanding target audiences and tailoring messages, media, and formats accordingly are highlighted. Using examples and case studies, we demonstrate why such efforts are worth it and how they can contribute not only to increased acceptance and funding support for HCM, but also to building public trust in animal research. The goal of this chapter is to help the reader understand that for any technical or scientific development *to have an impact*, efficient sharing of the new knowledge with relevant audiences is a prerequisite. We will explain in detail in the following subchapters:

1. The effects efficient communication can have on stakeholders, and what are the negative consequences of inadequate communication (see section "Consequences of Inadequate Communication")
2. What dissemination channels are available and how to use them strategically

M. Čater (✉)
University of Ljubljana, Biotechnical Faculty, Ljubljana, Slovenia
e-mail: Masa.Cater@bf.uni-lj.si

S. M. Hölter
Helmholtz Munich, German Research Centre for Environmental Health, Neuherberg, Germany

S. Gaburro, S. Mandillo (eds.), *Home Cage Monitoring in Rodents: A Global Effort*,
https://doi.org/10.1007/978-3-032-19781-8_12

3. The importance of identifying relevant target audiences, understanding their needs, and tailoring messages and communication channels to every single one of them
4. Which communication tools and techniques are most effective
5. Typical challenges encountered in communication
6. Examples of successful communication strategies
7. How to use collaboration as multiplier
8. How to monitor the effectiveness of communication
9. What are the next steps for HCM communication

Keywords

Stakeholders · Target audience · Message framing · Outreach · Public trust

1 Importance of Communication of HCM

Technological advances such as home cage monitoring (HCM) systems represent a paradigm shift in the way we study, understand, and care for laboratory animals. However, the potential of these systems cannot be fully realised without effective communication and dissemination strategies. At a time when scientific transparency, ethical responsibility, and interdisciplinary collaboration are increasingly coming to the fore, communication around HCM plays a central role in driving scientific progress, improving animal welfare, and increasing public confidence (Hölter et al. 2023; Hurst and West 2010).

1.1 Promoting Animal Welfare by Raising Awareness

One of the most immediate and impactful contributions of HCM systems is their ability to improve animal welfare. Through continuous, non-invasive observation of animal behaviour in their familiar environment, HCM reduces the stress caused by human intervention and repetitive handling (Spruijt and Devisser 2006; Richardson 2015). In addition, early detection of abnormal behaviour or health problems facilitates rapid intervention, minimizing animal suffering and improving experimental outcomes (Voikar and Gaburro 2020). However, the potential of HCM for animal welfare can only be fully realised if its capabilities and benefits are clearly communicated to those responsible for the care and supervision of animals—veterinarians, animal technicians, researchers, and institutional animal care and use committees (Fig. 1). If these stakeholders understand how HCM contributes to improvement, they are more likely to advocate for its implementation and integration into standard practice (Morton 2000).

In addition, it is crucial to communicate the improvements in animal welfare obtainable by HCM outside the laboratory. The public is increasingly demanding higher ethical standards in animal research, as evidenced by the "Modernise science" demand in the recent

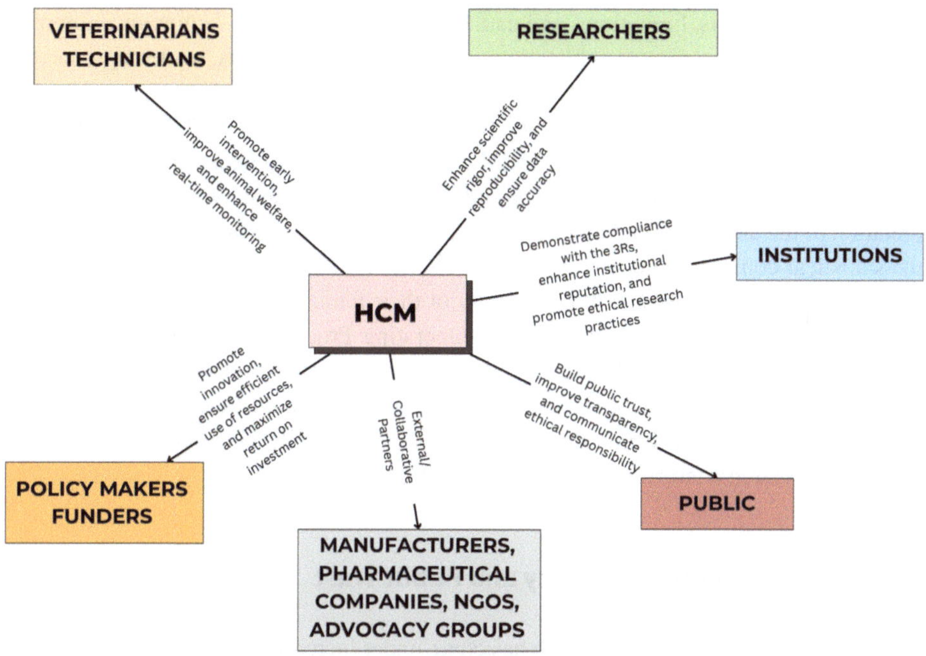

Fig. 1 Stakeholder communication benefits of HCM systems. HCM—home cage monitoring

European Citizen Initiative Save Cruelty Free Cosmetics—Commit to a Europe Without Animal Testing (Initiative 2023). Demonstrating the potential for improvement of HCM systems through transparent and proactive communication can help address societal concerns and promote a more informed dialog about the role of animal models in biomedical research (Pound and Blaug 2016). Most importantly, it helps to build public trust (see Fig. 1), which is also important for policy makers and funders, as they prefer to act in line with the perceived public opinion. Moreover, if the latter understand the innovative technological advances of HCM and how its use can enhance the efficient use of resources and maximise their return on investment, they are more incentivised to support and fund it.

1.2 Promoting Scientific Progress and Reproducibility

Scientific progress depends on accurate data, reproducibility, and innovation. HCM systems provide comprehensive and detailed behavioural data that can reveal previously undetectable phenotypic differences, enable longitudinal studies, and reduce observer bias. They enable more reliable behavioural and physiological measurements, particularly in areas such as circadian rhythms, social interactions, and subtle disease progression (Kahnau et al. 2023). However, for these innovations to be widely adopted and effectively applied, researchers need to be made aware not only of the existence of HCM technology, but also of its benefits, limitations, and data handling requirements. Communication plays a key role here: peer-reviewed publications, conference presentations, workshops, and collaborative networks (such as the COST Action 20,135 TEATIME) help to disseminate best practice and promote knowledge sharing (Prescott and Lidster 2017; COST 2021).

Inadequate communication about HCM can not only lead to underutilisation and thus stall scientific progress, but also to reproducibility issues because of misuse or misinterpretation of the data generated by these systems. For example, researchers unfamiliar with the statistical considerations of continuous behavioural data may draw incorrect conclusions, which could undermine the credibility of their findings (Voelkl and Würbel 2016). A lack of communication about Standard Operating Procedures for HCM can lead to reproducibility issues due to different vendor implementations, inconsistent parameter settings, or varied analysis approaches. Efficient communication, training resources, and open dialog can mitigate these risks and support the responsible and effective use of HCM in various research contexts (Hohlbaum et al. 2017).

1.3 Improving Transparency and Public Trust

The ethical use of animals in research has come under increasing scrutiny in recent years. Mistrust can easily arise when the public perceives a lack of transparency, unnecessary harm to animals, or a reliance on outdated practices (Ormandy et al. 2013). One way to address these concerns is through clear, open communication about technological advances, such as the use of HCM systems. HCM technology plays a critical role in minimizing stress, improving animal welfare, and improving the quality of scientific data, which directly aligns with the 3Rs principle (Russell and Burch 1959). HCM systems specifically support the principle of refinement by reducing the need for repeated animal testing, enabling earlier humane endpoints and improving the overall welfare of animals involved in research. Institutions can demonstrate these ethical improvements with concrete examples of how HCM systems contribute to more humane and effective research practices (Spruijt and Devisser 2006; Pound and Blaug 2016). It is important that researchers and institutions disseminate these advances not only through traditional scientific channels, such as peer-reviewed journals, but also through more accessible platforms. Social media, blogs, institutional websites, newsletters, and outreach campaigns provide opportunities to reach a wider audience and inform the public about ethical advances in animal research. In this way, researchers can promote a more balanced and evidence-based understanding of the ethical considerations in animal research (EARA 2025).

Moreover, communication should not be limited to a reactive response to criticism. Waiting until concerns arise can lead to misunderstandings that ultimately damage public trust. Instead, it is important to be proactive and engage in consistent, transparent, and honest dialog. This includes acknowledging the challenges and limitations of animal research, which helps to build long-term credibility and strengthen trust in the scientific community (Pound and Blaug 2016; Mcleod and Hobson-West 2016).

1.4 Consequences of Inadequate Communication

Inadequate communication about HCM systems can have several negative consequences for both scientific progress and public perception. One important problem is the risk of mistrust and misunderstanding. If stakeholders or the public are not properly informed about how and why HCM systems are used, they may perceive them as intrusive surveillance tools. This misunderstanding could lead people to view HCM systems as contributing to depersonalised animal care, rather than seeing them as technologies designed to improve animal welfare and research outcomes (Ormandy et al. 2013).

In addition to risking mistrust, poor communication can also lead to missed opportunities. Institutions that fail to clearly articulate the value and impact of their public health work may miss out on important funding, collaborative partnerships, or valuable scientific insights that could accelerate progress in animal welfare and research practices (Collins and Tabak 2014). Without clear communication, researchers are less likely to use HCM systems in their work. If the benefits of HCM are not well communicated or researchers do not know how to interpret the data or how to use the associated software, they may remain hesitant or sceptical about incorporating these systems into their experimental protocols (Kahnau et al. 2023).

Finally, there is the potential risk of ethical backlash. Misconceptions about animal monitoring technologies such as the HCM may contribute to broader public opinion about unethical animal treatment. If the public is under the impression that HCM is replacing human observation and care, rather than supporting these efforts, this may fuel concerns about the ethical implications of such technologies and undermine trust in animal research overall (Pound and Blaug 2016). Therefore, effective communication about the purpose and benefits of HCM is crucial to ensure ethical acceptance, promote scientific progress, and secure support from key stakeholders.

1.5 Communicating the 3Rs

The principles of the 3Rs in animal research, replacement, reduction, and refinement, have first been articulated by Russell and Burch in 1959 (Russell and Burch 1959). They provide a framework for performing more humane animal research that has been codified in Europe in Directive 2010/63/EU on the protection of animals used for scientific purposes (see (Directive 2010)). The Directive demands the replacement of the use of animals by other methods wherever possible, and where this is not possible, the minimisation of the number of animals used (reduction) as well as the minimisation of their distress or pain (refinement). According to the website of NC3Rs, "Opinion polls of public attitudes consistently show that support for animal research is conditional on the 3Rs being put into practice" (Nc3rs 2025). Thus, compliance with the 3Rs is not only a legal requirement in animal research, but communication about it also promotes public acceptance.

HCM is a clear example of how refinement, often the biggest challenge in implementing the 3Rs, can be realised through technological innovation. By reducing the need for invasive procedures, enabling humane endpoints, and providing 24/7 insights into animal welfare, HCM supports multiple dimensions of refinement (Spruijt and Devisser 2006; Voikar and Gaburro 2020). In addition, more accurate data and reduced variability may lead to a reduction in animal numbers as fewer animals are required to achieve statistical significance (Kahnau et al. 2023). While HCM does not directly contribute to animal replacement, the rich behavioural data it provides can complement or enhance in silico and in vitro modelling efforts and ultimately contribute to the overall need for fewer animal models and fewer experiments with live animals, as explained in more detail in (Sillito et al. 2025). To ensure that these benefits are understood, it is critical to integrate the information how HCM contributes to the 3Rs into all communications about HCM, whether directed at funders, ethics committees, or the general public.

2 Dissemination Channels

Effective dissemination of the applications and benefits of HCM systems necessitates a thoughtful, multi-faceted dissemination strategy. A single medium cannot reach all the stakeholders (scientists and veterinarians, policy makers, funders, and the public) so one needs to utilise multiple platforms. Choosing the right dissemination medium depends on the audience, the degree of complexity of the message, the degree of interaction sought, and available resources.

2.1 Traditional Academic Channels

Peer-reviewed journals continue to be the cornerstone of scientific communication because they are essential to the reproducibility and credibility of research results. Publishing research in reputable journals not only guarantees research is rigorously reviewed, but also guarantees transparency and best-practice development and is key to secure future funding. For HCM systems, publication in reputable journals guarantees standards for consistent and reliable use. Particularly, open access journals bear a crucial burden because they allow the dissemination of research results at no cost to a wider spectrum of people like researchers, practitioners, and ethics administrators. Laboratory animal science, animal behaviour, or biomedical innovation journals are particularly important for engaging the scientific community and inspiring ethical use of animals (Kilkenny et al. 2010).

Symposia and congresses, such as those organised by FELASA (Federation of European Laboratory Animal Science Associations), AALAS (American Association for Laboratory Animal Science), LASA (Laboratory Animal Science Association), FENS (Federation of European Neuroscience Societies), and the Society for Neuroscience, are a great platform for face-to-face communication, networking, and real-time feedback. These conferences bring together experts, researchers, and practitioners and offer the opportunity to exchange novel findings, protocols, or innovative applications related to HCM technologies. Oral presentations, posters, and panel debates offer the opportunity to communicate novel research findings, provoke critical discussion, and demonstrate the practical impact of HCM systems on animal welfare and research quality.

Workshops and webinars are invaluable training and education resources. They provide an interactive platform where the participants can discuss at length, witness practical demonstrations, and interact directly with experts and users. These platforms fill the gap between theory and practice and facilitate the transfer of skills and knowledge. For example, the COST Action 20,135 TEATIME regularly held workshops that not only disseminated the latest information on HCM technologies but also facilitated interdisciplinary collaboration (COST 2021). Such events provide researchers across disciplines the opportunity to share experiences, share challenges, and exchange best practices, thereby opening the doors to the wider implementation and proper use of HCM systems.

2.2 Digital and Open Access Platforms

Preprint servers such as bioRxiv and Research Square provide an effective means for researchers to quickly share their findings with the scientific community before being formally peer-reviewed. This model accelerates release of new data and facilitates early comment by the wider scientific community. In allowing researchers to make their work openly available, preprint servers enable promotion of transparency of research and encourage collaborative refinement. Such servers are particularly beneficial in communicating interim results or material that could benefit from community suggestions prior to formal publication, accelerating overall advance of scientific research (Tennant et al. 2016; Piwowar et al. 2007).

Project web sites and institutional repositories are necessary for archiving and making available important resources such as protocols, SOPs, and datasets related to HCM systems. These web sites are not only a repository of knowledge, but also an open and trustworthy source of information for researchers, regulators, and other stakeholders. They prove particularly valuable within joint or state-funded research due to the fact that they guarantee protocols and information are freely provided for inspection, replication, and further analysis, therefore ensuring research reproducibility and integrity (Piwowar et al. 2007; re3data.org 2025).

Further on, computer training modules and teaching videos, either offered by research institutions, equipment manufacturers, or consortia, present a cost-effective means of overcoming knowledge gaps and providing for uniform application of HCM technologies among various research facilities. These digital materials enable scientists to learn in their own timeframe, enabling the standardisation of the application of HCM systems within institutions. Through provision of simple, accessible instructions and demonstrations, web platforms enable a more knowledgeable and capable research base and ensure proper and consistent utilisation of HCM technologies.

2.3 Outreach and Social Media

The application of social media platforms to scientific dissemination has increasingly expanded over the past several years. Platforms such as X (formerly Twitter), LinkedIn, Mastodon, BlueSky, and ResearchGate give scientists the means to disseminate short messages, mention new publications, or inform others about upcoming events. These websites have become useful tools for reaching a wide audience beyond the traditional scientific circles. For example, a short blog post outlining how HCM technology can be used to improve early disease detection with a link to a full research paper can stimulate debate and encourage readers to engage with the original study. This direct link encourages interaction and gives researchers the chance to engage a wider audience, both experts and those outside the immediate research community (Van Dijck 2013).

Hashtags as #AnimalWelfare, #3Rs (Replacement, Reduction, Refinement), #HCM, #homecage, #behaviour, #AnimalResearch, and #refinement play an important role in increasing the reach and categorisation of posts. They allow scientists to reach individuals interested in specific subjects and provide ease for the concerned public to locate research findings regarding animal welfare and ethical practice. Also, tagging institutions, lead researchers, or organisations (e.g. @EARA, @FELASAorg) can increase engagement by attracting the followers of these institutions and thus increasing the reach and visibility of the post. This approach can also initiate interaction with new and diverse groups, provoking cross-disciplinary and international discussions of important research topics.

Visual contents, such as infographics (see Figs. 2 and 3) or short video segments, are particularly popular on social media since they make it easier to share complex ideas in an accessible and engaging format (Li and Xie 2020). Such images not only get noticed, but also ease comprehension and dissemination of information. For example, an infographic showing the benefits of HCM technology used in animal testing or a short video clip demonstrating how HCM works might be more persuasive than written texts. To show the same thing in the same manner on every platform is necessary because it keeps the message the same and clear and professional. Being readable but not dry is vital to credibility building and encouraging greater audience engagement, either insiders or outsiders to the subject.

2.4 Popular Science Mechanisms, Blogs, and Newsletters

Not all the stakeholders, such as policy makers, the public, or non-specialists, read scientific papers or go to conferences. Research consortia-targeted newsletters from lab animal societies or institutional publicity offices, therefore, provide an efficient and quick way of

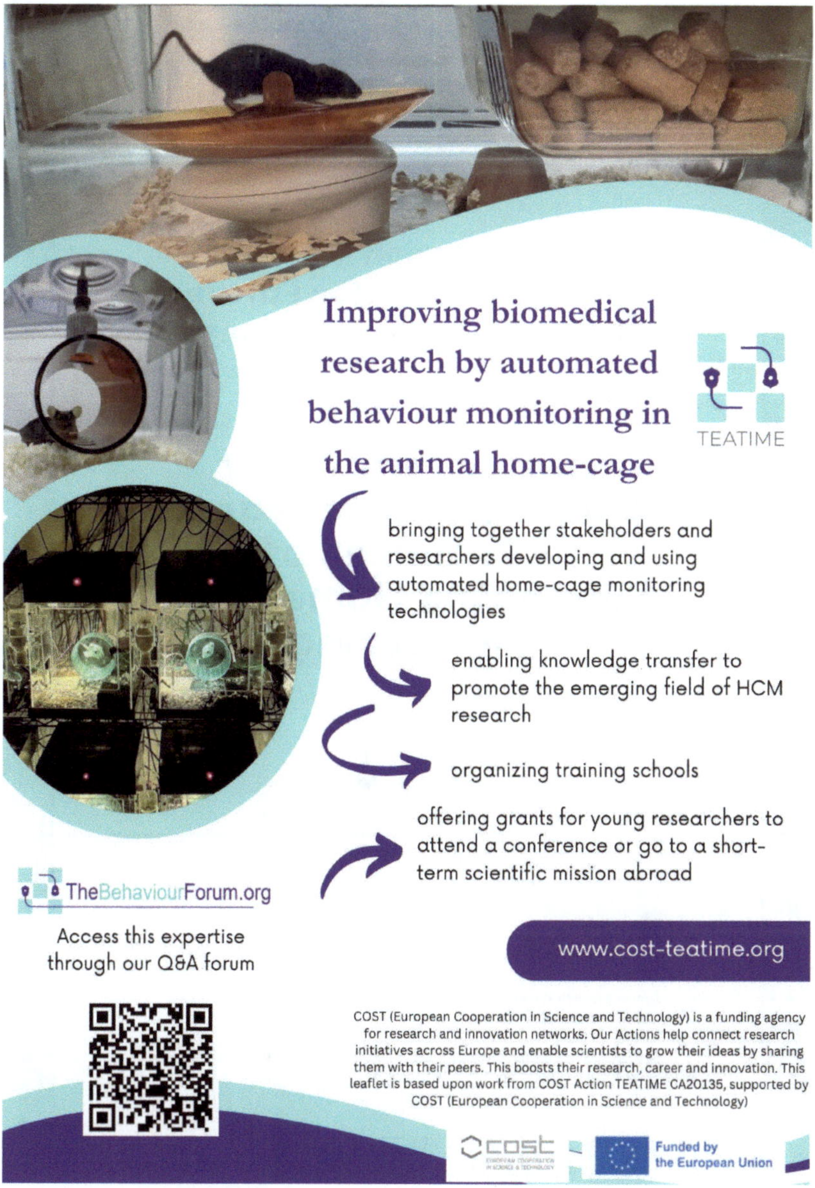

Fig. 2 An example of an infographic made to promote the COST Action 20135 TEATIME activities on social media

keeping such relevant stakeholders informed. They can inform the stakeholders of fresh developments, the results of new research, and utilisation of HCM systems in practice and also ensure that relevant information reaches parties with no opportunity to access more technical sources or who do not visit scientific conventions.

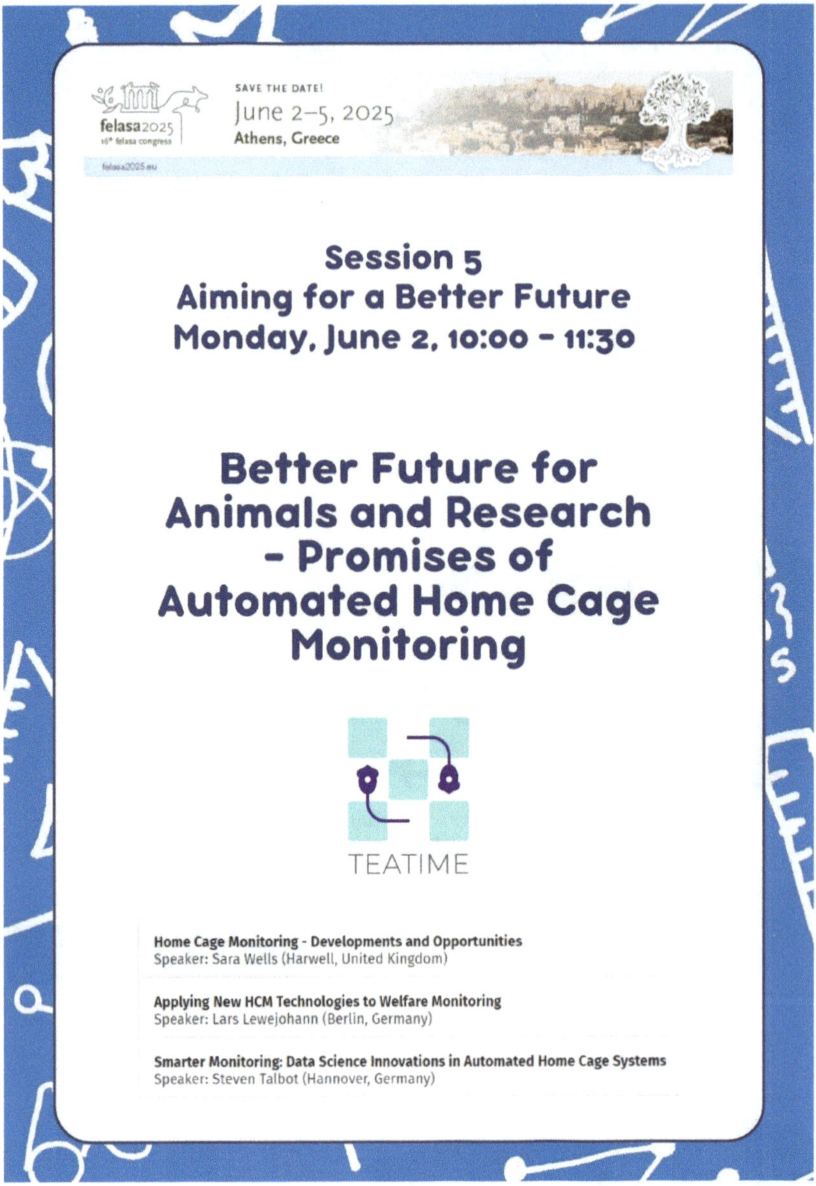
felasa2025
16th felasa congress
felasa2025.eu
SAVE THE DATE!
June 2–5, 2025
Athens, Greece
Session 5
Aiming for a Better Future
Monday, June 2, 10:00 - 11:30
Better Future for Animals and Research - Promises of Automated Home Cage Monitoring
TEATIME
Home Cage Monitoring - Developments and Opportunities
Speaker: Sara Wells (Harwell, United Kingdom)
Applying New HCM Technologies to Welfare Monitoring
Speaker: Lars Lewejohann (Berlin, Germany)
Smarter Monitoring: Data Science Innovations in Automated Home Cage Systems
Speaker: Steven Talbot (Hannover, Germany)

Fig. 3 Another example of an infographic made to inform about the HCM-related session at a FELASA2025 conference

Institutional websites and research blogs are publicly accessible hubs for disseminating news, detailed descriptions, and case studies. These websites provide less formal and more accessible information dissemination and place the use of HCM technology in a broader ethical and scientific context. By providing clear descriptions of how HCM improves animal welfare or helps research efficiency, these websites help to enhance transparency and assist stakeholders in having a clearer idea of the impact and significance of such technology in the lab setting.

Utilizing mass science media such as YouTube, science podcasts, and science magazines can significantly increase the reach of HCM-associated material (Velho et al. 2020). These media have extensive coverage and are ideally suited to communicate to a larger section, even beyond the scientific fraternity. For instance, interviews of scientists or animal welfare officers, laboratory behind-the-scenes visits, or cartoon videos demonstrating the advantages of HCM in animal husbandry can de-mystify the technology. By making complex scientific concepts more understandable, these media forms not only create awareness but also establish trust in the technologies by illustrating how they are being used to benefit animal welfare and research excellence.

2.5 Channel Comparison

When considering the various content distribution channels for information about HCM, one should consider their individual strengths and target market (Fig. 4). Peer-reviewed publications and conferences, however, continue to need to provide solid scientific evidence to researchers and ethics authorities to remain credible and promote professional collaboration. Online tools such as webinars, preprint servers, and institutional repositories provide instant access to information for speedy feedback and dissemination of information. Social media sites such as Twitter and LinkedIn are particularly well-suited for reaching a wider audience, including non-specialists and the public, via short messages and visual content. Science popularisation sites such as YouTube and podcasts extend reach by simplifying complex ideas into more accessible and comprehensible forms. By selecting the appropriate channel for each audience in a strategic manner, institutions can optimise the impact of their HCM-related content and promote both scientific progress and ethical practice.

Channel	Audience reach	Cost	Effort	Engagement	Recommended stakeholder	Sustainability
Peer-reviewed journals	high (academic)	medium-high	high	medium	researchers, funding bodies, policymakers	long-term visibility, static once published
Conferences/workshops	medium	high	high	high	researchers, industry, trainees	short-term event, medium-term follow-up
Webinars/online trainings	medium	low	medium	high	researchers, educators, students	medium-term (recordings extend reach)
Social media	high	low	medium	high	general public, journalists, peers	continuous, requires sustained engagement
Blogs/newsletters	medium	low	medium	medium-high	practitioners, policy, public	medium-term, refreshed periodically
Podcasts/YouTube	high (general public)	low-medium	high	high	students, educators, public	long-term if archived, medium effort to maintain
Preprint servers	medium	low	low	medium	researchers, collaborators	medium-term (until formal publication)
Institutional repositories	low-medium	low	medium	low	funders, institutional partners	long-term archival

Fig. 4 Comparison of dissemination channels regarding their targeted audience, cost, effort, engagement, and suitability for different stakeholders. Ratings are qualitative and based on relative comparisons of the time, resources, and coordination typically required for each format. "Timeframe" reflects how long engagement or visibility is sustained—for instance, social media require ongoing activity, while journal papers or repositories remain static but visible long-term

2.6 Strategic Use of Channels

A successful dissemination plan for HCM-related content should utilise more than one communication channel, each carefully selected to reach specific audiences. Peer-reviewed journals and meetings are critical for disseminating new findings of research and methodological developments. These traditional devices are valued by the research community and ensure that research is subjected to rigorous examination, so the resultant findings are valid and reproducible. However, as Gustavson et al. (2025) pointed out, other modern platforms such as webinars, institutional repositories, and preprint servers offer great advantages (Gustavson et al. 2025). They allow researchers to share their data in a timely manner, even before peer review, which ensures knowledge sharing at an accelerated rate and invites early comment. It also invites continuous improvement and greater collaboration between the scientific community.

Apart from intellectual publications, social networking sites, blogs, and podcasts have emerged as excellent channels to gain a larger audience. These platforms are most ideal to address the public and other stakeholders, such as animal rights groups or policymakers. By conveying recent data, speaking of ethical improvement, and laying down the benefits of HCM systems *in simple terms*, researchers can generate awareness and support for their research. Such publicly available materials as infographics or videos offering a behind-the-scenes look also increase transparency and confidence in the process of animal testing.

By strategically using these different dissemination channels, organisations can build an ecosystem that not only fosters scientific knowledge, but also provides assurance that healthcare systems are used ethically and transparently. With this multi-channel approach, researchers can reach a wide audience, from peers to the general public, and help in the facilitation of understanding and acceptance of HCM systems both scientifically and ethically.

To enhance this approach further, researchers should also consider cross-platform coordination and timing (Fig. 4). Dissemination is most effective when channels are used in a complementary rather than isolated manner. For example, a research team might first share a preprint to invite early feedback, then post short updates or visual highlights on social media during the review process to maintain engagement, and finally celebrate publication through a press release, blog post, or webinar. A concise video summary or infographic can extend the reach to non-specialist audiences, while repository uploads ensure long-term accessibility.

Such strategic sequencing allows content to evolve naturally across platforms, from preliminary findings to public communication, while reinforcing key messages and maintaining audience interest. Coordinated planning across these dissemination channels maximises visibility, engagement, and transparency, ensuring that research on HCM systems reaches the right people at the right time and with the right level of detail.

3 Target Audiences and Tailored Communication

The previous chapters have outlined the main dissemination channels for communicating about HCM and highlighted the general importance of sharing knowledge through different formats and platforms. However, effective communication is not just about where we share information, but also about how and to whom. Different target groups have different expertise, expectations, and concerns. To ensure our message is received, understood, and trusted, we need to tailor it to each stakeholder group; whether we are addressing fellow scientists, animal caretakers, funders, policy makers, or the general public (Europeancommission 2020).

This chapter builds on the foundations of the previous sections by taking a closer look at target group-oriented communication. It explores how to shape messages, adjust tone and content, and address different groups in an ethical and thoughtful way; ultimately helping to build understanding, trust, and support.

3.1 Understanding the Needs of Different Target Groups

Each stakeholder group involved in or affected by animal research with HCM systems has its own priorities and concerns. Understanding these is the first step to effective communication. Scientists and researchers value rigor, reproducibility, and innovative methods. They expect detailed explanations, validation data, and citations to back up their claims and they are more likely to engage through scientific journals, conferences, or collaborative networks. Veterinarians and animal caretakers focus on animal welfare and the practical integration of new technologies into daily care routines. They need evidence of how HCM benefits animals and how it fits with standard operating procedures (SOPs) and animal welfare protocols. Moreover, funders and facility managers value innovation, profitability, and alignment with strategic goals or the 3Rs. Thus, clear, concise summaries that demonstrate outcomes, impact, and feasibility are essential. Regulators and policy makers focus on compliance with ethical principles, transparency, and alignment with laws or directives (e.g. EU Directive 2010/63). They emphasise briefs, case studies, and documented improvements in refinement and reporting standards. General public and media are often not familiar with the details of laboratory animal research. Their concerns tend to focus on the translatability of results, ethics, transparency, and humane treatment. Thus, communication with this target group needs to be emotionally intelligent, clear, and understandable. If communication is not tailored to these groups, it can lead to confusion, mistrust, or missed opportunities for support and collaboration.

3.2 Message Framing: The Art of Shaping Perceptions

Framing is about how we present a message to emphasise certain aspects of an issue that resonate with the values and concerns of the target audience. A message about HCM can be framed as follows:

- A scientific breakthrough (for researchers)
- A refinement in animal care (for veterinarians)
- A cost-saving innovation (for investors)
- An aid to regulatory compliance (for regulators)
- Or as a humane improvement in the treatment of animals (for the public)

Research in the field of science communication has shown that the way people interpret and respond to information matters more than the facts alone (Nisbet 2009). The same HCM system can be seen as either "monitoring" or "continuous, stress-free care".

3.3 Language Level and Technical Complexity

Once the message is formulated, the next important decision is the level of language. Scientists can interpret statistical results, acronyms, and methods, but the general public cannot. The Flesch–Kincaid readability test or plain language guidelines (Plain 2011) can help calibrate text for different levels of expertise. Consider the difference:

- Technical language: "HCM enables longitudinal high-throughput analysis of spontaneous behaviour in undisturbed environments."
- Plain language: "HCM allows researchers to observe the behaviour of animals in their familiar environment over an extended period of time without disturbing them."

Clarity improves understanding and creates trust, especially when it comes to emotionally or ethically sensitive topics such as animal research.

3.4 Ethical Storytelling and Emotional Resonance

Facts are important, but stories move people. Storytelling offers a way to humanise HCM and illustrate its impact in practice. Rather than focusing on abstract data, ethical storytelling offers relatable stories that emphasise care, compassion, and curiosity. For example: "Before HCM, we could only examine the mice once or twice a day. Now we can detect early signs of disease without touching them—it's more comfortable for them and gives us better data." This story combines emotional appeal (comfort), ethical values (non-invasiveness), and scientific benefit (better data); a powerful trifecta for the public and policy makers alike. However, storytelling must be truthful and respectful. Avoid overly dramatic language or emotional manipulation. Ethical storytelling builds a bridge between scientific goals and public values.

3.5 Practical Example: One Message, Three Target Groups

A scientific result from an HCM study can be adapted to different target groups:

> Key message: "A novel HCM system detected subtle changes in circadian rhythms and social behaviour in group-housed mice exposed to chronic stress."

Scientific summary (researchers)

"We report the use of a high-resolution, automated home cage monitoring system to assess circadian and social behavioural changes in C57BL/6 mice following chronic mild stress. This method allows longitudinal tracking without observer intervention and reveals previously undetectable micro-behavioural changes."

- Press release (media professionals/general public)

"Researchers have developed an intelligent system that observes how laboratory mice eat, sleep and interact—without the need for handling. It helped detect early signs of stress in mice, giving scientists a better way to study mental health while improving animal welfare."

- Tweet (wider public, laypersons, stakeholders)

Stressed mice behave differently—but we caught it early with smart monitoring! No touching, no stress, just real behaviour. Better science, better care. #AnimalResearch #Refinement #HCM

This example illustrates how tone of voice, vocabulary, and focus are important and can change across different platforms, and why one message is not suitable for every audience.

3.6 Involve Stakeholders: Tailored Tactics

Different stakeholders respond best to specific formats and tactics (Fig. 5). Knowing not only what to say, but also how and where to say it, is the key to meaningful communication. Adapting communication to different target groups is not only a technique, but also a responsibility. As advocates for scientific progress and animal welfare, we need to ensure that our messages are clear, contextual, and ethically based. HCM offers many benefits, but whether it gains support and acceptance depends on how well we communicate its value—to scientists, animal caretakers, policy makers, and the society on whose trust we depend.

When resources are limited, focus on stakeholders who are most critical to your objectives. For example, prioritise scientists and veterinarians for scientific validation and implementation and policymakers or the public for ethical acceptance and broader support. Other audiences can be addressed as resources allow. Communication effectiveness can be monitored through engagement metrics (e.g. workshop attendance, social media

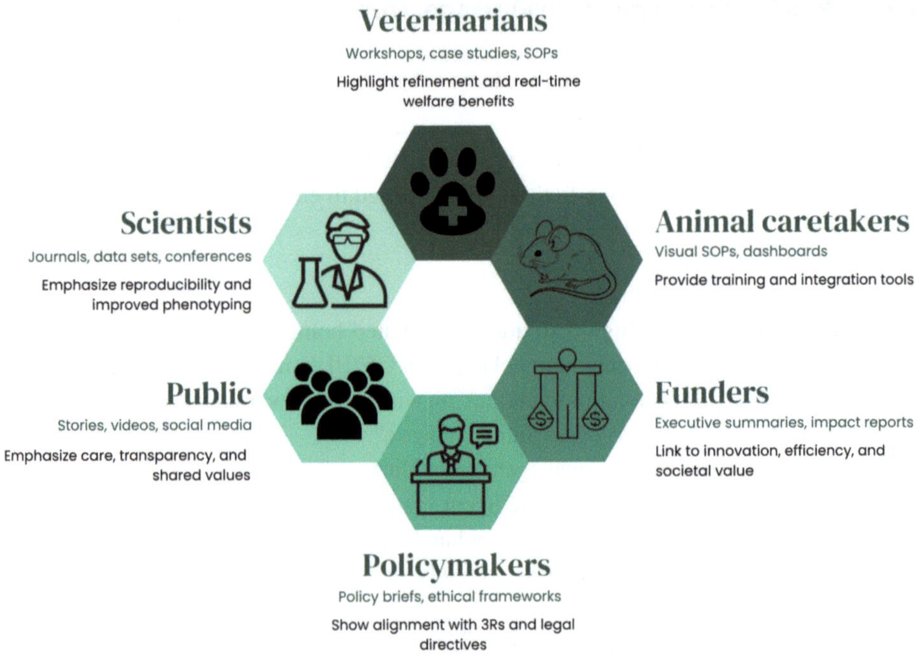

Fig. 5 Effective engagement strategies for diverse HCM audiences

interactions), qualitative feedback (comments, surveys), and outcomes (adoption of HCM methods, inclusion in policy or funding decisions).

4 Effective Tools and Techniques

In the modern landscape of science communication, not only in the field of HCM, visual and interactive content is essential to engage different audiences. This chapter will cover practical tools and techniques for creating effective content, from infographics to AI-driven storytelling, in order to improve the understanding, accessibility, and dissemination of complex topics.

4.1 Creating Infographics and Explainer Videos

Infographics and explainer videos can simplify complex processes, such as how HCM systems work or how they measure behavioural changes in laboratory animals. These formats allow different audiences to quickly grasp key messages (Mcinerny et al. 2014). Infographics are particularly valuable when it comes to summarizing workflows, illustrating behavioural data collection, or explaining the benefits of animal welfare. User-friendly platforms like Canva allow users to create visually coherent diagrams, posters, and slide decks with intuitive tools. For scientifically accurate visualisations, BioRender offers an extensive library of life science illustrations and templates that are especially helpful when depicting the anatomy of lab animals, cage components, or experimental setups. Doodly is another useful tool that allows users to create whiteboard animations that explain scientific concepts step-by-step in an understandable format. These resources help visualise ideas in a way that static text often cannot (Recall 2016).

Further on, explainer videos and short animated clips provide an additional level of engagement. For example, a 90-s video showing how chronic stress alters the circadian rhythms of group-housed mice, as detected by HCM systems, can convey technical insights more effectively than lengthy written descriptions. These materials are especially useful for training, conference presentations, and public awareness campaigns.

Recent studies support the effectiveness of these formats in enhancing public awareness. The majority of studies reported that infographics improved knowledge or changed behaviours, with many participants preferring them over other mediums (Kong et al. 2025). Similarly, animated explainer videos have been shown to significantly improve short-term recall of health information among adult patients across various healthcare settings (Hansen et al. 2024). These findings underscore the value of incorporating infographics and explainer videos into dissemination strategies to effectively communicate complex information to the public.

4.2 Using AI for Content Creation and Engagement

New digital tools, some of which are powered by AI, make it easier than ever to communicate science clearly and creatively. These tools can create content quickly, adapt it to different audiences, and enhance it with engaging visual elements. One example is ChatGPT, which allows researchers to rephrase technical data, create scripts, or simulate interviews for learning materials. When used wisely, these tools can save time and improve clarity, without compromising scientific accuracy.

Moreover, imaging tools like DALL-E can be useful for creating unique images, such as drawings of mice in home cages or artistic impressions of behavioural changes. Another tool, Lumen5, turns written content into short videos, complete with simple animations, subtitles, and background music. This is particularly helpful when it comes to presenting research summaries or blog posts in a more dynamic format, whether to funders or followers on social media. Jasper AI also helps with the creation of public-facing materials, such as social media posts, newsletters, or campaign updates, and guides users through the process.

However, it is important to remember that AI tools cannot replace human expertise. All content created by an AI user should be carefully reviewed to avoid misinterpretation or oversimplified messages. When used critically and with clear goals, AI tools can be valuable partners in helping scientists reach a wider audience and make their messages accurate and engaging (Van Dijck et al. 2018; Reinhardt 2023).

4.3 Designing Engaging Presentations: Practical Considerations and Best Practices

Modern communication tools can significantly enhance how data and messages about HCM are shared across stakeholder groups. As illustrated in Fig. 5, scientists, animal caretakers, funders, and the public have distinct information needs and expectations. Presentations designed with these audiences in mind, and supported by appropriate tools, can significantly improve understanding, engagement, and trust.

Clear, professional, and engaging presentations are essential in both academic and public communication. Presentations created with platforms such as Canva, Google Slides, or Microsoft PowerPoint benefit from consistent colour palettes, fonts, and icons. When including HCM-specific data, it is helpful to use screenshots of real dashboards or longitudinal charts to illustrate trends and results (Mcinerny et al. 2014). For technical or internal presentations aimed at researchers or caretakers, such visuals can demonstrate the practical value of monitoring systems and support data-driven decisions.

Interactive features such as clickable charts, embedded videos, and QR codes can further increase audience engagement. Moreover, tools such as Prezi add dynamic movement and flow to presentations, which can be especially effective when explaining research processes or navigating through multi-step experimental designs. Engaging visuals not only improve retention, but also help to emphasise important welfare and ethical considerations related to HCM, key aspects for both scientific and public audiences.

Regardless of the tools used, the basic principles of effective communication remain the same. The content must be tailored to the target audience, whether it is researchers, caretakers, funders, or the public. Visual and narrative coherence strengthens the message and builds trust. In addition, content should be tested before dissemination, through peer feedback, stakeholder input, or small focus groups, to ensure clarity and relevance. It is also important to consider accessibility. Ensuring that infographics are colourblind-friendly, videos are captioned, and text content is free of jargon will contribute to inclusive communication. Facility tours (virtual or in-person) are another valuable communication tool that fosters transparency and helps demystify HCM systems. Finally, freely accessible dissemination platforms such as institutional websites, social media, and preprint servers can help ensure that content reaches the intended audiences efficiently and effectively.

4.4 Adapting Messages: A Side-By-Side Example Using AI

One of the most effective ways to illustrate how communication strategies differ by audience is to take a single piece of scientific content and customise it using AI tools such as

ChatGPT or Jasper. These tools can help translate dense scientific knowledge into formats that are both engaging and accessible to non-specialist audiences, including journalists, policy makers, and the public. Take, for example, the abstract of a scientific study using HCM to detect behavioural changes in stressed mice. The original abstract, written for a research audience, reads:

> Title: Automated home cage monitoring reveals stress-induced changes in circadian and social behaviour in mice
>
> **Summary**
> Using an automated, high-resolution home cage monitoring (HCM) system, we investigated the effects of chronic mild stress on the circadian and social behaviour of group-housed C57BL/6 mice. The system enabled continuous, non-invasive tracking of activity patterns and social interactions over several weeks. Stressed mice showed a phase shift in activity rhythms, reduced locomotion in the dark phase, and decreased affiliative behaviour. These subtle behavioural changes were not detectable with conventional observational methods. Our results highlight the value of HCM in detecting early stress-related behavioural phenotypes and support its use in welfare assessment and neurobehavioural research.

Processed through an AI tool such as ChatGPT and adapted for the public, the same message can be presented as follows:

> Title: Intelligent system recognises early signs of stress in mice—without touching them
>
> **Summary**
> Scientists have developed a smart cage that monitors how mice eat, sleep, and socialise—all without being handled. When mice were exposed to prolonged, mild stress, the system noticed changes in their daily activity and social behaviour. These early warning signs of stress would have been missed with conventional methods. This new approach can improve mental health research and make the lives of animals in research easier.

The prompt that was used to generate this version was: "Rewrite the following scientific abstract for a general audience, such as readers of a science news article or press release. Use clear and engaging language, avoid jargon, and emphasise the relevance to human and animal welfare. Keep it concise."

Moreover, the prompt used to validate the output was: "Evaluate this rewritten text for factual accuracy, readability, and tone. Suggest any improvements to ensure it remains scientifically accurate while understandable to a general audience."

This comparison highlights several key differences. The original summary uses formal, technical terms such as "circadian rhythms", "affiliative behaviour", and "non-invasive tracking" and is aimed at researchers in the neurosciences or behavioural sciences. The emphasis is on methodological rigor and detailed data interpretation, with little emphasis on accessibility. In contrast, the summary produced by the AI is written in a colloquial tone and is better suited for press releases, public relations materials, or social media posts. It uses simple terms such as "daily activity", "social behaviour", and "smart cage", which makes it understandable to a wider audience. The focus is on real-world relevance (mental health, animal welfare, and innovation) and is presented in a concise, reader-friendly format.

When using AI tools for longer or more complex traits, it is advisable to combine automated assistance with human oversight to ensure output quality. This can include a human review by a subject-matter expert or communicator to ensure factual and ethical accuracy; cross-checking with another AI model or grammar/style assistant to detect inconsistencies; and iterative prompting, asking the AI to self-critique or rephrase unclear segments.

In summary, using AI tools to reformulate a single scientific message can help communicate its value to different audiences. This approach not only saves time but also ensures a consistent message that is tailored to the level of knowledge and interests of different stakeholders.

5 Challenges in Dissemination

The dissemination of information about HCM systems in laboratory animal research poses a particular challenge, as an effective communication must strike a balance between scientific accuracy and accessibility for various audiences, including researchers from other disciplines, funding agencies, regulators, ethics committees, policy makers, and the general public. In addition, ethical concerns and misinformation about monitoring technologies and animal testing can influence perceptions of HCM systems, emphasizing the need for thoughtful and strategic dissemination. These challenges highlight the need for a structured communication strategy, aligned with the framework in Fig. 5, where messages, tools, and stakeholders are matched according to communication goals such as awareness, understanding, and trust.

5.1 Balancing Between Technical Accuracy and Accessibility

HCM systems are often described in highly technical language (data streams, automated algorithms, behavioural clusters, telemetry, circadian rhythm mapping, etc.) which, while precise, can be off-putting to a non-specialist audience. On the other hand, oversimplification risks losing the core scientific and ethical value of these tools. Communicators must walk a fine line, making the content understandable while maintaining the rigor and nuance of the information.

One useful strategy is to take a layered approach to communication, adapting the same core message for different formats and audiences while maintaining factual integrity. For example, the scientific core message "HCM enables continuous, non-invasive monitoring of animal welfare" can be expressed differently depending on the channel. A scientific paper will focus on algorithms, validation, and reproducibility. A conference presentation will emphasise on methodological innovation and application. For creating an infographic or video, a simplification of terminology and highlighting welfare benefits will be used. For a public outreach or media post, connection of findings to societal relevance will be needed, such as "smarter ways to care for research animals". This approach links directly to the communication tools described in earlier sections (AI-assisted writing, visual storytelling, interactive dashboards) and supports consistent messaging across all stakeholders. The FAIR principles (Wilkinson et al. 2016), originally designed for data management, also provide a conceptual guide for communication: scientific information should not only be accessible and reusable but also interpretable by its intended audience. Infographics, short explanatory videos, and narrative case studies are effective tools to bridge this gap. These formats allow researchers to communicate the key findings and implications without neglecting the essence of their work. Importantly, such tools should be co-developed or tested with the target audience to ensure clarity and engagement (Illingworth and Allen 2016).

5.2 Dealing with Ethical Concerns

Although HCM systems improve animal welfare by enabling non-invasive, continuous monitoring and early detection of distress, ethical concerns remain. Critics sometimes refer to automated monitoring as surveillance and equate it with invasive or privacy-invading technologies. Such concerns are particularly prevalent among animal rights activists or laypeople who are unfamiliar with how these systems work. To counter these perceptions, communication must demonstrate how the HCM is consistent with the 3R principles (Russell and Burch 1959). Refinement is particularly important: HCM allows researchers to reduce handling stress, refine behavioural analyses, and detect subtle signs of pain or stress earlier than traditional methods (Balcombe 2006). Communicating these benefits using understandable language (for example "early warning system for animal discomfort") can help reshape the picture, for example, in animal license requests addressed at ethics committees and licensing authorities.

Another ethical issue concerns data protection and algorithmic decision-making. As AI-driven behavioural analysis gains traction, transparency about how data are collected, processed, and interpreted becomes increasingly important. Stakeholders, including animal welfare officers and ethics committees, need to be confident that the decisions made by automated tools are scientifically validated and ethically justified.

To manage ethical and reputational risks effectively, communicators should prioritise issues based on their likelihood and potential impact. For example, misconceptions about surveillance or data privacy are more likely to arise than concerns about algorithmic validations. Early warning indicators include increased public or media attention, stakeholder queries, or negative social media sentiment. Regularly tracking these signals through website analytics, comment monitoring, or informal feedback loops can guide timely responses and mitigation.

5.3 Combating Misinformation

Misinformation about HCM systems can result from a lack of understanding, sensationalist media coverage, or targeted disinformation campaigns. Misconceptions include the belief that animals are constantly monitored by cameras, that these systems replace human care, or that they lead to more animal testing. A proactive approach to counter misinformation involves open and transparent communication supported by data and imagery. Virtual or in-person tours of facilities, frequently asked questions on facility websites, and publishing lay summaries alongside scientific papers can demystify the use of HCM. Dedicated social media campaigns, ideally created in collaboration with communications experts, can also help debunk myths and shape public opinion. In addition, working with veterinarians, animal technologists, and ethics committees is essential for building trust. These stakeholders are often more trusted by the public than researchers and can serve as effective intermediaries in communication (Bubela et al. 2009). Educating and empowering these stakeholders to speak confidently about HCM is thus important and can increase the reach and credibility of dissemination efforts.

Disseminating information about HCM systems is therefore not just about sharing data, but also about promoting understanding, building trust, and addressing public concerns. Balancing accuracy and accessibility, addressing ethical perceptions, and combating misinformation are critical to ensuring that the benefits of HCM are recognised and responsibly embraced throughout the biomedical community.

Clear communication pathways are essential for effective dissemination and risk management. Within research institutions, responsibilities are typically shared across several roles. Researchers communicate primarily with peers, funding agencies, and regulators, ensuring that scientific accuracy and methodological transparency are maintained. Animal welfare officers and ethics committee members serve as intermediaries between research teams and oversight bodies, translating complex information into ethical and welfare-focused language. Facility managers and technologists often act as practical communicators, relaying operational insights to caretakers and technicians, while institutional communication officers or press teams engage with external audiences, including policymakers, journalists, and the public. Coordination among these roles ensures that messages remain consistent, timely, and audience-appropriate. Prioritisation depends on context: ethical concerns and public misconceptions typically require higher and more immediate attention than technical clarifications, while regular internal updates, feedback meetings, and media monitoring can function as early warning systems to detect emerging communication risks.

6 Case Studies

Case studies provide practical examples of how communication and dissemination strategies related to HCM can raise awareness, increase understanding, and promote acceptance. By analysing these efforts, we can gain important insights for future campaigns, both within the scientific community and beyond.

6.1 COST Action TEATIME: Building a Community of HCM Advocates

The COST Action CA20135—TEATIME (Improving Biomedical Research by Automated Behaviour Monitoring in the Animal Home-Cage) provides a practical example of how a coordinated communications strategy can build visibility, trust, and use of HCM systems across diverse stakeholder groups. Framed according to the communication framework in Fig. 5, TEATIME activities can be described in terms of the who, why, how, and what was achieved.

6.1.1 Who (Targeted Stakeholders)

TEATIME primarily targeted four stakeholder groups: researchers (to encourage uptake and cross-laboratory collaboration), animal caretakers and facility managers (to support operational use and welfare gains), policy makers and ethics committees (to inform regulatory and licensing conversations), and the interested public and media (to build transparency and social licence). Roles were distributed: researchers and working group led generated content, communication officers and COST handled press and outreach, welfare officers and technologists validated operational messaging.

6.1.2 Why (Objectives)

Objectives followed the framework goals of awareness (introduce HCM concepts), understanding (explain methods and welfare benefits), and trust/acceptance (address ethical concerns and transparency). Each objective guided the choice of tool and channel: peer-reviewed outputs and technical webinars for understanding; infographics and lay summaries for awareness and trust; and policy briefs for regulators.

6.1.3 How (Strategies and Tools Linked to Fig. 5)

TEATIME used a mixture of strategies mapped to stakeholder needs: technical webinars and recorded demonstrations for researchers; short training modules and dashboard screenshots for caretakers; targeted policy briefs and meetings for regulators; and infographics, social posts, and short videos for public audiences. A shared communications toolkit (templates for slides, posters, and contact cards for TheBehaviourForum.org, which is a web-based animal behaviour knowledge transfer platform created by TEATIME) ensured consistent branding and message fidelity across channels and members, turning participants into local ambassadors. When researchers have the right tools at their disposal to communicate their work, their messages are spread further and reach more people. Common branding and coordinated messages between institutions add weight and increase the overall impact. Online formats are great for bringing people together across borders, especially when supported by collateral materials and recordings. And perhaps most importantly, personal stories, such as what drives researchers or how HCM has improved animal welfare, can make science more tangible and inspire real empathy and engagement.

Various online events on HCM technologies and studies and a series of animal research communication webinars were organised, which trained early career scientists and communicators on how to use tools such as social media, explainer videos, and AI-powered platforms. Their webinars reached a diverse audience across the world and encouraged a cultural shift towards more open and strategic communication of animal research. Moreover, the hashtag #homecage and associated content on X (formerly Twitter), LinkedIn, BlueSky, and YouTube created a digital space for the dissemination of publications on HCM, upcoming events, member spotlights, and infographics. Posts that combined visual elements with clear, concise language generated higher engagement and were frequently shared by partner networks such as EARA (European Animal Research Association) and ALBA Network for Diversity, Equity and Inclusion in Brain Sciences.

6.1.4 What (Outcomes, Metrics, and Timeframe)

TEATIME activities ran from 2021 to 2025, with measurable results including webinar attendance and geographic reach, social media impressions and engagement rates (shares/comments), downloads of toolkits and lay summaries, and number of partner press releases coordinated via university press offices. Where possible, specific impact metrics were tracked (e.g. webinar registrants vs. attendees, toolkit downloads, hashtag impressions, number of policy briefings delivered). These metrics demonstrated increased awareness and network growth, and qualitative feedback from members reported improved confidence in communicating HCM to ethics committees and funders.

6.1.5 Challenges, Mitigation, and Comparative Impact

TEATIME work also revealed common problems: limited staff time for communications, variable institutional support for public outreach, and occasional public misunderstandings about monitoring (surveillance concerns). Mitigation included centralised templates to reduce workload, training sessions to upskill members in plain-language writing, and proactive transparency measures to address misconceptions early. TEATIME's coordinated, multi-channel approach, combining technical training, shared templates, and proactive transparency, contrasts with organisations that focused solely on academic outputs; the latter often produced high-quality science but limited public reach or policy uptake. The breadth of TEATIME stakeholder engagement and the adoption of shared materials across member institutions support the claim that it is a leading recent initiative for HCM dissemination (COST 2021, 2025).

The communications work relied on modest dedicated time from the Communication & Dissemination working group and contributions from member labs. A realistic timeframe for a campaign of similar scope is 12–24 months from planning to consolidated outputs, while smaller activities like single webinars or social media campaigns can deliver impact within weeks.

6.2 ALBA Network and EARA Campaigns for Transparency in Animal Research

Both the ALBA Network, which aims to promote equity and diversity in the brain sciences, and EARA run campaigns addressing the overlapping issues of ethical animal use, technological innovation, and transparency and can thus be used as a successful case study for animal research communication. By promoting the importance of openness in animal research, EARA provides examples of how complex technologies such as HCM can be presented in a positive ethical context. Campaigns that include testimonials from technicians and veterinarians emphasise the refinement aspect of HCM and thus resonate with broader societal values. Moreover, ALBA's visual identity, inclusive language, and downloadable resources are an excellent example of how clarity and accessibility can be maintained even in highly technical fields. Their communication around equitable research practices intersects with HCM-related topics, such as minimizing animal stress and ensuring quality data.

Messages that emphasise shared values, such as the association of HCM with refinement and ethical animal care, tend to resonate with both the public and policy makers. Images of HCM-equipped cages or simple graphics showing how the technology reduces handling are far more memorable than long, text-heavy explanations. For campaigns involving multiple partners, a consistent approach across all platforms (in terms of language, tone of voice, and imagery) really helps to deliver a clearer, stronger message. In conclusion, a successful communication of HCM depends not only on the message itself, but also on who delivers it, how it is formulated, and which tools are used. Whether through large-scale networks like TEATIME, cross-sector advocacy like EARA, or local initiatives, the key to effective dissemination lies in transparency, empathy, visual engagement, and empowering a broad coalition of communicators. As the field of HCM grows, so must our ability to explain its value to a world increasingly concerned with scientific rigor and animal welfare.

7 Role of Collaboration

Effective communication about HCM systems goes beyond the laboratory. To truly reach the various audiences of stakeholders, collaboration is essential. Coordinated cross-sector efforts allow for more effective communication, wider dissemination, and greater credibility. This subchapter examines how partnerships with manufacturers, pharmaceutical companies, non-governmental organisations (NGOs), and advocacy groups contribute to successful communication about HCM, using both practical examples and collaborative models such as the TEATIME COST Action.

7.1 Cooperation with Manufacturers and Pharmaceutical Partners

HCM manufacturers are often the first port of call for innovations and the practical use of monitoring technologies. Working with these companies not only ensures technical accuracy in communications but also reinforces messages with practical examples and visual content, such as product demonstrations, case studies, or user reports. Pharmaceutical companies, especially those using HCM in preclinical research, can serve as strong allies in communicating how such technologies improve data reproducibility, animal welfare, and regulatory compliance. Jointly authored white papers, joint conference presentations, or joint webinars can greatly enhance the credibility and reach of HCM messages. In addition, pharma partners often have access to global networks, making them valuable channels for disseminating best practices and success stories, as this recent publication demonstrates (Sillito et al. 2025).

7.2 Partnership with Non-Governmental Organisations and Advocacy Organisations

NGOs that advocate for animal welfare and responsible research play an important role in shaping public opinion. Groups such as the NC3Rs (National Centre for the Replacement, Refinement and Reduction of Animals in Research) have long advocated for the adoption of automated and less invasive techniques, including HCM. Their guidance documents, funding programs, and case studies help to validate the ethical benefits of HCM systems. Moreover, other NGOs such as EARA (2025) and ART (2025) address the public directly when it comes to animal experimentation. Working with such organisations ensures that the messages about HCM are in line with the public's values, highlighting how it reduces stress, minimises intervention, and improves animal welfare. These collaborations can help change public opinion on transparency and ethics in animal research.

7.3 TEATIME Action: A Model for European Cooperation

The COST Action TEATIME is an example of how international and interdisciplinary cooperation can strengthen communication on HCM. TEATIME brings together researchers, technology developers, communicators, and policy experts to promote the adoption and understanding of automated behavioural monitoring in laboratory animals. Through TEATIME, coordinated dissemination efforts, including webinars, joint publications, infographics, and social media campaigns, have shown that collective messages can be more effective than isolated efforts. TEATIME has also facilitated links between academia and industry and enabled the joint development of communication materials tailored to different stakeholder groups (see e.g. Figs. 2 and 3 and the TEATIME website under News (TEATIME 2025)). Importantly, the Action includes a Communications and Dissemination Working Group specifically focused on increasing the visibility and accessibility of HCM in Europe and beyond.

7.4 Advocacy and Public Engagement

In addition to the technical benefits, HCM also represents a step forward in making animal research more humane and transparent. Working with advocacy organisations allows researchers and developers to address public concerns openly and honestly. This can include organizing events for the public, participating in school or university outreach programs, or contributing to scientific communication platforms and media. In such endeavours, it is critical to speak a language that resonates with any audience: For scientists, it's about reproducibility and data; for the public, it's about ethics and animal welfare; and for funders, it's about innovation and cost-effectiveness (see Fig. 1). Collaborations make it possible to formulate and communicate these different messages appropriately using the credibility and trust that each partner brings to the table.

Strategic collaboration is a cornerstone of effective communication about HCM technology. By combining the efforts of manufacturers, pharmaceutical companies, NGOs, and advocacy groups, we not only expand our reach, but also ensure that our message is well-rounded, credible, and impactful. Initiatives like TEATIME show how such partnerships can work in practice and provide a replicable model for the future of research communication (COST 2025). In a landscape where public trust and scientific progress go hand in hand, collaboration is essential.

8 Monitoring the Impact of Communication

Good communication is more than just composing and transmitting messages. It is about ensuring that those messages are received, understood, and acted upon. In the context of HCM technology, monitoring the impact of communication helps to determine whether outreach is achieving its intended goals: raising awareness, improving understanding, and promoting acceptance of HCM systems. Several tools and strategies can be used for evaluating the effectiveness of communication, using both quantitative and qualitative methods. Investing time and resources in communication only makes sense if we can track the results.

Measuring impact helps us to understand the effectiveness of our dissemination efforts—it shows us what works and what needs to be improved. It also provides evidence to justify funding and the use of resources to stakeholders. We can use audience participation and feedback to refine our future strategies. Just as importantly, measuring impact allows us to demonstrate transparency and accountability in our communications with the public. Whether it is informing researchers, engaging regulators, or building public trust, impact monitoring provides the evidence base to improve and refine our strategies.

8.1 Metrics and Analytics: Quantifying Reach and Engagement

There are several tools you can use to determine how far your communication has spread. Altmetrics track the online attention that scientific publications receive, including mentions in newspapers, blogs, and policy documents, shares on platforms such as Twitter/X, LinkedIn, and Facebook, and saves and reads on platforms such as Mendeley or ResearchGate. For example, an open access article on HCM published in a neuroscience journal may receive strong altmetric attention if it is picked up by advocacy organisations or presented in a webinar. These numbers provide insight into how often and where your work is seen and discussed outside of traditional academic citations.

For social media analysis, each platform offers built-in analytics. Twitter/X analyses impressions, engagement rate, retweets, and likes. LinkedIn tracks post views, link clicks, and demographic data of viewers. YouTube tracks viewing time, viewer engagement, and traffic sources. You can use these data to identify which posts resonate with your target audience and which channels are most effective. For example, a short video explaining the benefits of HCM for animal welfare may have high engagement and distribution, indicating its success as a communication tool.

If your communications campaign includes a dedicated website or newsletter, it is advisable to track page visits, bounce rate (the percentage of visitors who leave a website without interacting further, such as clicking a link or viewing another page), time spent on page, newsletter open rates and click-through rates, and downloads of resources (e.g. infographics, white papers).

Together, these metrics provide a picture of who is engaging with your content and which aspects are attracting the most attention.

8.2 Surveys and Feedback: Capturing Audience Perceptions

Quantitative metrics are important, but they rarely reflect the whole truth. For this purpose, surveys offer a valuable way to measure changes in awareness, attitudes, and intentions, especially among researchers, students, policy makers, or the public. Tools such as Google Forms and SurveyMonkey can be used to collect such feedback. Google Forms are free and easy to use and allow for customizable charts to visualise responses. SurveyMonkey offers more advanced features, such as anonymous submissions and branching logic that allow questions to be customised based on previous responses.

When designing a survey, it makes sense to focus on a few key areas. First, assess basic awareness by asking respondents if they have heard of HCM. Then, assess understanding by exploring their thoughts on the benefits of HCM systems. Attitudes can be assessed by asking if they would consider using or supporting HCM in their own research or institution. Finally, behaviour change can be explored by asking if exposure to communication materials (webinars or articles) makes them more likely to recommend or adopt HCM technology. These types of questions can be asked in post-event feedback forms, incorporated into newsletters, or shared via social media to assess the longer-term impact of communication efforts.

Example

After organizing a TEATIME webinar on "Automated Behaviour Monitoring", a short post-event survey using Google forms asked participants how clear the information was, whether they felt more confident explaining HCM to others, and whether they planned to explore its use. The results showed a significant increase in perceived knowledge and several requests for further materials—evidence of successful knowledge transfer.

8.3 Mixed Methods Evaluation

The best picture of communication success can be achieved by a combination of quantitative metrics (views, clicks, shares, altmetric ratings) and qualitative feedback (survey comments, open-ended responses). To evaluate communication results using mixed methods, you should create a simple evaluation framework (Fig. 6). This type of systematic tracking is also helpful when writing grant reports, applying for future funding, or publishing your communication strategies. Monitoring the impact of communication is not an afterthought but should be an integral part of any dissemination plan. By using tools such as altmetrics, analytics, and feedback surveys, we can ensure that our efforts to explain and promote HCM technology are making a real difference. Communication is not just about disseminating information, but also about building a feedback loop with our target audiences.

Communication channel	Metrics tracked	Outcome
Webinar	Attendee count, feedback survey	85% reported increased understanding
Social media campaign	Impressions, link clicks	2,500 views, 130 clicks to HCM explainer
Article publication	Altmetric score, citations	Altmetric score: 47; Cited 3 times in 6 months
Public talk	Survey after event	90% said they now support automated monitoring

Fig. 6 Example of an evaluation framework for monitoring the impact of communication across different channels

Only by listening, measuring, and adapting can we ensure that our messages are not only heard, but also understood and remembered.

9 Future Directions

As scientific communication evolves, new opportunities are emerging that can help communicate HCM technology more effectively and reach a wider audience. These developments are changing not only the tools and strategies we use, but also the values that underpin collaboration between science and society. The future of HCM communication lies in adopting these innovations, particularly those associated with open science, transparency, and collaborative dissemination.

9.1 Open Science and Data Sharing

Open science is no longer a niche ideal—it is fast becoming a standard requirement across all disciplines. This movement promotes the sharing of research data, protocols, and results in accessible, reproducible formats, often in advance of formal, peer-reviewed publication. In the context of HCM, open science offers unique advantages. By making raw behavioural datasets, analysis pipelines, and validation studies openly available, researchers can accelerate replication, cross-laboratory validation, and ultimately broader adoption of the technology. Platforms such as the Open Science Framework (OSF), Zenodo, or protocols.io enable teams working with HCM systems to share methods and results in a transparent way. Preprints and open access publications lower the barrier for other researchers, students, industry partners, and even the public to engage with the topic. Data sharing and transparency are also in line with ethical principles in animal research, as the value of each dataset is maximised and unnecessary repetition is minimised. In addition, open communication builds public trust. For example, when facilities explain how continuous monitoring systems reduce animal stress and improve animal welfare, and back this up with openly available data or videos, they send a strong message of accountability and commitment to ethical science.

9.2 Interactive and Immersive Communication Tools

As technology advances, the formats for effective science communication are also changing. The future of HCM dissemination will likely include more interactive content: explanatory animations, real-time dashboards with anonymised animal activity data, virtual reality tours of HCM-equipped facilities, and even game-based learning tools for students or trainees. Infographics and short videos tailored for mobile use are particularly effective when it comes to reaching young scientists and the public, while interactive webinars or live Q&A sessions with HCM experts can create more direct contact and knowledge transfer. Moreover, the use of AI-powered tools now makes it easier than ever to transform complex data into readable summaries, visual representations, and multilingual content, promoting inclusion and accessibility for different audiences.

9.3 Building Communities Around HCM

The future of HCM communication will also benefit from stronger community building efforts. Initiatives such as the COST TEATIME Action have already demonstrated the value of bringing together researchers, manufacturers, ethicists, and communicators from across Europe. As the field grows, dedicated networks or working groups focused on HCM-related data standards, communication strategies, and public engagement could further increase both visibility and credibility. Crowdsourcing and citizen science could also find a place in the future of HCM, especially for high-profile projects focused on animal welfare or behavioural neuroscience. Transparent, participatory research models can help bridge the gap between science and society, especially when it comes to concerns related to animal research.

9.4 From Awareness-Raising to Advocacy Work

Finally, future communication strategies must not only aim to inform, but also to encourage advocacy. As HCM technology continues to demonstrate its potential to improve animal welfare and scientific accuracy, there is an opportunity to engage wider stakeholders in promoting its use, from funding bodies and policy makers to NGOs and educational institutions. Positioning HCM as part of a forward-looking, responsible approach to animal research can be aligned with global policy trends that emphasise the 3Rs and promote institutional change.

The next decade of HCM communication will be characterised by openness, interactivity, collaboration, and ethical responsibility. By embracing these trends, the HCM community can move beyond traditional dissemination, build trust, promote acceptance, and ultimately make a meaningful contribution to science and society. The challenge is not only to keep pace with these changes, but to lead them.

References

Art (2025) Animal Research Tomorrow [Online]. Available: www.animalresearchtomorrow.org/en. Accessed 24 Oct 2025

Balcombe JP (2006) Laboratory environments and rodents' behavioural needs: a review. Lab Anim 40:217–235

Bubela T, Nisbet MC, Borchelt R, Brunger F, Critchley C, Einsiedel E, Geller G, Gupta A, Hampel J, Hyde-Lay R (2009) Science communication reconsidered. Nat Biotechnol 27:514–518

Collins FS, Tabak LA (2014) Policy: NIH plans to enhance reproducibility. Nature 505:612–613

COST (2021) CA20135 - Improving biomedical research by automated behaviour monitoring in the animal home-cage (TEATIME) [Online]. Available: https://www.cost.eu/actions/CA20135/. Accessed 20 May 2025

COST (2025) Shaping the future of lab animal monitoring COST Action TEATIME [Online]. Available: https://www.cost.eu/long-read-teatime/. Accessed 26 Oct 2025

Directive E (2010) 63/EU of the European Parliament and of the council of 22 September 2010 on the protection of animals used for scientific purposes. Off J Eur Union 276:33–79

Eara (2025) European Animal Research Association [Online]. Available: https://www.eara.eu/. Accessed 23 Oct 2025

Europeancommission (2020) Communication Toolkit for EU Research Projects [Online]. Available: https://eismea.ec.europa.eu/communication-toolkit_en. Accessed 21 May 2025

Gustavson AM, Urbanski DP, Mcmahon SK, Moone R (2025) Advancing the impact of research through a dissemination-focused special interest group. BMJ Open 15:E098130

Hansen S, Jensen TS, Schmidt AM, Strøm J, Vistisen P, Høybye MT (2024) The effectiveness of video animations as a tool to improve health information Recall for patients: systematic review. J Med Internet Res 26:E58306

Hohlbaum K, Bert B, Dietze S, Palme R, Fink H, Thöne-Reineke C (2017) Severity classification of repeated isoflurane anesthesia in C57bl/6jrj mice—assessing the degree of distress. PLoS One 12:E0179588

Hölter SM, Wells S, Voikar V, COST Action 20135 (2023) Improving biomedical research by automated behaviour monitoring in the animal home cage–action needed for networking. Lab Anim 57:79–83
Hurst JL, West RS (2010) Taming anxiety in laboratory mice. Nat Methods 7:825–826
Illingworth S, Allen G (2016) Effective science communication: a practical guide to surviving as a scientist. Iop Publishing
Initiative EC (2023) Save cruelty-free cosmetics—commit to a Europe without animal testing. ECI
Kahnau P, Mieske P, Wilzopolski J, Kalliokoski O, Mandillo S, Hölter SM, Voikar V, Amfim A, Badurek S, Bartelik A (2023) A systematic review of the development and application of home cage monitoring in laboratory mice and rats. BMC Biol 21:256
Kilkenny C, Browne WJ, Cuthill IC, Emerson M, Altman DG (2010) Improving bioscience research reporting: the arrive guidelines for reporting animal research. J Pharmacol Pharmacother 1:94–99
Kong H-K, Zainab F, Turner AM, Bekemeier B, Backonja U (2025) Trends in and effectiveness of infographics for health communication: a scoping review. Health Commun 40:222–232
Li Y, Xie Y (2020) Is A picture worth a thousand words? An empirical study of image content and social media engagement. J Mark Res 57:1–19
Mcinerny GJ, Chen M, Freeman R, Gavaghan D, Meyer M, Rowland F, Spiegelhalter DJ, Stefaner M, Tessarolo G, Hortal J (2014) Information visualisation for science and policy: engaging users and avoiding bias. Trends Ecol Evol 29:148–157
Mcleod C, Hobson-West P (2016) Opening up animal research and science–society relations? A thematic analysis of transparency discourses in the United Kingdom. Public Underst Sci 25:791–806
Morton DB (2000) A systematic approach for establishing humane endpoints. ILAR J 41:80–86
Nc3rs (2025) The 3rs [Online]. Available: nc3rs.org.uk/who-we-are/3rs. Accessed 24 Oct 2025
Nisbet MC (2009) Communicating climate change: why frames matter for public engagement. Environ Sci Policy Sustain Dev 51:12–23
Ormandy EH, Schuppli CA, Weary DM (2013) Public attitudes toward the use of animals in research: effects of invasiveness, genetic modification and regulation. Anthrozoös 26:165–184
Piwowar HA, Day RS, Fridsma DB (2007) Sharing detailed research data is associated with increased citation rate. PLoS One 2:E308
Plain (2011) Federal plain language guidelines [Online]. Available: https://www.plainlanguage.gov/media/FederalPLGuidelines.pdf. Accessed 21 May 2025
Pound P, Blaug R (2016) Transparency and public involvement in animal research. Altern Lab Anim 44:167–173
Prescott MJ, Lidster K (2017) Improving quality of science through better animal welfare: the Nc3rs strategy. Lab Anim 46:152–156
RE3DATA.ORG (2025) Registry of research data repositories [Online]. Available: https://www.re3data.org/. Accessed 11 May 2025
Recall ER (2016) Beyond memorability: visualization recognition and recall. IEEE Trans Vis Comput Graph 22:519–528
Reinhardt K (2023) Trust and trustworthiness in Ai ethics. AI Ethics 3:735–744
Richardson CA (2015) The power of automated behavioural homecage technologies in characterizing disease progression in laboratory mice: a review. Appl Anim Behav Sci 163:19–27
Russell WMS, Burch RL (1959) The principles of humane experimental technique. Methuen
Sillito RR, Sutherland J, Milne A, Giuliano C, Sigfridsson C-G, Rolf M, Cherian AK, Mcclafferty ML, Rossman EI, Teuns G (2025) Rodent home cage monitoring for preclinical safety pharmacology assessment: results of a multi-company validation evaluating nonclinical and clinical data from three compounds. Front Toxicol 7:1655330
Spruijt BM, Devisser L (2006) Advanced behavioural screening: automated home cage ethology. Drug Discov Today Technol 3:231–237

TEATIME C (2025) Cost Teatime News [Online]. Available: www.cost-teatime.org/news/. Accessed 24 Oct 2025
Tennant JP, Waldner F, Jacques DC, Masuzzo P, Collister LB, Hartgerink CH (2016) The academic, economic and societal impacts of open access: an evidence-based review. F1000Res 5:632
Van Dijck J (2013) The culture of connectivity: a critical history of social media. Oxford University Press
Van Dijck J, Poell T, De Waal M (2018) The platform society: public values in a connective world. Oxford University Press
Velho RM, Mendes AMF, Azevedo CLN (2020) Communicating science with Youtube videos: how nine factors relate to and affect video views. Front Commun 5:567606
Voelkl B, Würbel H (2016) Reproducibility crisis: are we ignoring reaction norms? Trends Pharmacol Sci 37:509–510
Voikar V, Gaburro S (2020) Three pillars of automated home-cage phenotyping of mice: novel findings, refinement, and reproducibility based on literature and experience. Front Behav Neurosci 14:575434
Wilkinson MD, Dumontier M, Aalbersberg IJ, Appleton G, Axton M, Baak A, Blomberg N, Boiten J-W, Da Silva Santos LB, Bourne PE (2016) The fair guiding principles for scientific data management and stewardship. Sci Data 3:1–9

The Most Used Rodent Models in Home Cage Monitoring

Marion Rivalan, Arianna Novati, Stefano Gaburro, Lars Lewejohann, and Vootele Voikar

Abstract

Home cage monitoring (HCM) offers a transformative approach to understanding rodent behavior and physiology in biomedical research. This chapter reviews the most commonly used mouse and rat models in HCM. Mice, particularly the C57BL/6 inbred strain, dominate the field due to their genetic homogeneity, ease of breeding, and well-characterized genome. Despite their advantages, researchers must consider strain- (and substrain-) specific traits that can be either strengths or limitations of the model (such

M. Rivalan
Institute of Neuroscience Paris-Saclay, CNRS, University of Paris-Saclay, Saclay, France

A. Novati
Institute of Animal Welfare, Animal Behavior and Laboratory Animal Science, Department of Veterinary Medicine, Free University of Berlin, Berlin, Germany

Science of Intelligence, Research Cluster of Excellence, Berlin, Germany

S. Gaburro
Tecniplast S.p.A., Buguggiate, Italy

L. Lewejohann
Institute of Animal Welfare, Animal Behavior and Laboratory Animal Science, Department of Veterinary Medicine, Free University of Berlin, Berlin, Germany

Science of Intelligence, Research Cluster of Excellence, Berlin, Germany

German Federal Institute for Risk Assessment (BfR), German Center for the Protection of Laboratory Animals (Bf3R), Berlin, Germany

V. Voikar (✉)
Laboratory Animal Center, Helsinki Institute of Life Science, University of Helsinki, Helsinki, Finland
e-mail: vootele.voikar@helsinki.fi

S. Gaburro, S. Mandillo (eds.), *Home Cage Monitoring in Rodents: A Global Effort*,
https://doi.org/10.1007/978-3-032-19781-8_13

as susceptibility to diet-induced obesity, age-related hearing loss, retinal degeneration and visual impairment, and differences in locomotor and exploratory activity). HCM allows for the continuous monitoring of behaviors such as activity and feeding, providing insights into subtle phenotypes and genetic influences on behavior. Other mouse strains, including DBA/2, 129, BALB/c, and FVB/N, offer unique behavioral profiles useful for specific research applications. In rats, strains like the Long-Evans, Dark Agouti, and Spontaneously Hypertensive Rat (SHR) are highlighted for their relevance in cognitive, metabolic, and cardiovascular studies. This chapter underscores the importance of selecting appropriate strains for HCM studies, considering genetic background, behavioral traits, and experimental goals. The continuous, automated nature of HCM systems promises to advance our understanding of complex behaviors and physiological responses, paving the way for innovative approaches in biomedical research.

Keywords

Laboratory rodents · Inbred strains · Behavioral phenotyping · Genetic background

1 Introduction

In the EU research area, since 2015, after adoption of the Directive 2010/63/EU by the member states, precise statistics have been collected about how many animals and which species have been used in research and testing and for what purposes. All these data are reported yearly, albeit with a considerable delay, and are publicly available in the ALURES (ANIMALUSE REPORTING - EU SYSTEM) statistical EU-Database (ALURES database 2025).

In 2022, mice and rats composed approximately 55% of all animals used (4.7 million out of a total of approximately 8.5 million), making them the most commonly used mammalian species in biomedical research. They were used mostly for basic research (53%) but also in translational and applied research (28%) and regulatory use (17%).

In basic research, the main areas of use were the nervous system (28%), immune system, and oncology (18% both), whereas in translational research, mice and rats were used in studies on human cancer (35%), followed by human nervous and mental disorders (16%) and human infectious disorders (13%).

Any area of biomedical research, where the progression of disease symptoms or effect of the treatment is studied, can highly benefit from having continuous, 24/7 measurement of behavioral (activity, feeding, drinking, sleeping, etc.) and/or physiological (e.g., heart rate and body temperature) characteristics that can be collected through home-cage monitoring (HCM). Moreover, this approach would help in finding subtle phenotypes or completely new insights that could be not distinguished by short conventional tests, often affected by unspecific stressors or inappropriate timing during the circadian cycle. Thus, the measurements collected by HCMs can provide unique insights into the effects of genetic background on individual and group behavior not previously recognized.

There are several advantages that make mice and rats especially suitable for basic and applied research—genetic and biological similarity to humans, short lifespan and reproductive cycle along with small size, well-characterized genome, and long research history. Rats have traditionally been used more for behavioral, physiological, and pharmacological studies, whereas mouse strains were mostly developed for research in genetics and oncology. However, mice became a model of choice and almost a gold standard for all biomedical research in the 1990s, after the introduction of the technologies enabling genetic engineering to produce genetically modified (transgenic, knock-out) animals (Barinaga 1992), and ever since these technologies are evolving rapidly (conditional mutagenesis, optogenetics, and CRISPR-Cas9 technology).

In this chapter, we provide a short and nonexhaustive review of insights from the HCM with most common rodent models, based on the authors' personal experience and knowledge of the field.

2 Mouse Models Studied by the HCM

2.1 C57BL/6 and Other Inbred Strains; Spontaneous or Mutant Models

2.1.1 Name of the Model: C57BL/6 (BL6)

BL6 Strain Characteristics

Most biomedical research involving laboratory mice is conducted using BL6 mice. Advantages and disadvantages of the widespread use of this "gold-standard" strain will be discussed in the following section.

A quick PubMed search [Searchstring: "(c57) OR (c57BL) OR (C57BL/6) OR (c57BL*) OR (BL6) OR (B6)"] revealed over 369,000 results since the year 2000 compared to 155,000 results for the second most often used inbred strain, BALB/c. There are several reasons for the popularity of the BL6 mouse. Most prominent is that the strain is readily available, reproduces well, has a low susceptibility to tumors, and makes a "typical mouse" impression at first glance, including suitable behavioral phenotypes (escaping floor or ceiling effects) in most behavioral paradigms. BL6 is widely used as a 'general purpose strain' and was chosen as the background strain for the generation of most transgenic and knockout lines. In fact, BL6 has been shown to be an appropriate genetic background for many gene modifications. For these reasons, this strain was selected by the Mouse Genome Sequencing Consortium (MGSC) to represent the laboratory mouse reference genome, with sequencing completed in 2002. Thereafter, the C57BL/6 N substrain has been chosen as a background strain on which the International Mouse Phenotyping Consortium is creating and phenotyping null alleles for all protein-coding genes (Brown et al. 2018; Groza et al. 2023).

However, to be brutally honest, most of the reasons for choosing BL6 are based on the fact that almost everything we think we know about mice is based on the BL6 strain. The popularity of this model is caught in a positive feedback loop: many publications (including our own) contain statements such as "BL6 is the most commonly used mouse, so we conducted our research with BL6 to achieve the greatest possible relevance". It must be mentioned that BL6 is a family lineage with approximately 200 well-known and less well-known individual lines. There are subtle and sometimes striking differences between the substrains (Bryant 2011), which are beyond the scope of this chapter. However, knowing precisely which substrain is used (by adhering to international nomenclature) is crucial for reliable interpretation of data and reproducibility. You can find a good overview on the relevant pages of the major institutes for mouse production, such as The Jackson Laboratory (JAX Lab 2025).

BL6 mice can live up to 30 months (Brust et al. 2015), but it should be noted that significant signs of aging may become apparent at approximately 24 months, requiring close observation with regard to animal care and, if necessary, humane intervention (Kahnau et al. 2021). For an overview of the development of behavioral phenotypes in mice over the lifetime, see (Brust et al. 2015).

BL6 mice are usually considered relatively docile (Lidster et al. 2019). However, in some labs, BL6 has been found to show considerable amounts of aggressive behavior, possibly due to increased aggressiveness induced by corn cob bedding and other housing conditions (Theil et al. 2020).

Disadvantages and Caveats of the Model

Compared to other strains of mice, BL6 also carries disadvantages that must be considered when choosing this model. For example, BL6 mice have a high susceptibility to diet-induced obesity (Lang et al. 2019). For this reason, they are often used as a model for diet-related obesity, as they are comparatively similar to humans in this area. At the same time, for studies of a different nature, attention should be given to the diet so as not to bias the results. On a side note, it might be interesting to notice that the susceptibility to high-fat diet-induced obesity is strongly interacting with the microbiome and not as severe in BL6 mice with a wild-derived microbiome (Hild et al. 2021).

BL6 mice are known to be prone to age-related degeneration of hearing. It is worth noting that this also affects some other strains, but with BL6, this is one of the factors that is frequently mentioned when discussing the disadvantages of this model. Hearing begins to decline at approximately 3 months of age at high frequencies and is considered severely impaired at approximately 15 months of age. Most animals are tested at 60–90 days of age, and no or only mild impairments are expected at this age. However, if long-term studies are conducted into old age, it should be noted that social communication may be impaired. The cause is relatively well understood, and many BL6 carry a homozygous allele combination ($Cdh23^{ahl}$). However, there are differences between the various sublines, so it is advisable to use less susceptible lines when working with older animals in age-related studies (Newton et al. 2025).

It is to be noted that BL6 mice have peculiar immunological characteristics, as this strain was originally developed for the study of antitumor activity and immunology (Song and Hwang 2017). This strain presents increased immunological reactivity, which should be considered when aiming at modeling diseases such as obesity or depression, which are often characterized by low-grade inflammation. The progressive and multidimensional characteristics of such immunological factors are particularly relevant to follow longitudinally within the natural environment of the home cage.

BL6 in HCM

Because so many researchers use BL6, it is not surprising that there are numerous examples of this strain being used in HCM. In fact, in a recent systematic review, it was found that 49% of studies using mice in HCM were conducted with BL6 mice (Kahnau et al. 2023). Unfortunately, in many studies, the animals were kept individually for long periods of time in order to allow for detailed individual monitoring. Interestingly, it was found that BL6 mice showed a bimodal activity pattern when observed in the home cage, contrasted with a unimodal pattern in the strain C3H Adamah-Biassi et al. (2013). These data were derived from single-housed males using a camera-based system (HomeCageScan System 3.0, CleverSys Inc.). Such bimodal activity patterns of BL6 and C3H mice were also found in group housing using RFID and video data by Bains (2016, 2018) and in Tph2−/− and Tph2+/+ mice of BL6 background by Rivalan et al. (2024). They also found activity patterns to be different from another (less active) strain, FVB/NcrlBRH (Bains), or from a more active genotype of the same background (Rivalan). BL6 mice proved to be a suitable strain for measuring hippocampus-dependent learning in a home cage environment using the IntelliCage, whereas similar results would be difficult to achieve with the DBA/2 mouse strain under the same experimental conditions (Voikar et al. 2010). These and other studies (Voikar et al. 2018) also show that BL6 mice in a home cage setting are suitable for spatial memory tests, for which tests outside the home cage, such as the water maze task, are usually used.

Things to Consider with HCM and This Model

It will come as no surprise that BL6 mice have black fur. This makes the animals stand out clearly against the usually light-colored bedding in their home cage. This is good for video tracking, but the black fur is surprisingly resistant to any kind of marking. From personal experience, we know that simple H_2O_2 bleach does not work easily. Even prolonged exposure to bleaching chemicals under anesthesia only leads to mediocre results. Our recommendation for manual observations is marking the tail roots using a unique two-color code applied with lacquer painting pens (Kahnau et al. 2021), but this requires regular renewal about once a week. As a caveat, to our knowledge, there is currently no tracking software that can identify and distinguish individual BL6 mice solely based on visual cues.

2.2 Other Commonly Used Mouse Strains

2.2.1 Background

At the dawn of "transgenic revolution", the researchers also began to investigate (or rediscover) the differences between a vast number of inbred strains that were available Crawley et al. (1997), although the advantages of these genetically defined, homogeneous animals (as compared to heterogeneous, outbred stocks) were well known (Festing 1999). However, the suggested major strength of low variability has also been challenged by Tuttle et al. (2018), who compared coefficients of variation between inbred and outbred mice and did not find evidence of greater trait stability in inbred mice.

The effect of genetic background was recognized and acknowledged and recommendations provided Silva et al. (1997); in reality, it has been dealt with in a reductionistic manner—the cases where a mutation is studied in any background other than C57BL/6 are very rare. However, when it is performed, the results almost always confirm the dependence of the phenotype on the background in mutant animals (Holmes et al. 2003; Morice et al. 2004; Sittig et al. 2016). Therefore, for generalizing the experimental findings, it would be always good to study the treatment in more than one genetic background (aka systematic heterogenization, Voelkl et al. 2020).

The overwhelming popularity of the BL6 strain has been described in the previous section. However, even the gold standard needs some references and comparisons. The strain comparisons can be extremely valuable in studying the variation in behavioral and physiological responses under different experimental conditions, providing essential information for developing and validating new tasks and systems. The Mouse Phenome Database (MPD, initiated in 1999) identified 40 common inbred strains and divided them into groups of ten by priority (Mouse Phenome Database 2025). The need for such an initiative to collect comprehensive phenotypic information on inbred strains was justified by common belief and understanding that mouse models serve as the primary animal model for exploring genetic variation and human biology, and reliable phenotypic data are essential for realizing the full utility of genomic information emerging from sequencing the genome. By using a panel of inbred strains, one could establish the baselines that would be helpful in interpretation of the experimental data. These strain differences are rather stable if careful attention to the nomenclature and origin of the substrains is given, along with comparable testing conditions and other factors that may influence the Genotype X Environment interactions.

2.2.2 Characteristics of the Other Strains

The following inbred strains (all belonging to the priority group A of the MPD) have been most commonly used in basic research, along with the B6 model (also in HCM, according to Kahnau et al. (2023)) (Fig. 1).

DBA/2 (DBA/2 strain 2025) is the first inbred mouse strain in history, with breeding initiated in 1909. The DBA/2 mice are widely used in behavioral studies and often compared to the BL6 mice as some of their characteristics are often contrasted (particularly,

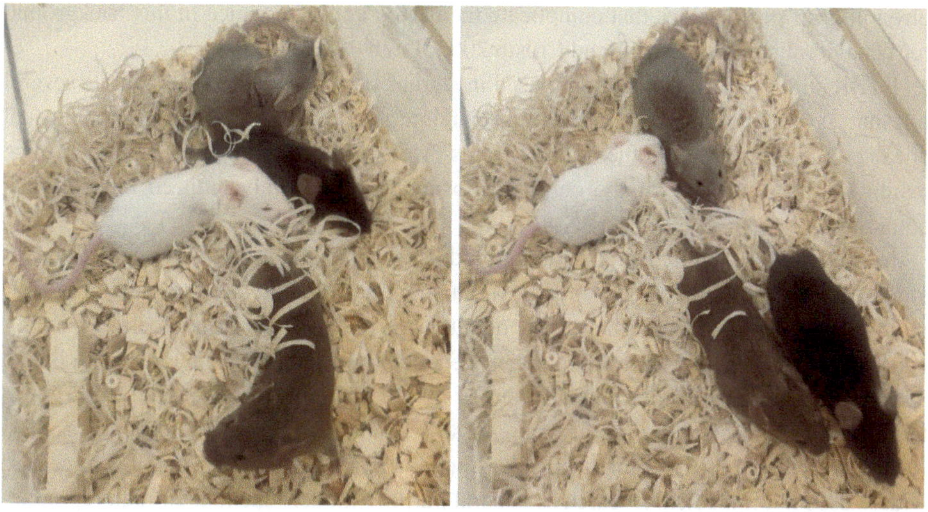

Fig. 1 Mouse strains can often be visually distinguished by their coat color—black (BL/6), agouti (129), white/Albino (BALB/c), and dilute-brown-agouti (DBA/2). In addition, they may have several strain-specific characteristics that need to be considered in planning the study and interpretation of the results, explained in this chapter

exhibiting poor spatial learning, avoiding alcohol in choice tests, impulsivity and anxiety-like behavior, susceptibility to audiogenic seizures, and high-frequency hearing loss). By crossing the DBA/2 and BL6 strains, followed by inbreeding, a number of recombinant inbred BXD strains have been created, which are extensively used for mapping genes related to physiological and behavioral traits like addiction, stress, metabolic disease, and cancer (Ashbrook et al. 2021).

129 family (129 strains 2025)—a number of peculiar substrains are available; therefore, following the proper nomenclature is even more important (Simpson et al. 1997; Festing et al. 1999). It has been the most widely used strain in the production of targeted mutations due to the availability of several lines of embryonic stem cells. However, the 129 substrains have a very complex and even confusing history (with genetic drift and contamination). Moreover, they display certain behavioral disadvantages (often poor spatial and motor learning, hypoactivity, and anxiety-like behavior) and neuroanatomical deficits (absent or deficient corpus callosum).

BALB/c (BALB/c strain 2025) is widely used as a general purpose inbred strain in various research areas (immunology, cancer, infectious disease, and behavioral research). Behaviorally, they have often been characterized as mice of high trait anxiety (Belzung and Berton 1997).

FVB/N (FVB strain 2025)—historically, the FVB/N strain has been used for producing transgenic mice. They have a vigorous reproductive performance with large litters. However, the strain suffers from retinal degeneration and has other behavioral and physiological peculiarities that complicate the use of transgenic mice in this background for behavioral studies (Mineur and Crusio 2002; Pugh et al. 2004).

BTBR strain (2025) is commonly used in studies of autism because it exhibits several relevant symptoms including reduced social interactions, impaired play, and unusual vocalizations compared to other inbred strains (Meyza and Blanchard 2017). BTBR mice exhibit a 100% absence of the corpus callosum and a severely reduced hippocampal commissure.

In contrast to the inbred strains, an outbred strain ("stock") is a closed population (for at least four generations) of genetically variable animals that are bred to maintain maximum heterozygosity. There is no genetic quality control system for these stocks; even their names provide little information about their genetic or phenotypic characteristics. It is also important to note that similar to substrains of inbred mice, the same outbred stock maintained at different breeding centers may possess significant phenotypic differences. The ICR (CD-1) and NMRI outbred mice, originally derived from Swiss albino mice, are widely used in biomedical research as general purpose models due to their high reproductive performance, rapid growth, and strong adaptability to the environment. They are albinos and may suffer from visual impairments (Serfilippi et al. 2004; Clapcote et al. 2005).

In summary, it should be emphasized that the selection of genetic background can impact the internal and external validity of research. This choice needs to be carefully weighed based on the research questions and outcome parameters, and strain names should be reported precisely according to international nomenclature. Using multiple inbred strains allows researchers to uncover strain-specific phenotypes, genetic interactions, and disease susceptibilities, thereby improving the robustness and translational relevance of biomedical studies. In contrast, relying solely on BL6 mice can limit the generalizability of research findings. The strengths and limitations of each strain depend heavily on the specific research question.

2.2.3 Differences Between the Strains Revealed by HCM

Next, we provide a short and not exhaustive overview of the studies, where the physiology and behavior (including locomotor activity and circadian rhythms; sleep and rest patterns; feeding and drinking; anxiety-related behavior; social behavior and interaction; and cognitive performance) of different mouse strains have been compared by using a variety of automated HCM systems.

By using radiotelemetry and measuring body temperature, heart rate, and locomotor activity, strain differences were found in the magnitude and duration of the stress responses and circadian activity between 129Sv/Ev, C57BL/6, and Swiss-Webster mice (Van Bogaert et al. 2006). However, the observed ranking in autonomic stress response did not match the behavioral stress responsivity of these strains, showing that simultaneous measurement of behavioral (activity) and autonomic parameters (heart rate and temperature) under stressful conditions contributes considerably to a better interpretation of anxiety and stress levels in mice.

Phenotyping spontaneous locomotor activity in inbred and outbred mouse strains by using Digital Ventilated Cages revealed significant differences in the circadian activity patterns of the three selected strains when comparing inbred versus outbred as well as inbred strains (C57BL/6NCrl; BALB/cAnNCrl; CRL:CD1(ICR) (Fuochi et al. 2021). These data corroborate the concept that each strain behaves under characteristic patterns (e.g., anticipation of the dark phase, peaks of activity, and behavior during the light period), which needs to be taken into consideration in the study design to ensure experimental reproducibility and comply with essential animal welfare principles. Strain-specific patterns of circadian activity were also revealed by using Home-Cage Analyzer (Bains et al. 2016).

Using the same dataset but novel and refined analysis tools, the authors were able to show that also when referring to space preference within the cage, C57BL/6NCrl has a high variability in the behavioral phenotypes from prepuberty until early adulthood compared to BALB/cAnNCrl, which is confirmed to be socially disaggregated, and CRL:CD1(ICR), which is conversely highly active and socially aggregated. These HCM data also suggest that a strain-oriented approach is needed when defining the frequency of cage change as well as the maximum allowed animal density, according to the physiological peculiarities of the strains, and always avoiding the "one size fits all" approach (Fuochi et al. 2023). Such findings can also inform evidence-based adjustments in animal husbandry, thereby contributing to improved animal welfare.

Spontaneous behavior in the social homecage can reliably discriminate strains, lesions, and mutations in mice, showing that mouse strains (BL6, DBA/2, 129S2, BALB/c, and B6D2F1) have unique and reproducible behavioral profiles in IntelliCage that help in interpretation of the results with models in the BL6 background. Moreover, monitoring of mutant mice with known deficits in hippocampus-dependent conventional tests produced profiles very similar to those of mice with hippocampal lesions (Vannoni et al. 2014). For developing new cognitive tasks in a fully automated HCM system, the combination of inbred strains (with known and contrasting characteristics) and brain lesions can be useful (Voikar et al. 2018). Multilaboratory studies add evidence for the generalisability and reliability of the new methods (Endo et al. 2011).

The problem of reproducibility of behavioral phenotyping results is well known (Crabbe et al. 1999), where experiments with experimental models may yield results that are idiosyncratic to a particular laboratory. Automated (and standardized) HCM systems have been shown to tackle this problem effectively. For instance, testing three strains of mice with divergent behavioral phenotypes (BL6, DBA/2, and B6D2F1) revealed consistent outcomes in four laboratories by using IntelliCage (Krackow et al. 2010). In another study, the ambulatory activity of BL6 and DBA/2 mice was tested by PhenoTyper in two laboratories under near identical housing and testing conditions, and similar circadian rhythms were observed across laboratories (Robinson et al. 2018).

One of the main benefits of several automated HCM systems is the possibility of tracking individual animals when group-housed. However, it is important to note that cohousing and social interaction between different strains can substantially affect their emotional phenotype (Kulesskaya et al. 2014; Heinla et al. 2018). Such information may also be important for interpreting the outcomes of research with disease models and genetically modified mice. Adherence to the PREPARE and ARRIVE guidelines cannot be emphasized enough when planning, conducting, and reporting preclinical studies involving animal models (Smith et al. 2018; Percie Du Sert et al. 2020).

2.3 Integrated Home-Cage and Circadian Monitoring in Mouse Models of Obesity and Diabetes

Escalating global prevalence of obesity and diabetes has prompted intensive use of rodent models for mechanistic and pre-clinical studies. A PubMed search combining "high-fat diet OR ob/ob OR db/db OR NOD" with "mouse" yields >75,000 articles since 2000, underlining the field's breadth. Automated home-cage technologies now allow for the continuous phenotyping of energy balance, while chronobiological tools reveal how circadian misalignment drives metabolic pathology. Commonly employed models include

- Diet-induced obesity (DIO) in C57BL/6 J mice: replicates human polygenic obesity with intact leptin signaling.
- ob/ob (leptin-deficient) and db/db (leptin-receptor-deficient) mice: severe hyperphagia, obesity, and insulin resistance.
- Non-obese diabetic (NOD) mice: autoimmune β-cell loss and hyperglycemia.
- High-fat diet plus streptozotocin models: combined insulin resistance and β-cell dysfunction.

2.3.1 Caveats When Interpreting Metabolic Read-Outs

Genetic models differ in basal locomotor activity and thermal conductance, which confound energy expenditure calculations. Hyperphagic strains (ob/ob and db/db) generate large bedding moisture volumes, necessitating bedding-specific calibration of capacitance-based sensors. Circadian damping in leptin-pathway mutants blunts locomotor rhythms, complicating phase-based analyses. Additionally, what is generally missing are environmental data (e.g., temperature, light, and housing), biological data (e.g., gender, age, and strain), and, ultimately, technical data (e.g., calorimetry assumption and cage effects).

2.3.2 Continuous Metabolic Phenotyping with Circadian Context

Timing and operant responding in group-housed mice via a feeder revealed that caloric-restricted C57BL/6 J mice voluntarily concentrate intake to the early dark phase, protecting glucose tolerance (Acosta-Rodríguez et al. 2017). Similarly, similar systems coupled infrared tracking with load-cell food hoppers, showing that a high-fat diet advances feeding onset by ≈2 h and fragments rest-activity rhythms (Nguyen et al. 2016). Wireless continuous glucose monitoring (CGM) in female NOD mice detects 24-h glucose waves inversely correlated with body temperature, capturing dawn hyperglycemia missed by single-time-point sampling (Korstanje et al. 2017). Tecniplast Digital Ventilated Cages (DVCs) use floor capacitance to flag polyuria episodes that align with CGM-verified hyperglycemic excursions, enabling noninvasive staging of diabetes progression (Brachs et al. 2025).

2.3.3 Circadian Disruption as a Pathogenic Driver

Shift-work simulations in mice (8-h phase advance every 3 days) accelerate weight gain despite unchanged caloric intake and elevate hepatic lipogenesis markers (Shi et al. 2013). Human laboratory studies corroborate that circadian misalignment reduces insulin sensitivity and elevates cortisol, predisposing to adiposity (Broussard and Van Cauter 2016). Sleep-corrected social jetlag in adolescents is associated with a higher BMI z-score and late-day snacking; meal-timing regularity interventions reduce weight and improve subjective well-being (Wilming et al. 2024).

2.3.4 Practical Considerations

- Combine infrared or RFID activity tracking with CGM or indirect calorimetry to disentangle energy expenditure from locomotor artifacts.
- Align data to zeitgeber time rather than clock time when diets differ in photoperiod alignment.
- Validate sensor accuracy after bedding changes or cage wash cycles.

2.3.5 Conclusion

Coupling home-cage analytics with circadian read-outs affords granular insight into how meal timing, activity, and endocrine rhythms converge to shape metabolic disease. These integrated platforms lay the groundwork for chrono-therapeutic strategies that restore temporal order to improve metabolic outcomes.

3 Rat Models Studied by the HCM

3.1 Long Evans (LE), Wistar (WI), Dark Agouti (DA), Spontaneously Hypertensive Rats (SHR), Sprague Dawley (SD)

3.1.1 Continuous Telemetry-Based Cardiovascular Characterization of Spontaneously Hypertensive Rats

The spontaneously hypertensive rat (SHR) is a genetically selected model that recapitulates the progressive elevation of systolic and diastolic blood pressure, vascular stiffness, and left-ventricular hypertrophy seen in essential hypertension. While conventional tail-cuff or catheter recordings provide isolated snapshots, implantable telemetry and other home-cage sensors permit 24-h cardiovascular surveillance in unhandled, freely moving animals.

Modern telemetry transducers implanted in the abdominal aorta (or carotid artery) or jacketed telemetry with less invasive allow beat-to-beat arterial pressure, electrocardiogram (ECG), heart-rate variability (HRV), and core temperature to be streamed wirelessly to receivers beneath standard cages. Coupling these signals with infrared or video activity tracking provides time-locked behavioral context with minimal investigator interference (Redfern et al. 2017; Voikar and Gaburro 2020).

Telemetry has confirmed that SHRs develop hypertension as early as 6–8 weeks of age, with mean arterial pressure exceeding 160 mmHg by 12 weeks (Lerman et al. 2019). Unlike normotensive Wistar–Kyoto rats, many adult SHRs fail to exhibit the normal nocturnal "dip" in blood pressure or show a reversed (non-dipping) profile, a pattern that correlates with greater end-organ damage in humans (Chen et al. 2017a). Pressure recordings also reveal exaggerated lability: transient surges of >40 mmHg occur during cage activity or startle responses, reflecting enhanced sympathetic reactivity.

Simultaneous ECG telemetry demonstrates shortened R–R intervals (baseline HR $\approx$ 380–420 bpm) and reduced HRV complexity across multiple time-scales in SHRs, indicating persistent sympathetic dominance and impaired vagal modulation (Silva et al. 2016). Baroreflex gain, calculated from spontaneous sequences of pressure–pulse interval coupling, is blunted by ~50% relative to controls, mirroring autonomic dysregulation in clinical hypertension.

Chronic stress paradigms applied in the home cage (e.g., unpredictable noise or restraint) exaggerate tachycardic and pressor responses in SHRs compared with normotensive rats. Repeated restraint elevates the basal heart rate and augments baroreflex-mediated tachycardia, effects captured only through continuous telemetry (Vieira et al. 2018).

When aligned with longitudinal echocardiography and vascular ultrasound, telemetry data show that sustained pressor load drives concentric left-ventricular hypertrophy, increased aortic wall thickness, and elevated vascular oscillatory shear index in SHRs by 24 weeks (Chen et al. 2017b). Pharmacological interventions such as angiotensin-II receptor blockers (losartan and telmisartan) normalize pressure rhythms and partially restore HRV within days, preceding regression of structural remodeling, underscoring the mechanistic value of continuous hemodynamic endpoints (Mulinari-Santos et al. 2018).

Continuous telemetry thus provides an integrative read-out of hemodynamic load, autonomic balance, and therapeutic efficacy in SHR. The approach enhances construct validity by capturing circadian, stress-induced, and drug-responsive changes and narrows the translational gap to human hypertension. Future work integrating pressure telemetry with optogenetic or calcium-imaging read-outs will further dissect central circuits governing sympathetic outflow.

The spontaneously hypertensive rat (SHR) has remained the work-horse model for essential hypertension for over five decades. A PubMed query ("spontaneously hypertensive rat" OR "SHR") returned >10,000 entries since 2000, underscoring its prominence in cardiovascular research. SHRs were derived from Wistar stock by selective breeding for elevated blood pressure; they reach systolic values ≥160 mmHg by 12 weeks and develop vascular stiffening, left-ventricular hypertrophy, and end-organ damage comparable to human hypertension (Doris 2017; Lerman et al. 2019). Under barrier conditions, SHRs live 24–30 months, yet clinically relevant cardiac and renal lesions often appear by 15 months, requiring close surveillance. Continuous telemetry assists in detecting early decompensation (e.g., sustained tachycardia or arrhythmia) and defines humane endpoints objectively. SHR displays greater locomotor activity and impulsivity than normotensive Wistar–Kyoto (WKY) rats. Group housing is generally compatible with implanted transmitters, although dominant aggression may surface in adolescent males; adequate cage space and enrichment mitigate these episodes.

Disadvantages and Caveats

Many colonies harbor the *Cdh23ahl* allele, resulting in progressive high-frequency hearing loss from approximately 3 months to virtual deafness at approximately 15 months (Brace et al. 2015). SHR also exhibits exaggerated sympathetic responses—brief restraint can raise mean arterial pressure (MAP) by more than 40 mmHg—so intermittent tail-cuff readings overestimate baseline MAP. Additionally, basal glucose levels are modestly elevated, and insulin sensitivity is reduced relative to WKY, factors relevant for cardiometabolic studies.

Continuous Cardiovascular Telemetry and Integration with HCMs

Implanted pressure transmitters (abdominal aorta or carotid) stream beat-to-beat MAP, ECG, and core temperature from freely moving SHR. Telemetry exposes a high prevalence of non-dipping or reverse-dipping BP rhythms that predict severe cardiac remodeling (Chen et al. 2017a). Heart-rate variability (HRV) shows reduced complexity and diminished vagal tone, and spontaneous baroreflex gain is $\approx$50% lower than in WKYs, reflecting autonomic dysfunction (Silva et al. 2016). Under chronic stress, telemetry captures exaggerated tachycardic and pressor responses unique to SHRs, as well as delayed baroreflex desensitization (Vieira et al. 2018). Several studies now combine telemetry with home-cage monitoring (HCM) to pair hemodynamic read-outs with continuous behavioral data. Azar et al. instrumented female SHRs with pressure transmitters and showed that environmental enrichment elevated dark-phase activity yet left basal MAP unchanged, demonstrating strain-specific cardiovascular resilience to enrichment (Azar et al. 2012). The same group reported that group-housing of SHRs reduced the resting heart rate and blunted stress-evoked tachycardia compared with singly housed counterparts (Azar et al. 2011). Another study used 72-h telemetric BP recording alongside RFID-based activity tracking to show that the dopamine-β-hydroxylase inhibitor etamicastat lowered BP without altering spontaneous cage activity, validating its antihypertensive efficacy in the absence of locomotor confounds (Igreja et al. 2015). Earlier telemetry work by van den Buuse mapped circadian BP, HR, and locomotor rhythms in unrestrained SHR, providing baseline chronobiological signatures still referenced today (Van Den Buuse 1994).

Structural Remodeling Endpoints

Coupling telemetry with echocardiography and vascular ultrasound reveals that sustained pressure load drives concentric left-ventricular hypertrophy, aortic wall thickening, and elevated oscillatory shear index by 24 weeks (Azar et al. 2012). Angiotensin-II receptor blockers (losartan and telmisartan) normalize BP rhythms within days, improve HRV, and precede hypertrophy regression (Azar et al. 2011). Thus, continuous telemetry plus heart failure with preserved ejection fraction (HCM) supplies sensitive biomarkers for therapeutic efficacy. Telemetry implants add ≈3 g and necessitate brief single housing post-surgery. Albino SHR coat color offers high video contrast, aiding automated tracking; infrared illumination permits dark-phase recording. Pressure sensors must be recalibrated periodically because fibrotic encapsulation can shift zero values over time.

Conclusion

Integrating telemetry with automated HCM refines cardiovascular phenotyping of SHRs, capturing dynamic links between behavior, circadian biology, and hemodynamics that static methods miss. These high-resolution datasets strengthen translational insight and support the development of next-generation antihypertensives.

3.2 Continuous Home Cage Monitoring of Social Interaction and Social Status in Dark Agouti (DA) Rats

3.2.1 DA Characteristics and Use

DA are pigmented inbred rats with good vision that are mainly used in physiological and medical studies and have only rarely been tested for their cognitive abilities (Aggleton et al. 1996) and only recently for their executive functions and social skills (Alonso et al. 2020). DA rats are known to be susceptible to induced arthritis, autoimmune thyroiditis, and the spontaneous development of certain forms of cancers (e.g., urinary bladder). However, how those physiological susceptibilities may influence behavioral outcomes, particularly in long-term or translational studies, is currently unknown. Their behavioral phenotype is less explored, although a multidimensional analysis of their cognitive and social profile revealed interesting specificities compared to the outbred line of Wistar Han (WI(Han)) rats.

Comparing their cognitive abilities, natural behaviors, and physiological responses to those of WI(Han) rats revealed similarities between strains in their performances in most tests. WI(Han) and DA lines, however, differed to some degree in their sensitivity to reward and impulsivity in operant cages and in their locomotor activity and open space-occupation in HCM. Both strains presented large phenotypic variation in behaviors pertinent for the study of the underlying mechanisms of poor decision making and associated disorders. Both the interindividual and interstrain comparison approaches provided new insights for the preferential use of each strain in future neuropsychopharmacological studies.

3.2.2 Spontaneous Profile of DA Compared to WI(Han) in HC

In a large automated home cage environment designed and named after the Visible Burrow System developed 30 years ago (Blanchard et al. 1995), the spontaneous and continuous recording of general activity, space use, and social and nonsocial behaviors was carried out for each individual in groups of male rats. The automated VBS consisted of an open area extended to the top by high walls and connected through transparent tunnels to a burrow system placed into a second cage. A grid of 32 RFID detectors was placed below the VBS in order to automatically detect individual animal positions. The behaviors expressed by the animals were scored from continuous video recordings following a list of typical affiliative, aggression, defensive, and maintenance behaviors (Rademacher et al. 2002; Burman et al. 2008; Alonso et al. 2020). The activity, place preference, and time spent in the open area of the VBS were measured using the data collected from the grid RFID detectors. Thanks to the RFID tracking of each individual of the group, we did not need any physical marking of the fur of the animal, simplifying data collection and resulting in minimal disturbance of the animal.

In both strains, the behaviors most frequently observed in the VBS were huddling (lying in contact with another rat), eating, and struggling at the feeder. The 19 other scored behaviors (e.g., allogrooming, embracing, following, mounting, flight, freezing, and upright defense) were seen more rarely in both strains. Considering the three most frequent behaviors, DA rats huddled more but struggled (at the feeder) less than WI(Han) rats and did not differ in eating behavior. Both DA and WI(Han) rats changed their activity (i.e., distance traveled) with the light/dark phase and were more active during the dark phase. Over all days, locomotion in WI(Han) rats was higher than in DA rats during both dark and light phases. DA rats preferred to stay more in the burrow area than the WI(Han) and, from Day 3, spent significantly less time in the open area, indicating a more defensive and anxious phenotype than the WI(Han) rats. These original results provided new insights for the preferential use of each strain in future neuropsychopharmacological studies. The WI(Han) and DA strains could be preferentially selected to study pathologies related to reward sensitivity and impulsivity on one side (WI(Han)) and compulsivity and anxiety-related behaviors (DA) on the other side (Alonso et al. 2020).

3.2.3 HC Profiling of DA and Model of Anxiety-Related Disorders

In this study, it was found that DA rats were more affiliative in the VBS, although they preferred hiding in the burrows than being exposed to the open space of the cage. This was consistent with their more fearful reaction to other classical tests (elevated plus maze and avoidance of the center of the open field), which is also an argument for the added ecological validity of the VBS (with its open area) with some shorter conventional assays. These results could validate, in different contexts, a specific fear of the open spaces. With DA rats presenting a more anxious and prosocial phenotype in both the VBS and classical out-of-the-cage tests, this strain could be interesting to use for studies on anxiety-related disorders. For example, patients diagnosed with anxiety disorder are extremely fearful/anxious of real-life threats (as opposed to unreal life-threatening concerns of OCD patients) and can express unritualized compulsive behaviors. In the case of social anxiety disorder (social phobia), a subcategory of anxiety disorder, they show strong social contact avoidance and/or seek to reduce their social fear. Anxiety indeed appears to be a trait often witnessed in inbred lines of mice (Belzung and Berton 1997; Tuttle et al. 2018). Biological substrates could support the inter-strain behavioral differences. It seemed that DA and WI(Han) shared traits that have been associated with the serotonergic system, especially hyposerotonergia. Mapping and quantifying the expression of the serotonin autoreceptor 5-HT1A and receptor 5-HT4 could support their anxiety (Donaldson et al. 2014) and reward sensitivity profiles, respectively (Rebholz et al. 2018). Additionally, the central levels of expression of SERT, which influence the 5-HT turnover, would be crucial to evaluate in DA. In DA, the lower sensitivity to reward, impulsivity, aggression, social preference, and higher anxiety might indicate a lower level of SERT expression compared to WI(Han) (Kalueff et al. 2010). Finally, and despite their marked differences, it is to be remembered that DA and WI(Han) rats also shared many similar traits, especially in the undisturbed environment of their social Home Cage Housing. The original approach to assess the spontaneous behaviors of rats, within the VBS as their HCM gave an unprecedented view on the richness of each strain specificity at multiple behavioral and temporal levels all at once.

3.2.4 Things to Consider with This Model and Advantages of HCM

The DA line is particularly sensitive and reactive to handling, requiring a longer and adapted procedure for habituation to handling by the experimenter and classical testing. The use of HCMs for the evaluation of their sensitive phenotype is a good alternative to control for the impact of human handling on their behaviors when using conventional tests. The VBS also offers the possibility of a multidimensional profiling in naturalistic conditions essential for improving high translational value to results.

The boom in the generation of genetically modified mice in the 1990s did not occur in rats, although they were previously the preferred species over the mice to study cognition and social behaviors in laboratory settings. Finding the background strain for generating transgenic rats and at a reasonable price was two of the main challenges (Meek et al. 2017). One successful transgenic rat with a DA background is the Tph2 −/− rat line (Kaplan et al. 2016). In this line, when DA rats were stripped off of their serotonin in the brain using a KO technology, blocking the production of the rate-limiting enzyme Tryptophan Hydroxylase 2 in the production of serotonin in the brain specifically (production of serotonin at normal levels outside of the brain), their behavioral phenotype was markedly impaired in their home cage environment. As described in the section above, combining the use of HCM with classical tests demonstrated that although brain serotonin depletion did not impact the animal's cognitive abilities in classical procedures, their everyday phenotype turned out to be particularly compromised in the home cage. The most critical behaviors of DA rats with no serotonin in the brain effectively resembled symptoms of impulse control and anxiety disorders (Alonso et al. 2023).

3.3 Wistar Han

A quick PubMed search [Searchstring: "(Wistar Han) OR (wistar han) OR (Wistar H) OR (WI(Han))"] revealed more than 49,000 results since 2000, with a peak of publications in 2012 followed by an accelerating decrease after 2021, underlining the relatively important but recessing use of this strain. Wistar Han rats are outbred albino rats. Docile, they are largely used in pharmacological and toxicity studies. Thanks to their good longevity, they are of interest for longitudinal and behavioral studies (Taylor and Mowat 2020). Rats in general but also WI(Han) are easily trained in operant conditioning boxes in contrast to mice. Since the 1930s, with the first created operant cages (or skinner box), hundreds of protocols have been developed and validated to be able to test various and subtle cognitive abilities in rats, neurobiologically mapped and similar to neuropsychological and batteries of cognitive tests used in humans. The advantages of testing a rat out of its homecage, alone in a highly controlled environment, following a strictly designed protocol are that the animal's memory, attention, impulsivity, sensitivity to reward, decision making, and so on, can be easily statistically analyzed and compared between individuals. Although cognitive abilities can also be assessed in some home cage set ups, specific conditions of tests easily implemented in stand-alone operant systems cannot be directly transferred to the continuous although intermittent testing of the animal's abilities and conditions of the Home Cage. To combine advantages of both testing and monitoring conditions set ups, and without the intervention of the experimenter, one idea has been to connect the home cage of group-housed rats to the operant cage via an automated animal gating or sorting system. In this configuration, the rats lived undisturbed and could decide when voluntarily entering the operant chamber (a touchscreen operant system) to perform one session of test and in comparable standardized conditions than if manually entering the testing box (Rivalan et al. 2017). Although mostly developed for mice, such an automated gating system works similarly well in rats, using radio-frequency identification (RFID) technology to replace the need for experimenter involvement. In this study, it was shown that WI(Han) rats readily learned to voluntarily and individually access the operant chamber and remained there solely for the duration of each experimental session and not to sleep or use the box as a simple extension of their Home Cage. Interestingly, these self-initiated sessions enabled the rats to acquire a complex touchscreen-based trial-unique nonmatching to location (TUNL) task in approximately half the time reported for manually placed animals, mainly due to the continuous access to the test cage. Task performance was comparable between the automated and manually handled groups, supporting the reliability of the approach. Overall, this fully automated, experimenter-independent platform represents a valuable tool for investigating a wide range of cognitive functions in future research.

3.3.1 Practical Considerations

To maintain a satisfying level of motivation by the rat for performing the task when entering the operant chamber, one critical aspect has been to implement a time out of several hours (from 1 to 3 h) between two visits of the operant box by the same animal. This would equally reduce the exclusive access of the test box by the dominant animal. Another key aspect is to ensure correct synchronization of times between the Gating device and the operating system of the test box to avoid mistakes in later analysis of results. For advice on synchronization of external modules with HCM, see chapter "Achieving Independence and Precision: A Guide for Do-It-Yourself (DIY): Home Cage Monitoring" on DIY HCM approaches.

3.4 Long Evans Rats

3.4.1 Name of the Model: Long Evans (LE)

LE Strain Characteristics

LE rats are a commonly used outbred strain of laboratory rats. A PubMed search using [Long Evans] keywords resulted in more than 26,000 studies since 1922. Even though less frequently used than Wistar (W) and Sprague–Dawley (SD) rats (ratio of studies: LE:W, 1:12 and LE:SD, 1:15), the LE rats are present in multiple research fields, including behavior, aging, addiction, and obesity, and are frequently chosen for cognitive studies. They are phenotypically characterized by a black hooded coat and a pigmented retina, conferring good visual function. Their visual acuity is reported to be superior to that of W, SD, and Fischer 344 rats (Prusky et al. 2002), which should make LE rats more suitable than albino rats for cognitive tasks that involve visual cues, such as spatial learning and visual discrimination tasks. Accordingly, LE rats were shown to perform better than albino rats in different spatial learning tasks (Tonkiss et al. 1992; Turner and Burne 2014; Raje et al. 2025). Even though mixed results have been found for the water maze, in a water maze place task, LE outperformed not only albino but also pigmented rats, including DA rats (Harker and Whishaw 2002) that have a comparable visual acuity to LE rats (Prusky et al. 2002), suggesting better cognitive abilities in the LE strain with respect to other pigmented rat strains in specific tasks. Furthermore, LE performed better than SD in operant and touchscreen paradigms involving signal detection and pairwise discrimination tasks, respectively (Turner and Burne 2014; Martis et al. 2018). It is not entirely clear to what extent the higher performance of LE over albino rats in the abovementioned tasks is driven primarily by their better visual function or, in part, by better cognitive skills. Comparing LE with other strains in different touch screen paradigms revealed that LE rats can outcompete SD and W rats in a visual discrimination task, but their performance is similar to that of the albino strains in an automated spatial search task, which is less dependent on visual skills (Kumar et al. 2015). In addition to visual acuity, other factors could play a role in the LE's better performance in cognitive tasks. Taken together, the results of studies comparing LE rats to SD rats for anxiety and other behavioral measures, as well as stress, do not provide a straightforward explanation for the superior performance of LE rats (Turner and Burne 2014; Sanchís-Ollé et al. 2021; Raje et al. 2025).

Recent investigations showed that the onset of cognitive decline in LE rats varies between different cognitive skills, with motor learning declining first by 21 months of age, followed by a decline in attention, spatial learning, and later, social cognition by the age of 34 months (Ernyey et al. 2023). LE rats show marked individual differences in the decline with age in the Morris water maze performance (Tran et al. 2018), and brain analyses in this strain pinpointed markers associated with either resistance or sensitivity to cognitive decline. For instance, cognitively impaired aged individuals show a decreased amplitude of miniature inhibitory currents in hippocampal granule cells, whereas cognitively unimpaired aged individuals display the opposite change, accompanied by increased tone inhibition in CA1 pyramidal cells. A strain that presents neuronal changes associated with individual differences in cognition allows for the identification of the neurobiological mechanisms underlying cognitive aging and the development of intervention options for aging-associated disease. Therefore, LE rats are a valuable strain to model human cognitive aging, as humans also exhibit marked individual differences in aging, with some having good cognitive skills at advanced age and others experiencing pronounced cognitive decline earlier on.

If fed a high-fat diet, LE rats develop an obese phenotype with increased body weight and body fat as well as insulin resistance (Woods et al. 2003), which means they are a model of diet-induced obesity. Furthermore, if given a liquid ethanol diet or exposed to binge-like drinking procedures, LE rats show a higher alcohol intake than albino rats (Horowitz et al. 1999; Sauton et al. 2021). Consequently, research on alcohol addiction is often performed in LE rats. They are also a common strain in research on addiction to other substances, because, like SD rats, they display individual differences in drug-induced locomotor responses, which can be informative but also limit reproducibility. Given the impact of drugs on cognitive parameters and the good performance of LE rats on cognitive paradigms, they may be a suitable strain to assess the cognitive effects of addiction.

Sensorimotor gating has been well characterized in LE rats and frequently compared between LE and SD rats. One of the reasons is that prepulse inhibition (PPI) of the startle response, a validated index of sensorimotor gating, is differentially affected by dopamine agonists in the LE and SD strains (Swerdlow et al. 2003; Qu et al. 2009). The different PPI sensitivities are a valuable feature to investigate the neurobiological and regulatory mechanisms at the base of sensorimotor gating and its deficits in schizophrenia and other disorders. In Brattleboro rats, a vasopressin-deficient strain spontaneously originated from LE rats, and the PPI is lower than in albino and LE rats (Feifel and Priebe 2001). This phenotype is present along with other behavioral abnormalities, e.g., social deficits. Hence, the Brattleboro LE strain is ideal to study schizophrenia-related phenotypes. Despite their value in research, however, the use of Brattleboro rats has largely declined compared to the past (Zelena and Engelmann 2018).

3.4.2 Disadvantages of the Model

Like other strains, for example, F344/Brown Norway rats (Basken et al. 2012), LE rats' ultrasonic vocalizations (USVs) have been shown to change with increasing age. In LE rats, vocal changes have been observed by 18 months of age along with structural laryngeal alterations and include decreased USV peak frequency, maximum frequency, and bandwidth (Peterson et al. 2013). While age-related vocal changes in rats may be useful for studying mechanisms of vocal deterioration relevant to human aging, they can also be a disadvantage for experiments that measure USVs as readouts in LE rats or rat models with an LE genetic background, for example, studies in animal models of disease. It is then important to select appropriate-age animal cohorts when measuring USVs as a disease phenotype.

3.4.3 LE in HCM

LE rats have been used in different types of HCM systems to measure basic home-cage behaviors such as locomotor activity and decision making and to develop setups for cognitive assessment (Kaupert et al. 2017; Bruinsma et al. 2019; Hasanpour et al. 2021; Lapp et al. 2023; Puls et al. 2024). In some HCM systems, the animals were monitored in social groups. One study used the Home Cage Analyzer, combining radio frequency identification (RFID) and video recordings, and obtained automated measurements of activity, drinking, rearing, body temperature, and social interaction during development until early adulthood in female and male rats of multiple strains. Interestingly, the analyses identified circatidal-like rhythms in locomotor activity, which were more pronounced in LE than in SD and W rats (Hasanpour et al. 2021). Circatidal rhythms occur every 12 h and are best known for marine animals, although 12 h rhythms have also been identified in mice and humans. In the mouse liver, genes that follow a 12-h rhythm have been associated with metabolic homeostasis (Zhu et al. 2017). In the human brain, 12 h rhythms in transcript expression were associated with fundamental cellular functions, and their disruption was linked with psychopathology (Scott et al. 2023). An animal strain with distinct circatidal-like rhythms could therefore be relevant for translational research, which should encourage further investigation of these rhythms in LE rats.

Lapp and coworkers developed a pipeline for the automated scoring of maternal behaviors (automated maternal behavior during early life in rodents) using DeepLabCut on video recordings of LE dams and their pups during the first 10 postnatal days (Lapp et al. 2023). Combined with automated video recordings, the automated maternal behavior scoring reduces measurement time and allows the scoring of multiple cages simultaneously for extended time periods. Adapting the maternal care pipeline to other rodent strains will be useful for its validation and enable between-strain comparisons of maternal care measurements.

Since LE rats are frequently used in cognitive studies and perform well in learning tasks, the LE strain is an ideal candidate for developing and validating new cognitive tasks. In this strain, HCM systems have been tested, in which animals have access to virtual reality environments or to operant chambers as an extension of their home cage, thereby minimizing the experimenter's intervention and avoiding the repeated transferring of the animals outside their housing environment. However, there is limited information on the performance of LE rats in comparison to other strains or in relation to specific research questions. Comparing the LE strain with other commonly used strains is especially relevant in terms of behavioral aspects such as impulsivity, visual discrimination, spatial learning, and other emotional and cognitive parameters, which serve as readouts in preclinical research.

In one study (Kaupert et al. 2017), LE rats were trained on virtual radial maze tasks using a virtual reality system connected to their home cage. The rats could voluntarily and individually enter the virtual system, with access controlled by RFID. Using a spherical treadmill, the virtual reality system Servoball allows for the assessment of cognition and behavior, combined with recordings of neuronal activity in freely moving animals. Permanently connected to the home cage, it allows continuous self-timed training sessions, which should reduce the long training times observed with conventional systems. A second study tested, in LE rats, a variant of the mouse CombiCage SP-5-CSRTT for motor impulsivity and attention, where an operant box is directly connected to the home cage via a tunnel (Bruinsma et al. 2019). This setup, with either unlimited access to start trials or time-restricted access (i.e., trials initiated only at the beginning of the dark cycle), largely decreased training time compared to conventional protocols. Regarding task validation, both protocols yielded results consistent with those previously observed in the conventional setup when varying task parameters. Variable intertrial intervals increased premature responding, whereas varying stimulus duration decreased accuracy. The time-restricted protocol also reproduced the known effects of scopolamine on attention and inhibitory control.

The development, validation, and use of similar types of systems connected to the home cage for cognitive assessment will be useful, among others, in the context of cognitive aging experiments (see section "LE Strain Characteristics"), as it would facilitate correlating various cognition measures such as spatial learning, attention, and social cognition with behavioral and physiological parameters e.g., motor and circadian activity or metabolic measures over long periods of time. This will help identify the shape and rate of aging trajectories of behavioral and physiological traits in animal models.

4 Summary

Automated home cage monitoring has brought valuable advances to the study of rodent behavior and physiology by enabling continuous, minimally intrusive observation under conditions that better capture the animals' biological rhythms. Importantly, handling, observer bias, and short testing times in potentially aversive environments are suggested to be the major concerns for reproducibility, to be alleviated by HCM. As reviewed in this chapter, different mouse and rat strains offer distinct advantages and present specific challenges when used in HCM studies, and these must be considered in addressing the research questions. Recognizing the influence of genetic background, age, housing conditions, and sensory traits is essential for meaningful interpretation of the HCM data. Moreover, investigations should be carried out in both male and female mice. While the approach holds promise for identifying subtle behavioral and physiological phenotypes that may not be evident in conventional testing, it also calls for careful consideration of methodological limitations and the need for standardized analytical tools. As the field evolves, combining HCM with complementary technologies and fostering cross-laboratory collaboration will be important steps toward improving reproducibility and refining preclinical models. Rather than replacing traditional methods, HCM offers a valuable extension, supporting a more nuanced and comprehensive understanding of rodent models in biomedical research.

References

129 strains (2025) Available at: https://www.jax.org/strain/002448. Accessed 3 Nov 2025

Acosta-Rodríguez VA et al (2017) Mice under caloric restriction self-impose a temporal restriction of food intake as revealed by an automated feeder system. Cell Metabolism 26(1):267–277.e2. Available at: https://doi.org/10.1016/j.cmet.2017.06.007

Adamah-Biassi EB et al (2013) Automated video analysis system reveals distinct diurnal behaviors in C57BL/6 and C3H/HeN mice. Behav Brain Res 243:306–312. Available at: https://doi.org/10.1016/j.bbr.2013.01.003

Aggleton JP et al (1996) The effects of selective lesions within the anterior thalamic nuclei on spatial memory in the rat. Behav Brain Res 81(1–2):189–198. Available at: https://doi.org/10.1016/S0166-4328(96)89080-2

Alonso L et al (2020) Inter-individual and inter-strain differences in cognitive and social abilities of Dark Agouti and Wistar Han rats. Behav Brain Res 377:112188. Available at: https://doi.org/10.1016/j.bbr.2019.112188

Alonso L et al (2023) Constitutive depletion of brain serotonin differentially affects rats' social and cognitive abilities. iScience 26(2):105998. Available at: https://doi.org/10.1016/j.isci.2023.105998

ALURES database (2025) Available at: https://webgate.ec.europa.eu/envdataportal/content/alures/section1_number-of-animals.html. Accessed 3 Nov 2025

Ashbrook DG et al (2021) A platform for experimental precision medicine: the extended BXD mouse family. Cell Syst 12(3):235–247.e9. Available at: https://doi.org/10.1016/j.cels.2020.12.002

Azar T, Sharp J, Lawson D (2011) Heart rates of male and female Sprague-Dawley and spontaneously hypertensive rats housed singly or in groups. J Am Assoc Lab Anim Sci 50(2):175–184

Azar TA, Sharp JL, Lawson DM (2012) Effects of cage enrichment on heart rate, blood pressure, and activity of female Sprague-Dawley and spontaneously hypertensive rats at rest and after acute challenges. J Am Assoc Lab Anim Sci 51(3):339–344

Bains RS et al (2016) Analysis of Individual mouse activity in group housed animals of different inbred strains using a novel automated home cage analysis system. Front Behav Neurosci 10. Available at: https://doi.org/10.3389/fnbeh.2016.00106

Bains RS et al (2018) Assessing mouse behaviour throughout the light/dark cycle using automated in-cage analysis tools. J Neurosci Methods 300:37–47. Available at: https://doi.org/10.1016/j.jneumeth.2017.04.014

BALB/c strain (2025) Available at: https://www.jax.org/strain/001026. Accessed 3 Nov 2025

Barinaga M (1992) Knockouts shed light on learning: mice missing certain kinase genes lack a process in the brain called long-term potentiation and have difficulty remembering spatial information. Science 257(5067):162–163. Available at: https://doi.org/10.1126/science.1321491

Basken JN, Connor NP, Ciucci MR (2012) Effect of aging on ultrasonic vocalizations and laryngeal sensorimotor neurons in rats. Exp Brain Res 219(3):351–361. Available at: https://doi.org/10.1007/s00221-012-3096-6

Belzung C, Berton F (1997) Further pharmacological validation of the BALB/c neophobia in the free exploratory paradigm as an animal model of trait anxiety. Behav Pharmacol 8(6):541–548. Available at: https://doi.org/10.1097/00008877-199711000-00012

Blanchard DC et al (1995) Visible burrow system as a model of chronic social stress: behavioral and neuroendocrine correlates. Psychoneuroendocrinology 20(2):117–134. Available at: https://doi.org/10.1016/0306-4530(94)E0045-B

Brace LR et al (2015) Auditory responses in a rodent model of attention deficit hyperactivity disorder. Brain Res 1629:10–25. Available at: https://doi.org/10.1016/j.brainres.2015.09.038

Brachs S et al (2025) Robust non-invasive detection of hyperglycemia in mouse models of metabolic dysregulation: the novel Urination Index biomarker. Available at: https://doi.org/10.1101/2025.04.02.646666

Broussard JL, Van Cauter E (2016) Disturbances of sleep and circadian rhythms: novel risk factors for obesity. Curr Opin Endocrinol Diabetes Obes 23(5):353–359. Available at: https://doi.org/10.1097/MED.0000000000000276

Brown SDM et al (2018) High-throughput mouse phenomics for characterizing mammalian gene function. Nat Rev Genet 19(6):357–370. Available at: https://doi.org/10.1038/s41576-018-0005-2

Bruinsma B et al (2019) An automated home-cage-based 5-choice serial reaction time task for rapid assessment of attention and impulsivity in rats. Psychopharmacology 236(7):2015–2026. Available at: https://doi.org/10.1007/s00213-019-05189-0

Brust V, Schindler PM, Lewejohann L (2015) Lifetime development of behavioural phenotype in the house mouse (Mus musculus). Front Zool 12(S1):S17. Available at: https://doi.org/10.1186/1742-9994-12-S1-S17

Bryant CD (2011) The blessings and curses of C57BL/6 substrains in mouse genetic studies. Ann NY Acad Sci 1245(1):31–33. Available at: https://doi.org/10.1111/j.1749-6632.2011.06325.x

BTBR strain (2025) Available at: https://www.jax.org/strain/002282. Accessed 3 Nov 2025

Burman O et al (2008) Removing individual rats affects indicators of welfare in the remaining group members. Physiol Behav 93(1–2):89–96. Available at: https://doi.org/10.1016/j.physbeh.2007.08.001

Chen C-W et al (2017a) Reduced capacity of autonomic and baroreflex control associated with sleep pattern in spontaneously hypertensive rats with a nondipping profile. J Hypertens. 35(3):558–570. Available at: https://doi.org/10.1097/HJH.0000000000001205

Chen Z et al (2017b) Vascular remodelling relates to an elevated oscillatory shear index and relative residence time in spontaneously hypertensive rats. Sci Rep 7(1):2007. Available at: https://doi.org/10.1038/s41598-017-01906-x

Clapcote SJ et al (2005) NIH Swiss and Black Swiss mice have retinal degeneration and performance deficits in cognitive tests. Comp Med 55(4):310–316

Crabbe JC, Wahlsten D, Dudek BC (1999) Genetics of mouse behavior: interactions with laboratory environment. Science 284(5420):1670–1672. Available at: https://doi.org/10.1126/science.284.5420.1670

Crawley JN et al (1997) Behavioral phenotypes of inbred mouse strains: implications and recommendations for molecular studies. Psychopharmacology 132(2):107–124. Available at: https://doi.org/10.1007/s002130050327

DBA/2 strain (2025) Available at: https://www.jax.org/strain/000671. Accessed 3 Nov 2025

Donaldson ZR et al (2014) Developmental effects of serotonin 1A autoreceptors on anxiety and social behavior. Neuropsychopharmacology 39(2):291–302. Available at: https://doi.org/10.1038/npp.2013.185

Doris PA (2017) Genetics of hypertension: an assessment of progress in the spontaneously hypertensive rat. Physiol Genomics 49(11):601–617. Available at: https://doi.org/10.1152/physiolgenomics.00065.2017

Endo T et al (2011) Automated test of behavioral flexibility in mice using a behavioral sequencing task in IntelliCage. Behav Brain Res 221(1):172–181. Available at: https://doi.org/10.1016/j.bbr.2011.02.037

Ernyey AJ et al (2023) Age-related decline of various cognitive functions in well-experienced male rats treated with the putative anti-aging compound (2R)-1-(1-benzofuran-2-yl)-N-propylpentane-2-amine ((-)BPAP). GeroScience 46(1):417–429. Available at: https://doi.org/10.1007/s11357-023-00821-6

Feifel D, Priebe K (2001) Vasopressin-deficient rats exhibit sensorimotor gating deficits that are reversed by subchronic haloperidol. Biol Psychiatry 50(6):425–433. Available at: https://doi.org/10.1016/S0006-3223(01)01100-3

Festing MF (1999) Warning: the use of heterogeneous mice may seriously damage your research. Neurobiol Aging 20(2):237–244. discussion 245–246. Available at: https://doi.org/10.1016/s0197-4580(99)00040-8

Festing MFW et al (1999) Revised nomenclature for strain 129 mice. Mamm Genome 10(8):836–836. Available at: https://doi.org/10.1007/s003359901099

Fuochi S et al (2021) Phenotyping spontaneous locomotor activity in inbred and outbred mouse strains by using Digital Ventilated Cages. Lab Anim 50(8):215–223. Available at: https://doi.org/10.1038/s41684-021-00793-0

Fuochi S et al (2023) Data repurposing from digital home cage monitoring enlightens new perspectives on mouse motor behaviour and reduction principle. Sci Rep 13(1):10851. Available at: https://doi.org/10.1038/s41598-023-37464-8

FVB strain (2025) Available at: https://www.jax.org/strain/001800. Accessed 3 Nov 2025

Groza T et al (2023) The International Mouse Phenotyping Consortium: comprehensive knockout phenotyping underpinning the study of human disease. Nucleic Acids Res 51(D1):D1038–D1045. Available at: https://doi.org/10.1093/nar/gkac972

Harker TK, Whishaw IQ (2002) Place and matching-to-place spatial learning affected by rat inbreeding (Dark–Agouti, Fischer 344) and albinism (Wistar, Sprague–Dawley) but not domestication (wild rat vs. Long–Evans, Fischer–Norway). Behav Brain Res 134(1–2):467–477. Available at: https://doi.org/10.1016/S0166-4328(02)00083-9

Hasanpour M et al (2021) Intensive longitudinal characterization of multidimensional biobehavioral dynamics in laboratory rats. Cell Rep 35(2):108987. Available at: https://doi.org/10.1016/j.celrep.2021.108987

Heinla I et al (2018) Behavioural characterization of C57BL/6N and BALB/c female mice in social home cage – Effect of mixed housing in complex environment. Physiol Behav 188:32–41. Available at: https://doi.org/10.1016/j.physbeh.2018.01.024

Hild B et al (2021) Neonatal exposure to a wild-derived microbiome protects mice against diet-induced obesity. Nat Metab 3(8):1042–1057. Available at: https://doi.org/10.1038/s42255-021-00439-y

Holmes A et al (2003) Abnormal anxiety-related behavior in serotonin transporter null mutant mice: the influence of genetic background. Genes Brain Behav 2(6):365–380. Available at: https://doi.org/10.1046/j.1601-1848.2003.00050.x

Horowitz JM et al (1999) Behavior and drug measurements in Long–Evans and Sprague–Dawley Rats After Ethanol–Cocaine Exposure. Pharmacol Biochem Behav 62(2):329–337. Available at: https://doi.org/10.1016/S0091-3057(98)00160-9

Igreja B et al (2015) Blood pressure-decreasing effect of etamicastat alone and in combination with antihypertensive drugs in the spontaneously hypertensive rat. Hypertens Res 38(1):30–38. Available at: https://doi.org/10.1038/hr.2014.143

JAX Lab (2025) Available at: https://www.jax.org/. Accessed 3 Nov 2025
Kahnau P et al (2021) Lifetime observation of cognition and physiological parameters in male mice. Front Behav Neurosci 15:709775. Available at: https://doi.org/10.3389/fnbeh.2021.709775
Kahnau P et al (2023) A systematic review of the development and application of home cage monitoring in laboratory mice and rats. BMC Biol 21(1):256. Available at: https://doi.org/10.1186/s12915-023-01751-7
Kalueff AV et al (2010) Conserved role for the serotonin transporter gene in rat and mouse neurobehavioral endophenotypes. Neurosci Biobehav Rev 34(3):373–386. Available at: https://doi.org/10.1016/j.neubiorev.2009.08.003
Kaplan K et al (2016) Chronic central serotonin depletion attenuates ventilation and body temperature in young but not adult Tph2 knockout rats. J Appl Physiol 120(9):1070–1081. Available at: https://doi.org/10.1152/japplphysiol.01015.2015
Kaupert U et al (2017) Spatial cognition in a virtual reality home-cage extension for freely moving rodents. J Neurophysiol 117(4):1736–1748. Available at: https://doi.org/10.1152/jn.00630.2016
Korstanje R et al (2017) Continuous glucose monitoring in female NOD mice reveals daily rhythms and a negative correlation with body temperature. Endocrinology 158(9):2707–2712. Available at: https://doi.org/10.1210/en.2017-00266
Krackow S et al (2010) Consistent behavioral phenotype differences between inbred mouse strains in the IntelliCage. Genes Brain Behav 9(7):722–731. Available at: https://doi.org/10.1111/j.1601-183X.2010.00606.x
Kulesskaya N et al (2014) Mixed housing with DBA/2 mice induces stress in C57BL/6 mice: implications for interventions based on social enrichment. Front Behav Neurosci 8. Available at: https://doi.org/10.3389/fnbeh.2014.00257
Kumar G, Talpos J, Steckler T (2015) Strain-dependent effects on acquisition and reversal of visual and spatial tasks in a rat touchscreen battery of cognition. Physiol Behav 144:26–36. Available at: https://doi.org/10.1016/j.physbeh.2015.03.001
Lang P et al (2019) Effects of different diets used in diet-induced obesity models on insulin resistance and vascular dysfunction in C57BL/6 mice. Sci Rep 9(1):19556. Available at: https://doi.org/10.1038/s41598-019-55987-x
Lapp HE, Salazar MG, Champagne FA (2023) Automated maternal behavior during early life in rodents (AMBER) pipeline. Sci Rep 13(1):18277. Available at: https://doi.org/10.1038/s41598-023-45495-4
Lerman LO et al (2019) Animal models of hypertension: a scientific statement from the American Heart Association. Hypertension 73(6). Available at: https://doi.org/10.1161/HYP.0000000000000090
Lidster K et al (2019) Cage aggression in group-housed laboratory male mice: an international data crowdsourcing project. Sci Rep 9(1):15211. Available at: https://doi.org/10.1038/s41598-019-51674-z
Martis L-S et al (2018) The effect of rat strain and stress exposure on performance in touchscreen tasks. Physiol Behav 184:83–90. Available at: https://doi.org/10.1016/j.physbeh.2017.11.010
Meek S, Mashimo T, Burdon T (2017) From engineering to editing the rat genome. Mamm Genome 28(7–8):302–314. Available at: https://doi.org/10.1007/s00335-017-9705-8
Meyza KZ, Blanchard DC (2017) The BTBR mouse model of idiopathic autism – current view on mechanisms. Neurosci Biobehav Rev 76:99–110. Available at: https://doi.org/10.1016/j.neubiorev.2016.12.037
Mineur YS, Crusio WE (2002) Behavioral and neuroanatomical characterization of FVB/N inbred mice. Brain Res Bull 57(1):41–47. Available at: https://doi.org/10.1016/S0361-9230(01)00635-9
Morice E et al (2004) Phenotypic expression of the targeted null-mutation in the dopamine transporter gene varies as a function of the genetic background. Eur J Neurosci 20(1):120–126. Available at: https://doi.org/10.1111/j.1460-9568.2004.03465.x

Mouse Phenome Database (2025) Available at: https://phenome.jax.org/. Accessed 3 Nov 2025
Mulinari-Santos G et al (2018) Losartan reverses impaired osseointegration in spontaneously hypertensive rats. Clin Oral Implants Res 29(11):1126–1134. Available at: https://doi.org/10.1111/clr.13376
Newton S, Aguilar C, Bowl MR (2025) C57BL/6-derived mice and the Cdh23 allele – background matters. Hear Res 462:109278. Available at: https://doi.org/10.1016/j.heares.2025.109278
Nguyen KP et al (2016) Feeding Experimentation Device (FED): a flexible open-source device for measuring feeding behavior. J Neurosci Methods 267:108–114. Available at: https://doi.org/10.1016/j.jneumeth.2016.04.003
Percie Du Sert N et al (2020) The ARRIVE guidelines 2.0: updated guidelines for reporting animal research. J Cereb Blood Flow Metab 40(9):1769–1777. Available at: https://doi.org/10.1371/journal.pbio.3000410
Peterson JR et al (2013) Laryngeal aging and acoustic changes in male rat ultrasonic vocalizations. Dev Psychobiol 55(8):818–828. Available at: https://doi.org/10.1002/dev.21072
Prusky GT et al (2002) Variation in visual acuity within pigmented, and between pigmented and albino rat strains. Behav Brain Res 136(2):339–348. Available at: https://doi.org/10.1016/S0166-4328(02)00126-2
Pugh PL et al (2004) A behavioural characterisation of the FVB/N mouse strain. Behav Brain Res 155(2):283–289. Available at: https://doi.org/10.1016/j.bbr.2004.04.021
Puls F et al (2024) Steps into a Small World: first glimpses on everyday moment-to-moment decision making in an ecologically meaningful multi-choice system for assessing animal preferences. Ethology 130(7):e13468. Available at: https://doi.org/10.1111/eth.13468
Qu Y et al (2009) Neural basis for a heritable phenotype: differences in the effects of apomorphine on startle gating and ventral pallidal GABA efflux in male Sprague–Dawley and Long–Evans rats. Psychopharmacology 207(2):271–280. Available at: https://doi.org/10.1007/s00213-009-1654-9
Rademacher DJ et al (2002) Effects of cocaine and putative atypical antipsychotics on rat social behavior. Pharmacol Biochem Behav 73(4):769–778. Available at: https://doi.org/10.1016/S0091-3057(02)00904-8
Raje KR, Williams MT, Vorhees CV (2025) Comparison of Sprague Dawley with Long Evans rats on a battery of widely used neurobehavioral tests. Physiol Behav 294:114860. Available at: https://doi.org/10.1016/j.physbeh.2025.114860
Rebholz H, Friedman E, Castello J (2018) Alterations of expression of the serotonin 5-HT4 receptor in brain disorders. Int J Mol Sci 19(11):3581. Available at: https://doi.org/10.3390/ijms19113581
Redfern WS et al (2017) Automated recording of home cage activity and temperature of individual rats housed in social groups: The Rodent Big Brother project. PloS One. Edited by J. Homberg 12(9):e0181068. Available at: https://doi.org/10.1371/journal.pone.0181068
Rivalan M et al (2017) An automated, experimenter-free method for the standardised, operant cognitive testing of rats. PloS One. Edited by J. Homberg 12(1):e0169476. Available at: https://doi.org/10.1371/journal.pone.0169476
Rivalan M et al (2024) Serotonin drives aggression and social behaviors of laboratory male mice in a semi-natural environment. Front Behav Neurosci 18. Available at: https://doi.org/10.3389/fnbeh.2024.1450540
Robinson L, Spruijt B, Riedel G (2018) Between and within laboratory reliability of mouse behaviour recorded in home-cage and open-field. J Neurosci Methods 300:10–19. Available at: https://doi.org/10.1016/j.jneumeth.2017.11.019
Sanchís-Ollé M et al (2021) Male long-Evans rats: an outbred model of marked hypothalamic-pituitary-adrenal hyperactivity. Neurobiol Stress 15:100355. Available at: https://doi.org/10.1016/j.ynstr.2021.100355

Sauton P et al (2021) Interstrain differences in voluntary binge-like drinking behavior and in two acute ethanol injections-induced synaptic plasticity deficits in rats. Addict Biol 26(4):e12992. Available at: https://doi.org/10.1111/adb.12992

Scott MR et al (2023) Twelve-hour rhythms in transcript expression within the human dorsolateral prefrontal cortex are altered in schizophrenia. PLOS Biol. Edited by G. Asher 21(1):e3001688. Available at: https://doi.org/10.1371/journal.pbio.3001688

Serfilippi LM et al (2004) Assessment of retinal degeneration in outbred albino mice. Comp Med 54(1):69–76

Shi S et al (2013) Circadian disruption leads to insulin resistance and obesity. Curr Biol 23(5):372–381. Available at: https://doi.org/10.1016/j.cub.2013.01.048

Silva AJ et al (1997) Mutant mice and neuroscience: recommendations concerning genetic background. Neuron 19(4):755–759. Available at: https://doi.org/10.1016/S0896-6273(00)80958-7

Silva LEV et al (2016) Multiscale entropy analysis of heart rate variability in heart failure, hypertensive, and sinoaortic-denervated rats: classical and refined approaches. Am J Physiol Regul Integr Comp Physiol 311(1):R150–R156. Available at: https://doi.org/10.1152/ajpregu.00076.2016

Simpson EM et al (1997) Genetic variation among 129 substrains and its importance for targeted mutagenesis in mice. Nat Genet 16(1):19–27. Available at: https://doi.org/10.1038/ng0597-19

Sittig LJ et al (2016) Genetic background limits generalizability of genotype-phenotype relationships. Neuron 91(6):1253–1259. Available at: https://doi.org/10.1016/j.neuron.2016.08.013

Smith AJ et al (2018) PREPARE: guidelines for planning animal research and testing. Lab Anim 52(2):135–141. Available at: https://doi.org/10.1177/0023677217724823

Song HK, Hwang DY (2017) Use of C57BL/6N mice on the variety of immunological researches. Lab Anim Res 33(2):119. Available at: https://doi.org/10.5625/lar.2017.33.2.119

Swerdlow NR et al (2003) Heritable differences in the effects of amphetamine but not DOI on startle gating in albino and hooded outbred rat strains. Pharmacol Biochem Behav 75(1):191–197. Available at: https://doi.org/10.1016/S0091-3057(03)00078-9

Taylor I, Mowat V (2020) Comparison of longevity and common tumor profiles between Sprague-Dawley and Han Wistar rats. J Toxicol Pathol 33(3):189–196. Available at: https://doi.org/10.1293/tox.2020-0005

Theil JH et al (2020) The epidemiology of fighting in group-housed laboratory mice. Sci Rep 10(1):16649. Available at: https://doi.org/10.1038/s41598-020-73620-0

Tonkiss J, Shultz P, Galler JR (1992) Long-evans and sprague-dawley rats differ in their spatial navigation performance during ontogeny and at maturity. Dev Psychobiol 25(8):567–579. Available at: https://doi.org/10.1002/dev.420250804

Tran T, Gallagher M, Kirkwood A (2018) Enhanced postsynaptic inhibitory strength in hippocampal principal cells in high-performing aged rats. Neurobiol Aging 70:92–101. Available at: https://doi.org/10.1016/j.neurobiolaging.2018.06.008

Turner KM, Burne THJ (2014) Comprehensive behavioural analysis of Long Evans and Sprague-Dawley rats reveals differential effects of housing conditions on tests relevant to neuropsychiatric disorders. PloS One. Edited by J. Homberg 9(3):e93411. Available at: https://doi.org/10.1371/journal.pone.0093411

Tuttle AH et al (2018) Comparing phenotypic variation between inbred and outbred mice. Nat Methods 15(12):994–996. Available at: https://doi.org/10.1038/s41592-018-0224-7

Van Bogaert MJV et al (2006) Mouse strain differences in autonomic responses to stress. Genes Brain Behav 5(2):139–149. Available at: https://doi.org/10.1111/j.1601-183X.2005.00143.x

Van Den Buuse M (1994) Circadian rhythms of blood pressure, heart rate, and locomotor activity in spontaneously hypertensive rats as measured with radio-telemetry. Physiol Behav 55(4):783–787. Available at: https://doi.org/10.1016/0031-9384(94)90060-4

Vannoni E et al (2014) Spontaneous behavior in the social homecage discriminates strains, lesions and mutations in mice. J Neurosci Methods 234:26–37. Available at: https://doi.org/10.1016/j.jneumeth.2014.04.026

Vieira JO et al (2018) Influence of pre-existing hypertension on neuroendocrine and cardiovascular changes evoked by chronic stress in female rats. Psychoneuroendocrinology 97:111–119. Available at: https://doi.org/10.1016/j.psyneuen.2018.07.014

Voelkl B et al (2020) Reproducibility of animal research in light of biological variation. Nat Rev Neurosci 21(7):384–393. Available at: https://doi.org/10.1038/s41583-020-0313-3

Voikar V, Gaburro S (2020) Three pillars of automated home-cage phenotyping of mice: novel findings, refinement, and reproducibility based on literature and experience. Front Behav Neurosci. 14:575434. Available at: https://doi.org/10.3389/fnbeh.2020.575434

Voikar V et al (2010) Conditioned response suppression in the IntelliCage: assessment of mouse strain differences and effects of hippocampal and striatal lesions on acquisition and retention of memory. Behav Brain Res 213(2):304–312. Available at: https://doi.org/10.1016/j.bbr.2010.05.019

Voikar V et al (2018) Automated dissection of permanent effects of hippocampal or prefrontal lesions on performance at spatial, working memory and circadian timing tasks of C57BL/6 mice in IntelliCage. Behav Brain Res 352:8–22. Available at: https://doi.org/10.1016/j.bbr.2017.08.048

Wilming I et al (2024) Time to eat - a personalized Circadian eating schedule leads to weight loss without imposing calorie restriction: a randomized controlled pilot study. Available at: https://doi.org/10.1101/2024.01.30.24301983

Woods SC et al (2003) A controlled high-fat diet induces an obese syndrome in rats. J Nutr 133(4):1081–1087. Available at: https://doi.org/10.1093/jn/133.4.1081

Zelena D, Engelmann M (2018) The brattleboro rat: the first and still up-to-date mutant rodent model for neuroendocrine research. In: Ludwig M, Levkowitz G (eds) Model animals in neuroendocrinology, 1st edn. Wiley, pp 279–296. Available at: https://doi.org/10.1002/9781119391128.ch12

Zhu B et al (2017) A cell-autonomous mammalian 12 hr clock coordinates metabolic and stress rhythms. Cell Metab 25(6):1305–1319.e9. Available at: https://doi.org/10.1016/j.cmet.2017.05.004

Index

S. Gaburro, S. Mandillo (eds.), *Home Cage Monitoring in Rodents: A Global Effort*,
https://doi.org/10.1007/978-3-032-19781-8

MIX
Papier aus verantwortungsvollen Quellen
Paper from responsible sources
FSC® C105338

If you have any concerns about our products,
you can contact us on
ProductSafety@springernature.com

In case Publisher is established outside the EU,
the EU authorized representative is:
Springer Nature Customer Service Center GmbH
Europaplatz 3, 69115 Heidelberg, Germany

Printed by Libri Plureos GmbH
in Hamburg, Germany